Velo-Cardio-Facial Syndrome
A Model for Understanding Microdeletion Disorders

Velo-cardio-facial syndrome (VCFS) is a genetic disorder associated with a deletion of the long arm of chromosome 22. It is the most common interstitial deletion disorder found in man and affects every major system in the body with more than 100 physical and behavioural phenotypic features reported. This book, written by leading international VCFS clinicians and scientists, attempts to summarise the rapid progress that has recently been made in understanding and treating people with VCFS. The focus is on clinical issues with chapters devoted to psychiatric disorders (with particular reference to the high rates of schizophrenia reported), neuroimaging, speech and language disorders, as well as cardiac, ENT, gastrointestinal, ophthalmic, and urological manifestations. Molecular genetics, immunodeficiency, and genetic counselling are also covered, and practical approaches to diagnosis and treatment described. As VCFS is seen as a paradigm for other microdeletion disorders, this book will appeal not just to clinicians who see VCFS patients, but also to those with interests in other genetic disorders.

Kieran C. Murphy is Professor and Chairman of the Department of Psychiatry at the Royal College of Surgeons in Ireland, Dublin

Peter J. Scambler is Professor of Molecular Medicine at the Institute of Child Health in London

Velo-Cardio-Facial Syndrome

A Model for Understanding Microdeletion Disorders

Edited by

Kieran C. Murphy
Department of Psychiatry, Royal College of Surgeons in Ireland, Dublin, Ireland

Peter J. Scambler
Molecular Medicine Unit, Institute of Child Health, London, UK

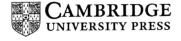

CAMBRIDGE
UNIVERSITY PRESS

CAMBRIDGE UNIVERSITY PRESS
Cambridge, New York, Melbourne, Madrid, Cape Town, Singapore,
São Paulo, Delhi, Dubai, Tokyo, Mexico City

Cambridge University Press
The Edinburgh Building, Cambridge CB2 8RU, UK

Published in the United States of America by Cambridge University Press, New York

www.cambridge.org
Information on this title: www.cambridge.org/9780521184328

First published 2005
First paperback edition 2010

A catalogue record for this publication is available from the British Library

ISBN 978-0-521-82185-8 Hardback
ISBN 978-0-521-18432-8 Paperback

Contents

v

Abbreviations

AAA	anomalies of the aortic arch
CCTCC	cortico-cerebellar-thalamic-circuit
COMT	catechol-O-methyltransferase
DTI	diffusion tensor imaging
FISH	fluorescence in situ hybridization
fMRI	functional MRI
FSIQ	full-scale IQ
IAA	interrupted aortic arch
MAPCA	major aorto-pulmonary collateral arteries
MRA	magnetic resonance angiography
NMDA	N-methyl-D-aspartate
NVLD	nonverbal learning disability
OSMCP	occult submucous cleft palate
PA-VSD	pulmonary atresia with ventricular septal defect
PTA	(persistent) truncus arteriosus
SLI	specific language impairment
SMG	supramarginal gyrus
TF	tetralogy of Fallot
VCFS	velo-cardio-facial syndrome
VDWS	van der Woude syndrome
VPI	velopharyngeal insufficiency
WMHI	white matter hyperintensities

Contributors

Therese van Amelsvoort
Department of Psychiatry
Academic Medical Centre
Tafelbergweg 25
1105 BC Amsterdam
Holland

Linda Campbell
P050 Section of Brain Maturation
Division of Psychological Medicine
Institute of Pscyhiatry
King's College London
De Crespigny Park
Denmark Hill
London SE5 8AF, UK

Adriano Carotti
Department of Pediatric Cardiac
Surgery
Bambino Gesù Hospital, Rome
Italy

Ingele Casteels
Department of Ophthalmology
University Hospital Gasthuisberg
Herestraat 49
B-3000 Leuven
Belgium

Koen Devriendt
Centre for Human Genetics
University Hospital Gasthuisberg
Herestraat 49
B-3000 Leuven
Belgium

Robert Di Donato
Department of Pediatric Cardiac Surgery
Bambino Gesù Hospital, Rome
Italy

Maria Cristina Digilio
Department of Clinical Genetics
Bambino Gesù Hospital, Rome
Italy

Stephan Eliez
Division of Child and Adolescent Psychiatry
41 Ch. Des Crets-de-Champel
Geneva
Switzerland

Karen J. Golding-Kushner
Velo-cardio-facial syndrome
Educational Foundation,
P.O. Box 874
Milltown
NJ 08850
USA

Richard E. Kirschner
Division of Plastic and Reconstructive
Surgery
The Children's Hospital Philadelphia
34th Street and Civic Center Boulevard
Philadelphia,
PA 19104
USA

Bruno Marino
Department of Pediatrics
University of Rome "La Sapienza"
V. le Regina Elena 324
00161 Rome
Italy

Donna M McDonald-McGinn
22q and You Center
The Children's Hospital of Philadelphia
34th Street and Civic Center Boulevard
Philadelphia,
PA 19104
USA

Federica Mileto
Department of Pediatric Cardiology
Institute of Pediatrics
University of Rome "La Sapienza"
Rome
Italy

Kieran C. Murphy
Department of Psychiatry
Royal College of Surgeons in Ireland
Education and Research Centre
Beaumont Hospital
Dublin 9
Ireland

Katrina Prescott
Molecular Medicine Unit
Institute of Child Health
30 Guilford Street
London WC1N 1EH, UK

Nathalie Rommel
Centre for Paediatric and Adolescent
Gastroenterology
Women's and Children's Hospital
Adelaide
Australia

Peter J. Scambler
Molecular Medicine Unit
Institute of Child Health
30 Guilford Street
London WC1N 1EH, UK

Robert J. Shprintzen
Center for Diagnosis, Teatment and Study
of Velo-Cardio-Facial Syndrome
Upstate Medical University
750 East Adams Street
Jacobsen Hall 714
Syracuse
NY 13210
USA

Julie Squair
The 22q11 Group
Milton Keynes
MK13 0LZ, UK

Angela F. Stevens
P050 Section and Brain Maturation
Division of Psychological Medicine
Institute of Psychiatry
King's College London
De Crespigny Park
Denmark Hill
London SE5 8AF, UK

Kathleen E. Sullivan
Department of Immunology
The Children's Hospital of Philadelphia
34th Street and Civic Center Boulevard
Philadelphia,
PA 19104
USA

Ann Swillen
Centre of Human Genetics
University Hospital Gasthuisberg
Herestraat 49
B-3000 Leuven
Belgium

Elaine H. Zackai
22q and You Center
The Children's Hospital of Philadelphia
34th Street and Civic and Center Boulevard
Philadelphia,
PA 19104
USA

Foreword

The term velo-cardio-facial syndrome (VCFS) was coined almost 30 years ago and at that time VCFS was thought to be a very rare congenital malformation. Molecular analysis subsequently revealed that VCFS is associated with deletions encompassing genes mapping to chromosome 22q11, and since that discovery VCFS has been studied intensively by clinicians, geneticists and developmental biologists. Part of this interest is sparked by the relative frequency of the deletion; at 1 in 4000 live births VCFS is the most common microdeletion syndrome known in man.

VCFS patients may present at many different clinics given the protean nature of the condition – over 100 different manifestations have been described in the literature. This book attempts to summarise the rapid progress that has recently been made in understanding and treating people with VCFS. We hope that publication of this book will be useful for several reasons: (1) professionals studying or treating one aspect of VCFS are often relatively unaware of the involvement of other systems and this book will assist them in obtaining a more holistic view of people with VCFS; (2) VCFS may been seen as a paradigm for other less common microdeletion disorders and experience with VCFS may help to direct research and treatment strategies across a range of other microdeletion disorders; (3) while this book emphasises the clinical issues relevant to VCFS, it also reflects the increasing recognition that an understanding of relatively rare disorders such as VCFS can tell us much about more common conditions, such as predisposition to psychiatric illness; (4) the study of the embryological basis for the structural malformations observed in VCFS is helping to uncover some basic mechanisms of developmental biology.

There has recently been considerable excitement at how rapidly our understanding of VCFS has evolved and we have sought to convey this excitement in this book. In addition, we have been privileged to meet numerous people with VCFS and their families over the past decade and have been inspired by the courage and dedication of affected individuals and their families. We dedicate this book to them.

Historical overview

Robert J. Shprintzen

Center for Diagnosis, Treatment and Study of Velo-Cardio-Facial Syndrome Syracuse, New York, USA

The recognition of velo-cardio-facial syndrome as a specific congenital malformation syndrome is a relatively recent development for so common a disorder. The syndrome has appeared in the medical literature either as a specific and distinct diagnostic entity or as part of a discussion of broader symptoms (such as immune compromise, heart anomalies, or speech disorders) since the 1950s, but the majority of interest in the disorder did not develop until the 1990s. The earliest descriptions of the disorder were based on specific symptomatic presentations to clinicians who found the problems to be common among their caseloads. In 1978, in collaboration with a number of my colleagues, I specifically described "velo-cardio-facial syndrome" (a label I personally constructed) as a genetically caused multiple anomaly syndrome in 12 unrelated cases and one mother–daughter pair (Shprintzen et al., 1978). However, an earlier paper had already reported VCFS as a distinct syndrome in a single family that drew interest because of the presence of congenital heart anomalies and cognitive impairment (Strong, 1968), and descriptions of patients with VCFS from a symptomatic perspective can be found nearly 50 years ago in the Czechoslovakian medical literature (Sedláčková, 1955).

Before going further, it would be useful for those readers who are not clinical geneticists or dysmorphologists to understand what the word "syndrome" connotes. *Syndrome* is defined as multiple anomalies in the same individual with all of those anomalies having a single cause (Smith, 1982; Shprintzen, 1997). This definition was agreed on by an International Working Group in order to differentiate the root causes of multiple anomaly disorders (Smith, 1982). Outside of the discipline of clinical genetics, the term "syndrome" is often applied in medicine to groupings of symptoms that do not meet the requirements for a multiple anomaly syndrome, such as postviral syndrome or AIDS (acquired immune deficiency syndrome). Familiar groupings of clinical findings are often referred to as syndromes consistent with the Greek roots for the word syndrome: *syn* meaning together and *dramein* meaning to run, or roughly translated as things that run together. However, as will be discussed later, not all things that run together meet the stricter criteria for syndrome in a genetic sense.

Velo-Cardial-Facial Syndrome: A Model for Understanding Microdeletion Disorders, ed. Kieran C. Murphy and Peter J. Scambler. Published by Cambridge University Press. ⓒ Cambridge University Press, 2005.

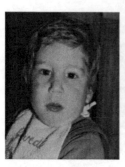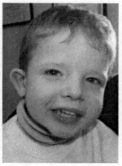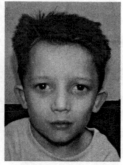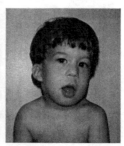

Figure 1.1 A variety of facial photos of children with VCFS, all of whom have the typical 3 megabase deletion at 22q11.2.

The failure to recognize velo-cardio-facial syndrome earlier is probably related to a number of factors. The first is that many children with VCFS who had more severe forms of heart anomalies associated with the syndrome, such as tetralogy of Fallot, interrupted aortic arch, and truncus arteriosus, did not survive the neonatal period or infancy. Because many of the findings in VCFS have a later onset (learning disabilities, speech disorders, cognitive impairment, etc.), there would not have been an opportunity to observe these differences in many cases, thus inhibiting syndromic differentiation and the number of cases available for study would have been far fewer. Because approximately 75% of patients with VCFS have congenital heart anomalies, and many are severe, it is possible that the population prevalence of individuals with VCFS may have been quite rare by comparison to today's figure of 1 : 2000 (Shprintzen, 2001).

Another factor that made recognition of VCFS difficult is that the large majority of children with VCFS are not truly dysmorphic. Although severe manifestations of the syndrome result in abnormal facial features, the large majority of individuals with VCFS are not at all unusual looking. It would be more appropriate to call the typical facial appearance of VCFS to be characteristic without being particularly abnormal. As can be seen in Figure 1.1, children with VCFS look alike without really standing out from the general population. Although individual facial features of VCFS may represent minor anomalies or variants of normal, these minor variations occur frequently enough in the general population so that they are not particularly distinctive. Although VCFS displays a pattern involving over 180 possible congenital anomalies, a high percentage of these anomalies are minor, many of them are behavioral, and many are not obvious nor detectable, such as a single missing or hypoplastic kidney, or a right-sided aortic arch in the absence of structural heart anomalies. Therefore, with many anomalies being difficult to detect without a detailed examination, it becomes more difficult to discern a syndromic pattern.

A third reason why VCFS may not have been recognized as a specific syndrome is that among its clinical presentations are a number of developmental sequences (to be defined and discussed later in this chapter). Sequences are etiologically nonspecific and can occur in association with more than one syndrome. The most common of these sequences that occur secondary to VCFS are Robin sequence and DiGeorge sequence, although several others also have been reported.

Therefore, with the larger pattern of anomalies going undetected as a syndromic association, many earlier clinicians and researchers reported on the individual components of the syndrome as the focus of investigation, such as the speech problems, immune deficiency, endocrine disorders, and heart anomalies.

Speech disorders and VCFS

Speech disorders were among the earliest noted problems to be published. In 1955, Sedlačková, a phoniatrist, published a series of 28 cases of a "syndrome" of congenitally short palate, and followed up that report with an additional 20 cases (Sedlačková, 1967). These cases represented children who had hypernasal speech in the absence of overt palatal clefts. Sedlačková noted a distinctive facial appearance among the children including flaccid facial musculature. The observation led Sedlačková to conclude that the constellation of anomalies was related to embryonic damage of the second branchial arch which was thought to be the origin of the muscles of the velum and the face. In reviewing the article, it is clear that some of the children shown had velo-cardio-facial syndrome while others did not. In these early publications, the intent was to describe the symptom of hypernasal speech that had been unexplained until that point in these cases. Sedlačková suggested that the palate was congenitally short without noting specific anomalies consistent with submucous cleft palate. Occult submucous cleft palate had not yet been described at that time, nor was nasopharyngoscopy in use to observe this anomaly, so Sedlačková's description was consistent with the state-of-the-art of the time. Few clinicians accept this nomenclature today and the term "congenitally short palate" is rarely applied because of more sophisticated assessments of the palate that followed in later years. Yet it is clear that Sedlačková recognized a difference in at least some children who had unexplained speech abnormality. It is also unfortunate that the publication of the first paper in 1955 was in a Czechoslovakian journal and published in Czech, thus limiting access to it by the large majority of the scientific community. However, Sedlačková's early reports clearly recognized the existence of VCFS and these early publications preceded the growth of clinical genetics by many years.

In 1975, Kaplan described a palatal anomaly in children with hypernasality but without overt clefts that he called the occult submucous cleft palate, a term still in use today. Kaplan, a plastic surgeon at Stanford in California reported on four children who had hypernasal speech of unknown origin, much like the cases reported by Sedlačková. Kaplan reported that his patients had normal-appearing palates on oral examination, but when he took them to surgery to correct their speech abnormality, he carefully dissected the soft palate in order to observe the muscle orientation. He found that the muscles of the velum were structurally abnormal, similar to patients with submucous cleft palate. He therefore called the abnormality in his patients the "occult submucous cleft palate" because of the mysterious nature of the defect. Kaplan indicated that the only way this abnormality could be detected was by surgical dissection, but his paper preceded the application of advanced diagnostic techniques that would be able to visualize the defect endoscopically in later years. In his article, Kaplan showed a series of four patients whose facial appearance clearly indicated that they had VCFS, and one patient who clearly did not. Of interest, Kaplan noted a flaccid-appearing facial musculature in his cases, also similar to Sedlačková's earlier papers. Kaplan's aim in this important paper was to describe a nettlesome surgical problem from a symptomatic standpoint rather than to describe a genetic syndrome, but he certainly added much to our understanding of the velar anomalies in VCFS and other disorders.

The reports of both Sedlačková and Kaplan are important for describing the unique nature of the speech problems in VCFS specifically related to hypernasality, although more detailed descriptions of the broader speech implications of VCFS would follow (Golding-Kushner et al., 1985; Shprintzen, 2000). Their early recognition that this was a special population has received too little attention, and they should be credited for providing valuable information in the process of syndrome identification.

Immune and endocrine disorders

The isolation of unusual symptoms in children with VCFS was not restricted to speech disorders. In 1965 when Angelo DiGeorge participated in a panel discussion of a colleague's paper relating to immune disorders in children, the proceedings of the meeting were published in the *Journal of Pediatrics*. DiGeorge described athymia and immune disorder in a child with a right-sided aortic arch during the question and answer session. Several years later, he published a series of cases in the birth defects literature that expanded the phenotype to include conotruncal heart anomalies (DiGeorge, 1968). The cases were described with the perspective of congenital absence of the thymus and its immunologic consequences, as well as the concurrence of congenital hypoparathyroidism, an uncommon finding in VCFS. The majority of the cases described by DiGeorge were infants, and many did not survive infancy because of the severity of their heart anomalies and the inability to repair many of these major malformations at the time. Therefore, these valuable observations of athymic neonates or infants with hypoparathyroidism could not account for the expansive phenotype in VCFS because of the absence of long-term follow-up. Photographs of the cases were not included in the early reports of DiGeorge. A pivotal article in the delineation of the phenotype came from Kretschmer *et al.* in 1968. Three cases of "DiGeorge's syndrome" were described, and one was shown in photographs with an obvious expression of VCFS. Kretschmer described a pattern of facial dysmorphism, although review of the photograph from this article shows a somewhat more severely affected individual than is typical in the syndrome. Of the three cases described, one died in the neonatal period and the other two were young children. The article described these cases in relation to the finding of absent thymus, but the finding of normal polymorphonuclear leukocyte function, normal immunoglobulins, and normal antibody formation. Of the two cases who survived, there were features that were clearly consistent with VCFS. Case 1, the case for whom photographs were published and who clearly had VCFS, a bifid uvula, umbilical hernia, hypotonia, right-sided aortic arch, and aberrant left subclavian were present. This case was reported as having frequent upper respiratory infections. Case 2, the other surviving infant, had what was reported as a bifid nose, high arched palate, and seizures that were reported to be hypocalcemic in origin. Although the article by Kretschmer focused on the immunologic and endocrine features of these three athymic children, this was the first paper to firmly link facial patterns to at least one, if not more, children with DiGeorge sequence.

Congenital heart anomalies

The earliest descriptions of VCFS came from Strong (1968) and Cayler (1969). Strong may have actually been the first person to truly describe VCFS as a distinct genetic syndrome. He reported a single family with an affected mother and three affected siblings (two girls and a boy) and two suspected cases amongst an anencephalic stillborn child and an infant who died at 10 months of complications from heart anomalies. Strong listed multiple anomalies in his sample including mental retardation, congenital heart disease, microcephaly, facial asymmetry, hypotonia, and inguinal hernias. Although there were a number of other incidental findings listed that are not considered typical in children with VCFS, review of the photos in Strong's article leaves no doubt that his cases represent VCFS. Conspicuously absent from Strong's list was cleft palate or submucous cleft palate. However, Dr. Strong indicated that although none of his cases had overt clefts, all of the children in the family "sounded as if they had clefts" (Strong, personal communication). Although not often credited for having delineated the syndrome, Strong's recognition of the pattern of anomalies is not sufficiently acknowledged.

Cayler published two articles describing a symptom complex he labeled *cardiofacial syndrome.* In his first paper (Cayler, 1969), a single case was shown in photographs and this patient did not appear to have the facial phenotype of VCFS, although asymmetric crying facies was present. In a follow-up article (Cayler *et al.*, 1971), Cayler showed a larger number of photographs of cases from among 30 described in the article. Of the cases shown, several clearly had VCFS, although others clearly did not, and in the review of the clinical features, it was obvious that some of the cases could not have had VCFS because some of the major anomalies reported are inconsistent with the diagnosis. Cayler's descriptions are based primarily on symptomatic associations in terms of focusing on asymmetric crying facies and congenital heart anomalies. Therefore, the article did not specifically delineate a new syndrome, but did include VCFS among the cases described.

Kinouchi *et al.* (1976) began the focus in Japan on the association between abnormal facial appearance and conotruncal heart anomalies, a focus that was refined in the Japanese literature in subsequent years with the label *conotruncal anomaly face syndrome* applied by other Japanese clinicians and researchers (Takao *et al.*, 1980; Momma *et al.*, 1996). Although some of the earliest cases described in the Japanese literature represented multiple anomaly syndromes other than VCFS, it is clear that the refinement of the phenotype over time has yielded a description in the Japanese literature of the same exact disorder described in the earliest reports from this author. This development ran essentially in parallel with the focus in the Japanese literature through the 1980s being on heart anomalies, while in the American literature the emphasis was on craniofacial disorders, communication disorders, and behavior. However, although the name for this disorder in the Japanese literature is different, the syndrome is exactly the same as VCFS.

Another probable description of VCFS was published by Stern *et al.* (1976). They described many cases with VCFS in a case report series published in the Birth Defects Original Articles Series. Although no photographs were shown in the published version of the presentation made at the annual March of Dimes Birth Defects meeting of 1975, it is very likely that many if not most of the cases described by Stern had VCFS. Stern described a series of 26 cases ascertained from a cardiology clinic with hypernasal speech in the absence of cleft palate (except for incomplete clefts of the palate in two cases). Nearly half of the cases had unusual cervical spine fusions, another anomaly that is probably common in VCFS, although it also occurs in other syndromes associated with conotruncal heart anomalies.

Several years after we had delineated VCFS, the pediatric cardiologist at our institution, Dennison Young reported on a series of 27 consecutive children with VCFS who were evaluated regardless of a past history of detectable heart anomalies (Young *et al.*, 1980). Of the 27 cases, 23 (85%) had heart anomalies. He reported that three of the subjects who had no apparent cardiac malformations (based on routine clinical examinations) had right-sided aortic arch that required imaging procedures for detection.

After the burst of interest in VCFS in 1992, a larger number of studies began to appear detailing the heart anomalies associated with VCFS, including a number of studies that screened populations of children with conotruncal heart anomalies in order to determine the frequency of 22q11.2 deletions in the population of children with congenital heart anomalies (Ryan *et al.*, 1997). Although statistics vary somewhat from study to study, it is clear that a high percentage of children with conotruncal heart anomalies have VCFS, and screening this population if conotruncal anomalies are present in the absence of other obvious diagnoses (such as Down syndrome) is certainly indicated.

As molecular genetics research moved forward, a number of candidate genes for the development of heart anomalies were identified. *UFD1L* generated significant excitement as a candidate gene for both heart and craniofacial malformations based on mouse studies (Yamagishi *et al.*, 1999), but more recently, *TBX1* has become the focus as the major candidate for the development of cardiovascular anomalies (Merscher *et al.*, 2001).

Development of interest in the 1990s

Prior to 1992, the majority of the scientific literature related to VCFS was coming from a small number of sources, but in 1992, two important events occurred that gave impetus to the study of VCFS in multiple locations around the world. The first was the confirmation that individuals with VCFS have deletions on chromosome 22 at the q11.2 band. This developed in two separate studies. The first was the outcome of a collaboration between several clinical programs including my own and the research laboratory of Peter Scambler in London (Scambler *et al.*, 1992; Kelly *et al.*, 1993). DiGeorge sequence had become associated with chromosome rearrangements at 22q11.2 in 1981 by de la Chapelle and in 1984 (Greenberg *et al.*, 1984). Both of these early identifications of chromosome rearrangements on 22q involved unbalanced translocations and focused on the heart anomalies and immune deficiencies. The family reported by de la Chapelle had a 20;22 translocation, while the Greenberg *et al.* (1984) cases had an unbalanced 4;22 translocation. However, the association between DiGeorge sequence and VCFS was first noted in 1985 (Goldberg *et al.*, 1985) and reported at the American Society of Human Genetics meeting that year. We noted that DiGeorge sequence was a clinical finding associated with VCFS in a minority of cases and our hypothesis was that the DiGeorge developmental sequence was triggered by the primary etiology of VCFS. We therefore initially contacted Dr. Scambler and provided him with DNA samples from a series of patients clinically diagnosed with VCFS. These samples were analyzed in Dr. Scambler's laboratory on a blind basis, and other samples from Newcastle and London were also analyzed. In all, 12 cases clinically diagnosed with VCFS were found to have deletions at 22q11.2. Two of the cases did not have congenital heart anomalies or other clinical findings consistent with DiGeorge sequence. This therefore supported the hypothesis that DiGeorge sequence was a secondary developmental field sequence caused by the deletion that was at the root of VCFS (Kelly et al., 1993). As a follow-up to this initial study, we later contributed a number of blood samples to the laboratory at the University of Pennsylvania in a study published shortly after (Driscoll et al., 1992). As in the previous study, the DNA contributed came from subjects with and without DiGeorge sequence, but all had VCFS. The findings from this second investigation confirmed the findings from Dr. Scambler's laboratory. The confirmation that DiGeorge sequence was a secondary developmental sequence in VCFS indicated that the expansive phenotype of VCFS was likely to result in a number of secondary developmental sequences, consistent with our earlier report of Robin sequence as a consequence of VCFS (Shprintzen et al., 1978).

Psychiatric manifestations

At the time researchers were focusing on the molecular genetics of VCFS, there was also the beginning of research interest into the psychiatric disorders associated with VCFS. The initial report documenting psychiatric illness in VCFS was actually a letter to the editor of Am. J. Med. Genet. that described the occurrence of psychiatric illness in individuals whom we had reported on many years earlier and who had been discharged from follow-up following the surgical resolution of their speech problems (Shprintzen et al., 1992). We labeled the onset of psychiatric illness as "late onset" only because we had been following these patients for many years without obvious evidence of their predisposition towards psychosis. Approximately one-third of the patients we contacted reported the onset of psychiatric illness in adolescence or early adult years. In this initial description of psychiatric illness in a small number of cases, we accepted the diagnoses from a number of private psychiatrists who had been assessing and treating these cases. The diagnosis of schizophrenia had been applied to a number of the cases and was reported in that article. Presuming that people with VCFS were prone to schizophrenia, we established a collaboration with Ann Pulver and her colleagues at Johns Hopkins to prospectively study 20 late adolescents and young adults with VCFS (Pulver et al., 1994). Of the 20 subjects studied, four were found to have either schizophrenia or schizoaffective disorder. As an extension of our collaboration with Dr. Pulver, we also reviewed a sample of 100 individuals who were being followed up longitudinally for schizophrenia in Maryland. Photos of these patients were examined for physical features that might be consistent with a diagnosis of VCFS. Molecular analysis showed that two of 100 cases studied had 22q11.2 deletions indicating that among people diagnosed as schizophrenic, there were likely to be individuals with VCFS.

We then established a collaboration with Demitri Papolos who was in our own institution and was conducting molecular genetics research on individuals with psychiatric illness. After examining a number of patients with VCFS, Dr. Papolos concluded that the psychiatric disorders observed in these cases were more consistent with a form of bipolar disorder rather than schizophrenia, and that the progression of the illness in the most severe cases resulted in schizoaffective disorder and symptoms that could be interpreted as consistent with schizophrenia. A second prospective study was implemented with 25 cases being examined with standardized tests and interviews. Papolos *et al.* (1996) reported that 16 of the 25 subjects studied met criteria for the spectrum of bipolar disorders.

In the years following these early publications, the debate over the nature of psychiatric disorders in VCFS ensued. It was also suggested that the psychiatric illness seen in individuals with VCFS was syndrome-specific and therefore was atypical for both schizophrenia and bipolar disorder (Vogels *et al.*, 2002). To date, there is no definitive answer to the debate, but it is clear that the study of psychiatric illness in a syndrome with a known genetic deletion continues to focus attention on the genes in the commonly deleted area as possible candidates for psychiatric illness.

Secondary sequences

As mentioned earlier, not every multiple anomaly disorder represents a syndrome. In true genetic syndromes, all of the anomalies seen in the individual are caused by some primary etiology that is in effect from the earliest stages of embryonic development. Therefore, the presence of chromosome rearrangements, genetic mutations, or teratogenic exposures will result in a series of anomalies that can all be traced back to their effects. Another type of multiple anomaly disorder is the sequence. Sequences are defined as the presence of multiple anomalies in a single individual, but many of the anomalies are secondary to the presence of an anomaly that interfered with the normal developmental process. For example, a genetic mutation may give rise to a tetralogy of Fallot. The presence of the tetralogy subsequently causes poor growth, poor peripheral perfusion, small stature, clubbing of the fingernails, circumoral cyanosis, and other anomalies. The small stature, clubbing, cyanosis, and other anomalies would not have been present

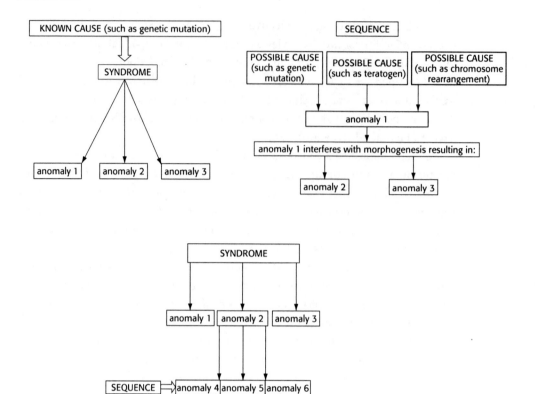

Figure 1.2   Schematic representation of the difference between a syndrome and a sequence. Syndromes (upper left) have a single known cause and all of the anomalies in the affected individual can be traced back to that cause. Sequences represent an interruption in the normal developmental process caused by the presence of an anomaly that causes other anomalies in a cascading manner (upper right). At lower center, it is shown that an individual feature of a syndrome can set a sequence into motion, so that sequences can occur secondary to syndromes.

were it not for the tetralogy, so the presence of the tetralogy was the structural anomaly that secondarily caused the other anomalies. However, tetralogy of Fallot is etiologically heterogeneous. Tetralogy of Fallot can be one of the features of VCFS, but it also occurs in fetal alcohol syndrome, CHARGE association, Down syndrome, and many other disorders. Therefore, sequences are etiologically heterogeneous, and sequences may be caused secondarily by syndromes. The difference between a syndrome and a sequence is demonstrated in Figure 1.2. VCFS has a number of developmental sequences that are set into motion as the result of its spectrum of anomalies. The finding of both Robin sequence and DiGeorge sequence in association with VCFS indicated that many early cases of VCFS were not diagnosed properly because they had a well-recognized malformation sequence as a secondary finding. Although DiGeorge is the secondary

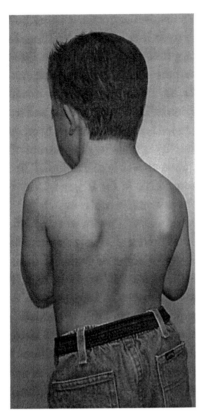

Figure 1.3   Webbing of the neck and low posterior hairline similar to that seen in Noonan syndrome
in a male patient with VCFS and the typical 3 megabase deletion at 22q11.2.

sequence most clinicians associated with VCFS, Robin sequence is actually more common (Shprintzen, 2001). It has been estimated that VCFS accounts for 11% of all cases of Robin sequence (Shprintzen & Singer, 1992), and that 17% of patients with VCFS initially present with Robin sequence (Shprintzen, 1997). DiGeorge sequence is known to be etiologically heterogeneous and is found in fetal alcohol syndrome, Down syndrome, 10p deletions, and a number of other syndromes.

The clinical features of VCFS also include Potter sequence (Devriendt *et al.*, 1997) and holoprosencephaly sequence (Wraith *et al.*, 1985). The clinical features of VCFS also have some significant overlap with other multiple anomaly disorders, including CHARGE association (Pagon, 1987) and oculo-auriculo-vertebral dysplasia spectrum (OAVS), Turner syndrome, and Noonan syndrome (Shprintzen, 2001). The phenotypic similarities to Noonan and Turner syndrome involve the association of webbing of the neck with heart anomalies (Figure 1.3). At our Center, we have had several prenatal detections of VCFS confirmed by FISH at the time of amniocentesis with the association of congenital heart anomalies and nuccal hygroma.

The phenotypic overlap with OAVS involves asymmetric facies, both structural and functional. A lower third facial paresis is common in VCFS and skeletal and soft tissue asymmetry is also seen in approximately 20% of cases. Orbital dystopia may also be seen, as well as asymmetric ear size, ear position, and even ear tags or pits in a small number of cases. We have also seen spine anomalies in VCFS, including cervical spine anomalies, spina bifida occulta, syrinx, and tethered cord. The cervical spine anomalies have included butterfly vertebrae, hemivertebrae, and vertebral fusions. All of these anomalies fit the phenotypic spectrum of OAVS, and congenital heart anomalies and renal anomalies may also be found. Because OAVS is etiologically heterogeneous and nonspecific in the large majority of cases, the phenotypic overlap with VCFS may be potentially confusing.

The overlap of the phenotypic spectrum of VCFS with so many other disorders is related at least in part to the fact that there are so many anomalies associated with VCFS (over 180) that the chances of some or many of them also being associated with other patterns of malformation is relatively high. In addition, many of these anomalies are common anomalies in humans, such as heart malformations, cleft palate or submucous cleft palate, minor craniofacial features, minor limb anomalies, renal anomalies, etc. Putting this into a historical framework, it is therefore likely that individuals with VCFS have been included in previous scientific reports that have described other disorders, as was previously mentioned in this chapter in relation to the publications of Kaplan, Sedlačková, and others.

Other syndromes associated with 22q11.2 deletions

As mentioned earlier, features common to individuals with VCFS are also found in a number of other common patterns of multiple anomalies, including Turner syndrome, Noonan syndrome, and oculo-auriculo-vertebral spectrum (OAVS). The expansive phenotype of VCFS has clinical features that overlap with a number of other syndromes leading some clinicians to mistake the phenotype for other diagnoses. Because some individuals with VCFS have mild orbital hypertelorism, feeding problems, cleft palate, heart malformations, and genital anomalies, several investigators have suggested that Opitz syndrome (also known as the G/BBB syndrome) is also caused by 22q11.2 deletions (Fryburg et al., 1996; McDonald-McGinn et al., 1996). The etiology of Opitz syndrome has been debated since its initial delineation in 1969 (Opitz et al., 1969a,b). Indeed, the association of orbital hypertelorism, swallowing problems, congenital heart anomalies, hypospadias, and cleft palate was described as two separate syndromes, the G syndrome and BBB syndrome (it was Opitz' convention to name syndromes after the initials of the affected family's surnames). Opitz initially reported the syndrome as X-linked recessive, but later reports suggested both autosomal dominant and X-linked recessive patterns. Robin *et al.* (1995, 1996) suggested that there are two disorders, one mapped to 22q11.2 and the other to Xp22. Robin *et al.* (1995) suggested that the anomalies found in Opitz syndrome might be related to mutations involving one of a number of zinc finger genes located in the distal portion of 22q11.2, and he emphasized that the phenotypes seen in Opitz syndrome are not similar to those seen in VCFS, even though the syndromes generically shared some common features.

A review of the photos of Opitz' original families (Opitz *et al.*, 1969a,b) and those shown by Robin *et al.* (1995) suggests that there is no resemblance whatsoever between these cases and VCFS. However, reviewing the photos presented by Fryburg *et al.* (1996) and McDonald-McGinn *et al.* (1996), those cases described as having Opitz syndrome clearly show facial phenotypes consistent with VCFS, but inconsistent with Opitz syndrome. It should also be pointed out that the swallowing problems associated with Opitz syndrome are not at all similar to those found in VCFS, nor are they caused by the same anatomical problems. Unfortunately, within the historical context of the study of VCFS, the linking of Opitz syndrome to VCFS has been a distraction to clinicians and researchers that may have impeded progress in the study of both disorders as emphasized by Wulfsberg (1996).

Nosology in the historical context

The process of naming genetic syndromes has been a hodge-podge of the application of terms to connote a specific disease from a large number of sources. We have already established that all disorders caused by deletions at 22q11.2 represent the same syndrome with marked variability of expression. Depending on the location of a clinician's training, their mentors, their field of study, and even geography, this single syndrome has had many names applied to it including velo-cardio-facial syndrome, conotruncal anomalies face syndrome (CAFS), DiGeorge sequence or DiGeorge syndrome, Shprintzen syndrome, Cayler syndrome, Sedláčková syndrome, velofacial hypoplasia, 22q11 deletion syndrome, Takao syndrome, or CATCH 22. These nosologic labels represent the influences of education, academic politics, and geography, something that is not unique to this disorder. Many genetic diseases are known by multiple names. Although the use of multiple labels is annoying, it only matters if the nosologic differences result in different perceptions of the syndrome. It should be pointed out that with the exception of CATCH 22, all of these appellations have some validity in the sense that they have been reported in the literature, and represent eponyms or symptomatic descriptions. The eponyms connote enormous contributions from people who had the foresight to recognize a population of individuals who had special symptoms requiring special attention. Although I personally prefer to avoid eponyms in the naming of syndromes, one cannot ignore the important contributions of

DiGeorge, Cayler, Sedlačková, Takao, Kinouchi, Momma, Strong, and others who have become so closely identified with this disorder. The problem develops when clinicians regard each of these separate labels as separate disorders. There have been many citations in the literature that have suggested that VCFS, DiGeorge, and CAFS are different disorders but all of them are caused by the same deletion. For example, the OMIM website (Online Mendelian Inheritance in Man) has two separate listings for VCFS (OMIM # 192430) and "DiGeorge syndrome" (OMIM # 188400). Under the listing for DiGeorge syndrome, the following is included in the description:

DiGeorge syndrome (DGS) comprises hypocalcemia arising from parathyroid hypoplasia, thymic hypoplasia, and outflow tract defects of the heart. Disturbance of cervical neural crest migration into the derivatives of the pharyngeal arches and pouches can account for the phenotype. Most cases result from a deletion of chromosome 22q11.2 (the DiGeorge syndrome chromosome region, or DGCR). Several genes are lost including the putative transcription factor TUPLE1 that is expressed in the appropriate distribution. This deletion may present with a variety of phenotypes: Shprintzen, or velocardiofacial, syndrome (VCFS; 192430); conotruncal anomaly face (or Takao syndrome); and isolated outflow tract defects of the heart including tetralogy of Fallot, truncus arteriosus, and interrupted aortic arch. A collective acronym CATCH22 has been proposed for these differing presentations.

Similarly, the description for VCFS is as follows:

A number sign (#) is used with this entry because of evidence suggesting that the velocardiofacial syndrome and DiGeorge syndrome (188400) may result from mutations in the same genes. The nature of the genes remains to be determined.

It is clear from both of these entries that both VCFS and DGS caused by 22q11.2 deletions are regarded as separate and distinct disorders, a concept that has been refuted on a number of occasions (Stevens *et al.*, 1990; Shprintzen, 1994, 1998, 2001). The worn and tired analogy of the four blind men and the elephant is actually quite appropriate in this case to demonstrate how the difference in names has prompted the confusion that has led some clinicians to believe that VCFS, DGS, CAFS, and other nosologic labels represent separate and distinct syndromes. DiGeorge's original description was based on immunologic patterns, our initial description of VCFS was published in the craniofacial literature, and CAFS was based on cardiologic findings. Although the descriptions were from different perspectives, the disorders studied were clearly the same. Some of the differences described in the early publications are related to variable expression, a common phenomenon well known to clinical geneticists and dysmorphologists. Differences in descriptions are also clearly related to the data derived from examinations of the cases published. Endocrinologists focus on some aspects, craniofacial dysmorphologists on others, and cardiologists on yet others. Readers and interpreters of the early research cannot assume that because some abnormalities were described that all abnormalities were described. Clearly, in our first article in 1978, we did not assess the cases as completely as we could have in subsequent years. If cases died as infants, there would have been no opportunity to observe speech, learning, or psychiatric problems.

The importance of the recognition that all of the syndromes described as associated with 22q11.2 deletions are the same will allow researchers to focus on what unifies the varying phenotypes. In 1997, we reported that it is possible that the varying presentations of 22q11.2 deletions may occur as secondary developmental sequences caused by vascular disruptions (Shprintzen et al., 1997). In other words, one of the primary effects of the deletion is to cause a disruption in the normal pattern, growth, and distribution of vascular supply in the developing embryo. If the vascular supply to the developing embryo is abnormal, then subsequent growth and development will be abnormal. This is an important concept, especially with researchers looking for gene effects in what is presumed to be a contiguous gene syndrome.

A final word about nosology; CATCH 22 should be, and in fact must be rejected as a diagnostic label because of its attempt at humor, something that patients affected with this disorder do not appreciate. CATCH 22 is a term that some clinicians still apply, although there have been published denouncements of the label (Wulfsberg et al., 1996; Shprintzen, 1998). CATCH is an acronym for Cardiac defects, Abnormal facies, Thymic hypoplasia, Cleft palate, and Hypocalcaemia, but the construction of this acronym is clearly meant to be humorous in its pairing with the number 22, as in chromosome 22. CATCH 22 refers to Joseph Heller's novel of the same name, a black comedy. The popular term **catch 22** refers to a paradoxical dilemma for which the solution is as big a problem as the dilemma. In other words, a catch 22 refers to a completely illogical or preposterous situation, thus invoking pejorative connotations; its application to individuals with a genetic syndrome as an attempt to be humorous is regrettable and has no place in our lexicon.

Spreading information

As will be seen in the chapters to follow, there has been an enormous amount of research into VCFS from many fronts. Because VCFS is only relatively recently delineated, information has not yet been disseminated to the entire professional community or the lay public. Therefore, in 1994, The Velo-Cardio-Facial Syndrome Educational Foundation was established to spread this information via annual meetings, newsletters, and a web site (www.vcfsef.org). The Foundation is mentioned here because it has been the impetus for bringing the public and professionals interested in studying the syndrome together. Indeed, several of the contributors to this text have been active participants in that process. Several fruitful collaborations have also been initiated at the Foundation meetings, and this has allowed research and the spread of information to flourish. As the first Executive Director of the Foundation, I would like to thank the Editors of this text, both of whom have presented at the Foundation annual meetings, and the many contributors who are active members of the Foundation for being so generous with their time, their collegiality, and graciousness in dealing with our lay members.

REFERENCES

Cayler, G. G. (1969) Cardiofacial syndrome. Congenital heart disease and facial weakness, a hitherto unrecognized association. *Arch. Dis. Childhood*, **44** (1), 69–75.

Cayler, G. G., Blumenfeld, C. M., & Anderson, R. L. (1971) Further studies of patients with the cardiofacial syndrome. *Chest*, **60** (2), 161–5.

de la Chapelle, A., Herva, R., Koivisto, M., & Aula, P. (1981) A deletion in chromosome 22 can cause DiGeorge syndrome. *Hum. Genet.*, **57** (3), 253–6.

Devriendt, K., Moerman, P., Van Schoubroeck, D. *et al.* (1997) Chromosome 22q11 deletion presenting as the Potter sequence. *J. Med. Genet.*, **34** (5), 423–5.

DiGeorge, A. M. (1965) Discussion on a new concept of the cellular nasis of immunology. *J. Pediatr.*, **67** (5) (Suppl.), 907–9.

(1968) Congenital absence of the thymus and its immunologic consequences: concurrence with congenital hypoparathyroidism. *Birth Defects Original Article Series*, **4** (1), 116–21.

Driscoll, D. A., Spinner, N. B., Budarf, M. L. *et al.* (1992) Deletions and microdeletions of 22q11.2 in velo-cardio-facial syndrome. *Am. J. Med. Genet.*, **44** (2), 261–8.

Fryburg, J. S., Lin, K. Y., & Golden, W. L. (1996) Chromosome 22q11.2 deletion in a boy with Opitz (G/BBB) syndrome. *Am. J. Med. Genet.*, **62** (3), 274–5.

Goldberg, R., Marion, R., Borderon, M. *et al.* (1985) Phenotypic overlap between velo-cardio-facial syndrome and the DiGeorge sequence. *Am. J. Hum. Genet.*, **37**, A54.

Golding-Kushner, K. J., Weller, G., & Shprintzen, R. J. (1985) Velo-cardio-facial syndrome: language and psychological profiles. *J. Craniofac. Genet. Devel. Biol.*, **5** (3), 259–66.

Greenberg, F., Crowder, W. E., Paschall, V. *et al.* (1984) Familial DiGeorge syndrome and associated partial monosomy of chromosome 22. *Hum. Genet.*, **65** (4), 317–19.

Kelly, D., Goldberg, R., Wilson, D. *et al.* (1993) Velo-cardio-facial syndrome associated with haplo-insufficiency of genes at chromosome 22q11. *Am. J. Med. Genet.*, **45** (3), 308–12.

Kinouchi, A., Mori, K., Ando, M. & Takao, A. (1976) Facial appearance of patients with conotruncal anomalies. *Pediatr. Jpn*, **17** (1), 84–7.

Kretschmer, R., Say, B., Brown, D. & Rosen, F. S. (1968) Congenital aplasia of the thymus gland (DiGeorge's syndrome). *N. Engl. J. Med.*, **279** (24), 1295–301.

McDonald-McGinn, D. M., Emanuel, B. S. & Zackai, E. H. (1996) Autosomal dominant "Opitz" GBBB syndrome due to a 22q11.2 deletion. *Am. J. Med. Genet.*, **64** (3), 525–6.

Merscher, S., Funke, B., Epstein, J. A. *et al.* (2001) TBX1 is responsible for cardiovascular defects in velo-cardio-facial/DiGeorge syndrome. *Cell*, **104** (4), 619–29.

Momma, K., Kondo, C., Matsuoka, R., & Takao, A. (1996) Cardiac anomalies associated with a chromosome 22q11 deletion in patients with conotruncal heart anomaly face syndrome. *Am. J. Cardiol.*, **78** (5), 591–4.

Opitz, J. M., Frias, J. L., Gutenberger, J. E., & Pellett, J. R. (1969a) The G syndrome of multiple congenital anomalies. *Birth Defects Original Article Series*, **5** (2), 95–101.

Opitz, J. M., Summitt, R. L., & Smith, D. W. (1969b) The BBB syndrome: familial telecanthus with associated congenital anomalies. *Birth Defects Original Article Series*, **5** (2), 86–94.

Pagon, R. A. (1987) Velo-cardio-facial syndrome vs. CHARGE "association." *Am. J. Med. Genet.*, **28** (3), 751–8.

Papolos, D. F., Faedda, G. L., Veit, S. *et al.* (1996) Bipolar spectrum disorders in patients diagnosed with velo-cardio-facial syndrome: does a hemizygous deletion of chromosome 22q11 result in bipolar affective disorder? *Am. J. Psychiatry*, **153** (12), 1541–7.

Pulver, A. E., Nestadt, G., Goldberg, R. *et al.* (1994) Psychotic illness in patients diagnosed with velo-cardio-facial syndrome and their relatives. *J. Nerv. Ment. Dis.*, **182** (8),476–8.

Robin, N. H., Feldman, G. J., Aronson, A. L. *et al.* (1995) Opitz syndrome is genetically heterogeneous, with one locus on Xp22, and a second locus on 22q11.2. *Nat. Genet.*, **11** (4), 459–61.

Robin, N. H., Opitz, J. M., & Muenke, M. (1996) Opitz G/BBB syndrome: clinical comparisons of families linked to Xp22 and 22q, and a review of the literature. *Am. J. Med. Genet.*, **62** (3), 305–17.

Ryan, A. K., Goodship, J. A., Wilson, D. I. *et al.* (1997) Spectrum of clinical features associated with interstitial chromosome 22q11 deletions: a European collaborative study. *J. Med. Genet.*, **34** (10), 798–804.

Scambler, P. J., Kelly, D., Lindsay, E. *et al.* (1992) Velo-cardio-facial syndrome associated with chromosome 22 deletions encompassing the DiGeorge locus. *Lancet*, **339** (8802), 1138–9.

Sedláčková, E. (1955) The syndrome of the congenitally shortening of the soft palate. *Cas. Lek. Ces.*, **94** (12), 1304–7.

(1967) The syndrome of the congenitally shortened velum: the dual innervation of the soft palate. *Folia Phoniatr.*, **19** (6), 441–50.

Shprintzen, R. J. (1994) Velocardiofacial syndrome and DiGeorge sequence. *J. Med. Genet.*, **31** (5), 423–4.

(1997) *Genetics, Syndromes, and Communication Disorders.* San Diego: Singular Publishing.

(1998) The name game. *The Velo-Cardio-Facial Syndrome Educational Foundation Newsletter*, **3**, 2–5.

(2000) Velo-cardio-facial syndrome: a distinctive behavioral phenotype. *Ment. Retard. Dev. Disabil. Res. Rev.*, **6** (2), 142–7.

(2001) Velo-cardio-facial syndrome. In Cassidy, S. B. & Allanson, J., eds., *Management of Genetic Syndromes.* New York: John Wiley & Sons, pp. 495–517.

Shprintzen, R. J. & Singer, L. (1992) Upper airway obstruction and the Robin sequence. *Int. Anesthesiol. Clin.*, **30** (4), 109–14.

Shprintzen, R. J., Goldberg, R. B., Lewin, M. L. *et al.* (1978) A new syndrome involving cleft palate, cardiac anomalies, typical facies, and learning disabilities: velo-cardio-facial syndrome. *Cleft Palate J.*, **15** (1), 56–62.

Shprintzen, R. J., Goldberg, R., Golding-Kushner, K. J., & Marion, R. (1992) Late-onset psychosis in the velo-cardio-facial syndrome. *Am. J. Med. Genet.*, **42** (1), 141–2.

Shprintzen, R. J., Morrow, B., & Kucherlapati, R. (1997) Vascular anomalies may explain many of the features of velo-cardio-facial syndrome (Abstract) *Am. J. Hum. Genet.*, **61**, A34.

Smith, D. W. (1982). *Recognizable Patterns of Human Malformation (3rd edn)*. Philadelphia: W.B. Saunders.

Stern, A. M., Sigmann, J. M., Perry, B. L. *et al.* (1976) An association of aorticotrunconal abnormalities, velopalatine incompetence, and unusual cervical spine fusion. *Birth Defects Original Article Series*, **13** (3B), 259.

Stevens, C. A., Carey, J. C., & Shigeoka, A. O. (1990) DiGeorge anomaly and velocardiofacial syndrome. *Pediatrics*, **85** (4), 526–30.

Strong, W. B. (1968) Familial syndrome of right-sided aortic arch, mental deficiency, and facial dysmorphism. *J. Pediatrics*, **73** (6), 882–8.

Takao, A., Ando, M., Cho, K. *et al.* (1980) Etiologic categorization of common congenital heart disease. In Van Praagh, R. & Takao, A. eds., *Etiology and Morphogenesis of Congenital Heart Disease*. Mount Kisco, NY: Futura, pp. 253–69.

Vogels, A., Verhoeven, W. M., Tuinier, S. *et al.* (2002) The psychopathological phenotype of velo-cardio-facial syndrome. *An. Genet.*, **45** (2), 89–95.

Wraith, J. E., Super, M., Watson, G. H., & Phillips, M. (1985) Velo-cardio-facial syndrome presenting as holoprosencephaly. *Clin. Genet.*, **27** (4), 408–10.

Wulfsberg, E. A. (1996) Is the autosomal dominant Optiz GBBB syndrome part of the DiGeorge/velocardiofacial syndrome with deletions of chromosome area 22q11.2? *Am. J. Med. Genet.*, **64** (3), 523–4.

Wulfsberg, E. A., Leana-Cox, J., & Neri, G. (1996) What's in a name? Chromosome 22q abnormalities and the DiGeorge, velocardiofacial, and conotruncal anomalies face syndromes. *Am. J. Med. Genet.*, **65** (4), 317–19.

Yamagishi, H., Garg, V., Matsuoka, R. *et al.* (1999) A molecular pathway revealing a genetic basis for human cardiac and craniofacial defects. *Science*, **283** (5405), 1158–61.

Young, D., Shprintzen, R. J., & Goldberg, R. (1980) Cardiac malformations in the velo-cardio-facial syndrome. *Am. J. Cardiol.*, **46** (4), 643–8.

2

Molecular genetics of velo-cardio-facial syndrome

Katrina Prescott and Peter J. Scambler

Molecular Medicine Unit, Institute of Child Health, London, UK

Introduction

It has been known for over a decade that the majority of cases of DiGeorge Syndrome (DGS) and velo-cardio-facial syndrome (VCFS) are caused by an interstitial deletion of chromosome 22q11 (Carey *et al.*, 1992). Rarely, terminal deletions and balanced translocations involving chromosome 22q11 may also cause the syndrome, and some cases appear to have a robust diagnosis but no deletion. Estimates of the frequency with which the deletions occur have been made from populations where ascertainment is thought to be particularly high and generally suggest an incidence of 1 : 4000 live births (Wilson *et al.*, 1994; Du Montcel *et al.*, 1996); 5–10% of deletions are inherited (Ryan *et al.*, 1997). Molecular studies have shown that most patients have a 3Mb interstitial deletion – the typically deleted region, or TDR – a minority having somewhat smaller (1.5–2Mb) deletions (Emanuel *et al.*, 1998). As will be evident from other chapters in this volume there is a great deal of variation in severity and type of malformation between patients. However, there is no evidence that the size or the precise endpoints of the deletion have any influence on phenotype. Variation of phenotype extends to individuals within the same family and, as molecular studies have shown that deletion size is stable in different members of the same family, this cannot be ascribed to subtle differences in the extent or position of the deletion. Moreover, phenotypic discordance between monozygotic twins has been described (Goodship *et al.*, 1995). Thus, the phenotypic variations observed are likely to be due to background genetic or stochastic effects. The term 22q11 deletion syndrome (22q11DS) is used in this review to encompass all these associated phenotypes.

Prenatal diagnosis of the 22q11 deletion

The occurrence of familial 22q11DS raises the possibility of prenatal diagnosis for those families at risk, and parents of any new case should be offered deletion

Velo-Cardial-Facial Syndrome: A Model for Understanding Microdeletion Disorders, ed. Kieran C. Murphy and Peter J. Scambler. Published by Cambridge University Press. © Cambridge University Press, 2005.

screening (Driscoll, 2001). The offer of prenatal testing would be indicated where a parent carries a deletion. Clearly, the recurrence risk where both parents have normal chromosomes 22 is low, but germinal mosaicism might be suspected where two sibs are affected and their parents unaffected. Germline mosaicism has been reported in 22q11DS, and should be borne in mind during genetic counseling (Hatchwell *et al.*, 1998; Sandrin-Garcia *et al.*, 2002). 22q11 deletion screening might be offered where an interrupted aortic arch or persistent truncus arteriosus has been detected on fetal echocardiography. Ultrasound examination might also detect a heart defect in association with a renal defect or cleft palate, a standard karyotype and fluorescence in situ hybridisation (FISH) being indicated in such circumstances. FISH-based preimplantation diagnosis of the deletion has been reported in one instance where a mother carried a deletion (Iwarsson *et al.*, 1998).

Embryology of main structures affected in 22q11DS

The structures primarily affected in 22q11DS – thymus gland, parathyroid gland, the branchial arch artery derivatives, and the face – are all at least partial derivatives of the branchial arch/pharyngeal pouch system. Indeed, DGS has been termed III–IV pharyngeal pouch syndrome in some discussions (Robinson, 1975). The rostral neural crest migrates from the neuroepithelium into the pharyngeal pouches and makes a major contribution to the structures affected by the deletion. Experiments which ablate the premigratory crest or otherwise perturb crest function can produce a good phenocopy of the main features of 22q11DS (Bockman & Kirby, 1984; Binder, 1985; Lammer *et al.*, 1986; Bockman *et al.*, 1987; Wilson *et al.*, 1993; Kirby, 1999). Natural or induced mutations of genes thought to have a role in controlling neural crest development can result in partial phenocopy of 22q11DS (Conway *et al.*, 1997; Takihara *et al.*, 1997; Thomas *et al.*, 1998; Clouthier *et al.*, 2000). These observations stimulated the hypothesis that the deletion of 22q11 disrupts the rostral neural crest cells, or the cells with which the neural crest interacts, at a critical phase of organogenesis. The endoderm is also required for formation of the pharyngeal structures, and the arches can form even in the absence of neural crest (Graham, 2001), and endoderm can also be affected by teratogens (Vermot *et al.*, 2003). Thus, in considering candidate genes for 22q11DS, investigators have favored genes which are expressed in the presumptive neural crest, the migrating neural crest, or the pharyngeal arches and cardiac outflow tract.

A molecular genetic approach

Several microdeletion syndromes are known where mutations within a single gene of nondeleted patients recapitulate the spectrum of defects observed in patients with a deletion. Examples include Rubenstein–Taybi syndrome, Angelman Syndrome, and Alagille syndrome. In other cases, major features of a deletion syndrome can be ascribed to haploinsufficiency of specific contiguous genes within the deletion interval. For instance, the supravalvular aortic stenosis of Williams syndrome is seen in patients with mutations in elastin. As a second example, Langer–Giedion syndrome comprises multiple cartilaginous exostoses, caused by mutations in the *EXT1* gene, and tricho-rhino-phalangeal syndrome, caused by mutations in a zinc-finger protein. Thus, a major question concerning the 22q11 deletion syndrome is whether the entire spectrum of defects is the result of haploinsufficiency of a single, key gene within the TDR, or whether the full syndrome results from a combined haploinsufficiency. Courtesy of the efforts of the University of Oklahoma laboratory of Prof. B. Roe, the TDR was one of the first regions of the human genome to be subject to megabase scale genomic sequencing, and the chromosome 22 sequence was the first to be published, in 1999 (Dunham *et al.*, 1999). There is, therefore, considerable literature concerning the genes mapping to the TDR and their potential relevance to the 22q11 deletion syndrome. As described below, haploinsufficiency of *TBX1* is likely to be the major determinant of the physical abnormalities observed in the syndrome. However, given the lack of *TBX1* mutations in humans, one or more of the other genes mapping to the TDR may play an independent or modifying role in the syndrome. Some TDR genes are mutated in other conditions, and there is as yet no evidence that physical abnormalities outwith the branchial arch derivatives, or the cognitive and behavioral aspects of the syndrome, are due to *TBX1* hemizygosity. In light of these considerations, and in the absence of a similar compilation, a short summary of other TDR genes is given below.

Genes mapping within the TDR

The TDR is a gene-rich region, and the following listing does not include several predicted transcripts or ESTs of uncertain significance. Genes are presented in a proximo-distal listing. As the genome sequence data and nomenclature changes with time, a current map is best viewed via the ENSEMBLE engine at http://www.ensembl.org/Homo_sapiens/mapview?chr = 22.

DGCR6

The function of *DGCR6* is still unknown. Based upon its sequence similarity to the *Drosophila melanogaster* gonadal protein and g-laminin protein *DGCR6* is thought to be involved in cellular adhesion. *Dgcr6* is expressed from the seventh embryonic day in the mouse, predominantly in the brain, spinal cord, and pharyngeal arches (Lindsay & Baldini, 1997). Both *DGCR6* and *PRODH* have pseudogenes located more distally within the DGCR.

PRODH

PRODH is a mitochondrial enzyme which metabolizes proline and is involved in the transfer of redox potential. Loss of PRODH causes hyperprolinaemia, a situation analogous to that seen in the sluggish-A mutation in *Drosophila melanogaster*. Proline itself may be a modulator of neuronal glutaminergic activity. Mice with the *ProRe* mutation (a premature translational termination in a conserved region of the carboxy terminus) have increased circulating and brain proline levels, and behavioral analysis indicates a decreased prepulse inhibition of startle reflex (PPI) suggestive of a defect in sensorineural gating in these mice (Gogos et al., 1999). This is significant, because individuals with schizophrenia-like psychosis are reported to have similar deficits. Thus, PRODH is a candidate predisposition gene for some of the behavioral problems seen in 22q11DS. One group has proposed that genetic variation in PRODH is a general schizophrenia predisposition gene based upon association analyses (Liu et al., 2002), but the significance levels of the study were not great. Interestingly, most PRODH variants are found in a neighbouring pseudogene for PRODH, a reflection of the recombination between low copy repeats in this region of the genome giving rise to gene conversion events. A heterozygous deletion of the entire PRODH gene was found in a study of 63 unrelated schizophrenic patients (Jacquet et al., 2002). The same study found heterozygous PRODH mutations in three other members of this cohort (but not in a control group). Both mutations (L441P and L289M) gave rise to increased circulating proline levels. Thus, while confirmatory studies are required, PRODH variants appear to modulate behavior.

DGCR5

DGCR5 is probably a pseudogene, with some sequence similarity to a seven-pass transmembrane receptor. It is of interest since the alternatively spliced transcripts are disrupted by the VCFS-associated 2;22 balanced translocation described below (Sutherland et al., 1996).

DGCR2 (aliases IDD, LAN, Sez 12)

DGCR2 encodes a protein with a single transmembrane domain, the extracellular region containing C-type lectin binding domains. DGCR2 is the closest protein-encoding gene to the 2;22 translocation mentioned below. DGCR2 was found to be downregulated in a cellular system designed to identify genes differentially expressed on exposure to anticonvulsants (Kajiwara et al., 1996; Taylor et al., 1997). The gene is ubiquitously expressed and targeted mutants of Dgcr2 appear to be normally viable and fertile (Saint-Jore, Puech, & Skoultchi, personal communication).

TSK

> *TSK* is a testes-specific serine-threonine kinase (Goldmuntz *et al.*, 1997). No additional functional data are available.

DGSI (alias Es2)

> The *DGSI* protein has no similarity to mammalian proteins of known function. However, GFP-tagged *DGSI* is detected in the nucleus (Lindsay *et al.*, 1998). *DGSI* appears to be the mammalian ortholog of yeast *Bis1*, similar genes also being found in *Drosophila melanogaster*, *Caenorhabditis elegans* and *Arabidopsis thaliana*. Overexpression of *Bis1* in yeast results in a cell elongation phenotype, whereas *bis1* cells exhibit a reduced viability in stationary phase (Taricani, Tejada, & Young, 2002). The *DGSI* homolog in *C. elegans* interacts with the MAP kinase MPK1 in a two-hybrid screen. In yeast, bis1 interacts with three classes of protein, each compatible with the nuclear localization seen in mouse and involved in RNA processing/modification, protein degradation and centromere/chromatin structure (Taricani, Tejada, & Young, 2002). Targeted mutations of *Dgsi* have been created, heterozygotes being apparently normal, and *Dgsi-/-*animals demonstrating prenatal lethality of unknown cause.

GSCL

> *GSCL* encodes a member of a family of Gooscoid-related proteins which interact with a RING protein known as rnf4 (Galili *et al.*, 2000). *Gsc* itself is known to be involved in the development of first and second branchial arch derivatives. *Gscl*, however, is expressed in the testes, and in the pons where it shares a zone of expression with *DGSI/ES2* (see above) (Galili *et al.*, 1998; Gottlieb *et al.*, 1998b). Two *GSCL* knockouts have been created and neither line has features suggesting a role in 22q11DS (Saint-Jore *et al.*, 1998; Wakamiya *et al.*, 1998). Embryos that lacked both *Gscl* and *Gsc* also appeared normal.

SCL25A1 (alias CTP)

> *SCL25A1* is a human mitochondrial citrate transporter protein with ubiquitous expression.

CLTCL1

> *CLTCL1* (alias *CLTD*) encodes a clathrin heavy chain polypeptide and is ubiquitously expressed (Gong *et al.*, 1996). This is the only gene from the 22q11 deletion interval not found in the mouse genome. One patient with dysmorphic features and congenital heart defect has a 21;22 translocation disrupting *CLTCL1*, but it is difficult to envisage how *CLTCL1* hemizygosity could cause 22q11DS (Holmes *et al.*, 1997). More likely, the translocation exerts an effect on the transcription of neighboring genes.

HIRA (alias TUPLE1, DGCR1)

The *Hira* gene encodes a nuclear WD40 domain protein homologous to the yeast transcriptional co-repressors Hir1p and Hir2p. The region C-terminal to the WD40 domains has no strong matches to known motifs, but is responsible for the biochemical interaction of Hira with paired homeodomains (Magnaghi *et al.*, 1998), Hirip3 (Lorain *et al.*, 1998) and core histones (Lorain *et al.*, 1998), the functional significance of which remains unknown. The interaction of Hira with Pax3 was provocative, given the conotruncal heart defects, absent thymus and absent parathyroids seen in *Pax3-/-* embryos. Hira protein is localized to the nucleus where a proportion is associated with the nuclear matrix (De Lucia *et al.*, 2001). Hira is a target for cdk2/cyclinE phosphorylation, and ectopic expression of *Hira* can block cells in the S phase of the cell cycle (Hall *et al.*, 2001). In *Xenopus* Hira is essential for a nucleosome assembly pathway (Ray-Gallet *et al.*, 2002). Taken together existing data suggest *Hira* may be involved in cell cycle-dependent transcriptional regulation of a wide range of target genes, possibly acting via altered chromatin structure.

Hira displays a dynamic expression pattern during murine and chick embryogenesis (Roberts *et al.*, 1995; Wilming *et al.*, 1997). At E8–9/st6–12 expression is detected in the neuroepithelium, pre- and migratory neural crest and head mesenchyme. At E9.5/st 18–23 expression is seen in neural crest-derived regions of the head and branchial arches and in a number of other tissues including the somites and forelimb bud. Antisense attenuation experiments in the chick cardiac crest resulted in an increased frequency of PTA in the experimental animals (Farrell *et al.*, 1999).

Targeted mutagenesis demonstrated that *Hira* is essential for murine embryogenesis, although heterozygotes were normal. Analysis of inbred 129Sv *Hira-/-* embryos revealed an initial requirement during gastrulation, with many mutant embryos having a distorted primitive streak. Later embryos have a range of malformations with axial and paraxial mesendoderm being particularly affected, consistent with the disruption of gastrulation seen earlier in development. This phenotype could be partially rescued by a CD1 genetic background, although the homozygous mutation was always lethal by E11, with death probably resulting from abnormal placentation and failure of cardiac morphogenesis. The heart did not loop correctly and chamber formation was disturbed (Roberts *et al.*, 2002).

NLVCF

NLVCF is a ubiquitously expressed gene encoding a protein with two consensus sequences for nuclear localization signals (Funke *et al.*, 1998).

UFD1l

UFD1l is a human ortholog of yeast *Ufd1* which is required for ubiquitin-dependent protein degradation. *Ufd1l* interacts with *Cdc48* and *Npl4*, a complex involved in the recognition of several polyubiquitin-tagged proteins and their presentation to the 26S proteasome for processive degradation (Rape *et al.*, 2001). *Ufd1l* complexes may also be involved in nuclear transport and endoplasmic reticulum protein export (Meyer *et al.*, 2000; Ye, Meyer, & Rapoport, 2001). *Ufd1l* is expressed in the pharyngeal arches of developing mouse embryos, and is downregulated in *Hand2-/-* mouse embryos (Yamagishi *et al.*, 1999). As these mutant mice have outflow tract as well as other heart defects, *Ufd1l* was proposed as a DGS/VCFS candidate gene. Functional attenuation of chick *Ufd1l* using retrovirally encoded antisense constructs resulted in an increased incidence of conotruncal septation defects (Yamagishi *et al.*, 2003a). However, human mutations of *UFD1l* have yet to be convincingly demonstrated, and *Ufd1l+/-* mice are normal (Lindsay *et al.*, 1999).

CDC45L

CDC45L is required for the initiation of DNA replication in yeast and functions as a DNA polymerase α loading factor in *Xenopus*. Protein interactions indicate that a similar function is likely in mammals. Mice with mutations in *Cdc45l* are normal as heterozygotes, but *Cdc45l-/-* embryos die shortly after implantation with deficient cell proliferation in the inner cell mass (Yoshida *et al.*, 2001).

CLDN5 (alias TMVCF)

CLDN5 is one of a family of four-transmembrane domain proteins which form components of tight junction strands (Morita *et al.*, 1999). *CLDN5* is found predominantly in blood vessel endothelium, but not in epithelium other than retinal epithelium, as its expression may be activated by sheer stress. It promotes activation of pro-matrix metalloproteinase-2 mediated by membrane-type matrix metalloproteinases (Miyamori *et al.*, 2001).

PNUTL1 (alias CDCREL1)

PNUTL1 is a member of the septin family of proteins which play a role in cytokinesis (McKie *et al.*, 1998). It co-purifies with SNAP-25 (see SNAP-29 below) and synaptophysin marked synaptosomes, suggesting the protein may function in synaptic vesicle transport, fusion, or recycling events (Caltagarone *et al.*, 1998). The gene is expressed during brain development, from mid-gestation stages onwards. Gene targeting of *Pnutl1* does not lead to any apparent phenotype (Lindsay & Baldini, personal communication).

GP1Bβ

GP1Bβ is a component of the platelet receptor for von Willebrand factor (vWF), mediating initial platelet adhesion and activation. Recessive mutations cause

Bernard Soulier syndrome, which may be uncovered by deletion 22q11 (Budarf *et al.*, 1995). Hemizygosity for this gene may be responsible for the large platelets sometimes observed in 22q11DS (Van Geet *et al.*, 1998).

GNB1L (alias WDR14)

GNB1L encodes a protein with WD40 domains (Gong *et al.*, 2000). The function of this protein is unknown, but unpublished data from our laboratory indicate that homozygous mutations in the mouse cause embryonic lethality, and that the gene is expressed strongly in the developing and postnatal brain.

TRXR2

TRXR2 encodes a thioredoxin reductase, an enzyme involved in protection against oxidant injury, cell growth and transformation, and the recycling of ascorbate from its oxidized form.

COMT

COMT (catechol-O-methyl transferase) is involved in the elimination of biologically active or toxic catechols and their metabolites. Polymorphism within the gene leads to high activity (Valine 158) or low activity (Met 158) alleles. Homozygosity for Met 158 leads to a 3–4-fold reduction in enzymatic activity, compared with Val 158 homozygotes. In 22q11DS an association between the low-activity allele and the development of bipolar spectrum disorder and, in particular, a rapid-cycling form of the disease has been reported (Lachman *et al.*, 1996). However, there is little evidence of a major role in predisposition to schizophrenia or depression in the general population, although there are some positive associations within the vast literature. Gene targeting has been used to generate null mice. *Comt*-null female mice show altered emotional reactivity in a dark/light exploratory situation, suggesting *Comt* has a role in controlling some aspects of emotionality in mice (Gogos *et al.*, 1998). Heterozygous male mice were said to be aggressive, but this phenotype was not observed in *Df1* animals (see below).

ARVCF

ARVCF is a catenin and is thought to contribute to the morphoregulatory function of the cadherin-catenin complexes. Intracellular localization may be at adherens junctions or within the nucleus depending upon protein interactions (Waibler *et al.*, 2001). ARVCF also interacts with Erbin, a member of the LAP (leucine-rich repeat and PDZ domain) protein family present at adherens junctions, and with M-cadherin via its armadillo domains (Mariner *et al.*, 2000; Laura *et al.*, 2002). Presumably, other catenins can compensate for loss of *Arvcf* function, as mice null for *Arvcf* are normal (Saint-Jore, Puech & Skoultchi, personal communication).

T10

Protein sequence predictions reveal little about *T10* function, although the gene is conserved during evolution with a similar gene discovered in the rice genome. Expression is ubiquitous (Halford *et al.*, 1993b).

DGCR8

DGCR8 encodes a 773 amino acid protein containing two double-stranded RNA-binding domains, and a WW domain. The function of this protein has not been tested.

RANBP1

RANBP1 is a binding partner of RAN, which has a central role in nucleocytoplasmic transport. RT-PCR and in situ hybridization studies demonstrate expression in the forebrain, hindbrain, branchial arches, limb and heart (Maynard *et al.*, 2002). Overexpression and RNAi experiments in the zebrafish did not induce any defects reminiscent of 22q11DS (Mangos *et al.*, 2001).

ZNF74

ZNF74 encodes a zinc finger transcription factor which interacts with a hyperphosphorylated form of the largest subunit of RNA polymerase II, and it is expressed in human neural crest-derived tissues and foregut endoderm epithelia (Grondin *et al.*, 1997; Ravassard *et al.*, 1999). Some splice variants associate with sc-35 nuclear speckles suggesting a role in mRNA processing (Cote *et al.*, 2001).

RTN4R

RTN4R was identified as the NOGO-66 receptor, but also acts as a receptor for Omgp and MAG (myelin-derived growth inhibitory proteins) in mediating the interactions between the neuronal growth cone and oligodendrocytes (McKerracher & Winton, 2002). RTN4R functions in axon-glial cell interactions, neuroregeneration and regulating neuronal plasticity. It will therefore be interesting to test the cognitive function of mice deficient for this gene product.

USP18 (UBP43)

USP18 is homologous to well characterized ubiquitin-specific proteases, but appears to efficiently cleave only ISG15-protein fusions. ISG15 is found conjugated to intracellular proteins via an isopeptide bond in a manner similar to ubiquitin, and can also act as a cytokine, induced by interferon, genotoxic stress, and viral infection. It is unknown whether ISG15-fusion proteins are targeted to proteosomes, or whether they are protected from this by a block to ubiquitin fusion (Malakhov *et al.*, 2002).

SREC2

SREC2 encodes a scavenger receptor expressed by endothelial cells which displays strong heterophilic trans-interaction with SREC1 through the extracellular epidermal growth factor-like repeat domains. It may modify SREC1's role in metabolism of low-density lipoproteins (Ishii *et al.*, 2002).

PCQAP

PCQAP encodes one subunit of a large protein complex which acts as a coactivator for RNA polymerase II driven transcription. *PCQAP* is expressed ubiquitously during development (Berti *et al.*, 2001).

PIK4CA

Phosphatidylinositol 4-kinase localizes to the plasma membrane of several tissues including brain, and catalyzes the first committed step in the biosynthesis of phosphatidylinositol 4,5-bisphosphate. The enzyme functions in the PKC1-mediated MAP kinase signaling cascade and may be involved in lipid-protein interactions with cytoskeletal proteins (Gehrmann & Heilmeyer, Jr. 1998).

HC-II

HC-II, or heparin cofactor II precursor, belongs to a subclass of the serpin protease inhibitors whose activity is greatly enhanced upon binding to glycosaminoglycans like heparin, heparan sulfate and dermatan sulfate which are found in vivo on cell surfaces and in extracellular matrix. Various mutations are present in patients with pro-coagulant states (Akhavan *et al.*, 2002; Baglin *et al.*, 2002).

SNAP 29

SNAP 29 is a synaptosomal-associated protein likely to be involved in vesicle-membrane fusion processes such as neurotransmission and hormone secretion (Su *et al.*, 2001).

CRKL

CRKL encodes an SH2–SH3–SH3 adapter protein which acts within several signaling pathways involved in growth and differentiation (Feller, 2001). CRKL adapter proteins play a critical role in the breakdown of adherens junctions and the spreading of sheets of epithelial cells (Lamorte *et al.*, 2002). Mice homozygous for a targeted null mutation at the *CrkL* locus (gene symbol *Crkol* in mice) show some of the defects seen in 22q11DS and in particular interrupted aortic arch (IAA) (Guris *et al.*, 2001). In addition, there is a low frequency of craniofacial dysmorphism, and defects within other cranial and cardiac neural crest derivatives including the cranial ganglia, thymus, parathyroid glands, although crest migration appears unaffected. It is important to emphasize that heterozygous animals were normal and that *CRKL* is not reduced to hemizygosity in all 22q11DS patients.

LZTR1 (alias TCFL2)

LZTR1 is a putative leucine zipper transcription factor (Kurahashi *et al.*, 1995).

P2X6

P2X6 encodes one of a family of purinoceptors expressed in the CNS where they mediate excitatory synaptic transmission and act presynaptically to modulate neurotransmitter release (Bobanovic *et al.*, 2002).

SLC7A4

SLC7A4 encodes a cationic amino acid transporter otherwise known as *CAT-4* expressed in the placental syncytiotrophoblast (Ayuk *et al.*, 2000).

Mechanism of deletion

Deletion of 22q11 is the most frequent interstitial chromosome deletion observed in man, begging the question as to whether there is any structural predisposition to chromosome rearrangements of this region. In addition to the deletion, non-random rearrangements of 22q11 are found in the recurrent constitutional abnormalities seen in cat eye syndrome (characterized by a supernumerary bisatellited marker chromosome), the supernumerary der 22t(11;22) chromosome, and various tumour-associated translocations e.g. the t(9;22) Philadelphia chromosome and the t(8;22) seen in Burkitt's lymphoma. There have been a few reports of mosaicism for the 22q11 deletion suggesting a degree of mitotic instability. Beginning with the observation that 22q11 contained a number of repeat sequences unique to this region of the genome (Halford *et al.*, 1993a), and culminating with detailed mapping and sequencing of these DNAs, a number of studies have provided evidence for the structural predisposition hypothesis (Edelmann *et al.*, 1999a, b; Shaikh *et al.*, 2000, 2001).

Four discrete blocks of chromosome 22q11 specific repeat sequences have now been identified and are referred to as low copy repeat (LCR) units A through D. Each is comprised of smaller repeat modules, different units having different representations and relative orientations of the constituent modules. The modules show sequence similarity to a number of previously described genes and markers, for instance *GGTL*, *NF1*, *BCR* and AT-rich regions. The LCRs are 100–400 kb long, the two largest being the most proximal (LCR-A) and most distal (LCR-D) units, which occur at the ends of the typical 3Mb deletion. These and the other repeat units are variously found at the ends of smaller atypical deletions and the other rearrangements involving 22q11 listed above. Two models have been proposed

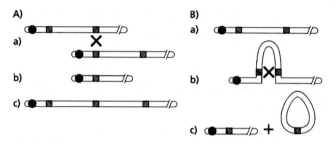

Figure 2.1   Possible mechanisms underlying 22q11 deletion. In A, two chromosome 22 homologues align with their low copy number repeats (LCNRs) offset. Interchromosomal recombination (a) results in two derivative chromosomes, one with a deletion (b) the other with a reciprocal duplication (c).
In B, looping within a single chromosome 22 aligns LCNR units which are in an inverse orientation (b), recombination giving an intrachromosomal deletion (c). The acentric fragment is lost.

to explain the origin of the deletion (Shaikh *et al.*, 2001), as shown in Figure 2.1. In one, an *inter*chromosomal misalignment of the two chromosome 22 homologs takes place during meiosis I, the modules of a more proximal LCR of one homolog aligning with identically orientated modules of more distal LCR. Recombination in this configuration produces a deletion and the reciprocal duplication. Reports of such duplications are very rare (Bergman & Blennow, 2000; Edelmann *et al.*, 1999a). It is possible that this is a result of ascertainment bias, since even in the reported cases the phenotype is mild and many instances may simply go unnoticed, or at least without a detailed chromosome analysis. The second model invokes an *intra*chromosomal recombination, where it is duplicated modules in an inverse orientation that align between the LCRs involved. Recombination at these points simply produces a deletion. The two models can be tested by tracing the inheritance of polymorphic markers flanking the deletion, with instances of both types of recombination event having been described.

It is interesting that there is no equivalent of these LCRs in rodents, and no report of any spontaneous deletion mutants of the relevant region of mouse chromosome 16. However, FISH studies demonstrate the presence of 22q11 repeat units in a range of apes and old world monkeys. Moreover, PCR is capable of amplifying repeat unit DNA from a range of apes, Old and New World monkeys, suggesting that the duplications arose at least 40 million years ago (mya) (Shaikh *et al.*, 2001).

It has been postulated that, as for Noonan syndrome (Osborne *et al.*, 2001), parental inversion polymorphism at 22q11 might predispose to the deletion. However, one study specifically investigated this issue and no evidence to support the theory was found (Gebhardt *et al.*, 2003).

Testing candidate genes

The single gene hypothesis predicted that a subset of those VCFS/DGS patients with no apparent deletion of 22q11 would have a small deletion or point mutation inactivating the major gene haploinsufficient in the condition. Initially, attempts to identify a candidate gene for mutation screening involved comparison of deletions of different patients on the basis that any major gene would be hemizygous in all deleted patients. As described above, most 22q11DS patients have a virtually identical 3 Mb deletion, making the construction of a shortest region of deletion overlap (SRDO) map difficult (Scambler, 2000). However, progress was apparently made comparing interstitial with terminal deletions, studies which suggested that the proximal third of the TDR was most important. Of particular interest was the presence of a chromosome 2;22 balanced translocation with a breakpoint within the proximal part of the TDR (Augusseau et al., 1986; Lindsay et al., 1993). It was anticipated that this translocation would directly disrupt the gene haploinsufficient in 22q11DS. However, cloning of the sequences disrupted by this translocation failed to identify any protein-encoding gene, and mutation screening of the closest gene (DGCR2) failed to identify any sequence changes likely to be associated with loss of function. Mutation screening then progressed through most of the genes of the proximal TDR (DGCR6-ARVCF) with similarly negative results.

Concurrently, efforts to refine the SRDO map produced conflicting data (Scambler, 2000). One deletion was similar to the TDR but did not extend so far proximally, and did not include the sequences disrupted by the 2;22 balanced translocation (Levy et al., 1995). Other deletions overlapped with different parts of the TDR, and one did not overlap but lay just distal to it (Kurahashi et al., 1996; O'Donnell et al., 1997; Amati et al., 1999; McQuade et al., 1999). How do these deletions cause the syndrome? One answer is that they do not, in the sense that one could question the diagnoses in most of these cases. A second explanation is that haploinsufficiency of different genes within 22q11 can produce a broadly similar phenotype. However, a favored explanation is that at least some of these rearrangements produce a long-range effect on the transcription of a critical gene (or genes) that mimics the effect of the deletion. Such effects have been described in other syndromes and can range over several hundreds of kbp (Pfeifer et al., 1999). Despite these intensive efforts, human SRDO mapping and gene mutation analyses failed to identify which gene or genes caused the syndrome.

Mouse models

The frustration at failure to find any loss of function mutations of DGCR genes in patients with no deletion prompted investigators to pursue animal models. Initially, this involved expression analysis of genes during murine and chick embryogenesis to enable prioritization of genes for further work on the basis of their expression pattern. Genes expressed in the branchial arches, outflow tract of the heart or neural crest were considered stronger candidates. These studies were followed by antisense attenuation experiments in the chick; for instance, "knock-down" of Hira expression in the cardiac neural crest was accompanied by an increased frequency of persistent truncus arteriosus in treated versus control embryos (Farrell *et al.*, 1999). However, murine gene targeting was the method of choice for probing mammalian gene function. Accordingly, several single gene mutants were made, but none represented a good model for 22q11DS.

At this stage it was not apparent whether 22q11DS was the result of haplo-insufficiency of one gene, or a combination of TDR genes. In order to allow for this second possibility, chromosome engineering experiments were conducted to mimic the human situation of multigene hemizygosity in the mouse. These experiments were feasible because the genes deleted in 22q11DS are all, bar one or two exceptions, clustered on proximal mouse chromosome 16, even though gene order is not perfectly conserved (Botta *et al.*, 1997; Puech *et al.*, 1997; Sutherland *et al.*, 1998). While one smaller deletion was created by a direct targeting strategy (Kimber *et al.*, 1999), all others reported to date have made use of the loxP Cre system. The first such targeted deletion was reported by Lindsay *et al.* (1999). This deletion was termed *Df1* (Deficiency 1), and establishes hemi-zygosity of 18 genes within a 1.2 Mb interval. Although hemizygous mice were viable and fertile, approximately 20% died in the perinatal period. Examination of late-gestation embryos revealed a series of congenital heart defects reminiscent of 22q11DS e.g. IAA-B and membranous ventricular septal defect (VSD). Analysis of mid-gestation embryos demonstrated full penetrance for hypo/aplasia of at least one of the fourth branchial arch arteries. These defects represent the class of heart defects most specific to 22q11DS. Most importantly, mice carrying a deleted chromosome 16 together with the reciprocal duplication on the corresponding homolog had no heart defects. This demonstrated that a gene or genes within the *Df1* interval was responsible for the observed phenotype, and that long-range effects on transcription such as those proposed to act in the human situation did not have a role. Similar experiments created a larger, 1.5 Mb, deletion termed *Lgdel* (Merscher *et al.*, 2001). The phenotype of +/*Lgdel* mice was similar to that seen in +/*df1*, although the perinatal mortality rate was higher, at around 40%.

Further examination of +/*df1* embryos at different stages of gestation revealed that a form of embryonic "recovery" takes places as time proceeds (Lindsay & Baldini, 2001). This recovery process could be influenced by the genetic back-ground of the +/*df1* mutation, although no evidence for a role of non-deleted TDR gene alleles could be shown (Taddei *et al.*, 2001). Parathyroid and thymic abnormal-ities could be also detected in +/*df1* embryos, albeit at a low frequency. The variable penetrance of thymic defects was also at least partly due to the presence of genetic modifiers.

Subsequently engineered deletions and duplications allowed a shortest region of deletion overlap map to be established in the mouse, and this in turn suggested that one or more of six genes in the *Arvcf–Ufd1l* interval had a haploinsufficient phenotype (Puech *et al.*, 2000; Lindsay *et al.*, 2001). Transgenic rescue experiments with either human or murine genes narrowed the region further, to just four genes. Based on its embryonic expression pattern in the mesodermal core of the pharyngeal arches the transcription factor *Tbx1* appeared the best candidate, and three teams independently created single gene-targeted mutants at this locus (Jerome & Papaioannou, 2001; Lindsay *et al.*, 2001; Merscher *et al.*, 2001). In each case, the heterozygous mice had the same cardiovascular malformations that had been observed in the *Df1* strain. The *Tbx1-/-* (*Tbx1* null) phenotype comprises defects of all the main structures affected in 22q11DS, and these mice can perhaps be viewed as having a severe form of the syndrome. Null mice die at birth, presumably as a result of their major heart malformations and other abnormalities. In particular, the null mice have persistence of the truncus arteriosus (PTA), absence of the thymus and parathyroids, a severely hypoplastic pharynx, a short neck and microtia together with other defects of the skull and vertebrae. *Tbx1-/-* embryos have severe hypo/aplasia of the pharyngeal arches, as shown in Figure 2.2.

Developmental genetics

Neural crest involvement

Aortic arch artery remodeling relies upon neural crest cells, and thus it is relevant to ask whether the *Df1* and *Tbx1* mutations affect these cells. Examination of *Tbx1* null embryos reveals a failure of development of the 2nd–6th pharyngeal arch arteries and the 2nd–4th pharyngeal pouches (Jerome & Papaioannou, 2001). Thus, the absence of normal pharyngeal pouches in null mutant embryos precludes the normal migration of neural crest cells and also results in disorganization in the development of some of the cranial nerves (Vitelli *et al.*, 2002a). Initial migration, proliferation and survival of neural crest cells appears normal in *Tbx1-/-* embryos and *Tbx1* is not expressed in the cardiac neural crest; therefore, a primary defect of these cells seems unlikely. However, there is evidence for a deficiency of the crest-derived vascular smooth muscle cell (VSMC) contribution to the fourth and possibly sixth pharyngeal arch artery in *+/df1* and *+/Lgdel* mice (Lindsay & Baldini, 2001; Kochilas *et al.*, 2002). Conditional targeting has been used to induce the *Lgdel* deletion in neural crest derivatives (Kochilas *et al.*, 2002). While the *Lgdel* could clearly be demonstrated in neural crest derivatives, no embryological defects were found. Thus, the secondary effects observed in neural crest cells suggest that they are the target of signals from pharyngeal endoderm, signals which are dependent upon *Tbx1*-driven transcription.

Fibroblast growth factors (Fgfs) represent one class of proteins which potentially mediates this activity. *Fgf8* and *Fgf10* expression is downregulated in certain expression zones within *Tbx1* null embryos (Vitelli *et al.*, 2002b). *Fgf8-/-* embryos demonstrate early embryonic lethality, but a hypomorphic allele has been used to show that Fgf8 signaling is vital for the formation of the structures affected in 22q11DS (Abu-Issa *et al.*, 2002; Frank *et al.*, 2002). Moreover, *Fgf8+/- Tbx1+/-* embryos have an increased frequency of IAA and other heart defects, providing compelling genetic evidence that these genes co-operate on the same developmental pathway (Vitelli *et al.*, 2002b).

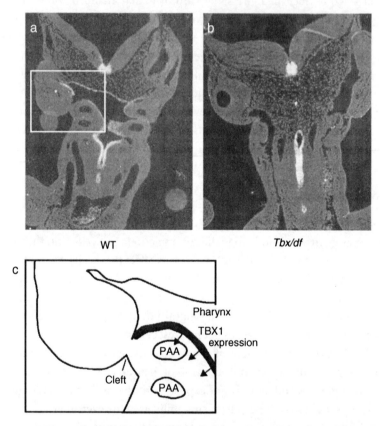

Figure 2.2   Loss of pharyngeal structures in *Tbx1-/-* embryos. Panel a shows a section through a day 10.5 embryo, which has well-developed branchial arches and pharyngeal arch arteries. In b the *Tbx1* null embryo has a narrow pharynx with absent caudal arches. In c a schematic of the boxed region of the section shown in a indicates how *Tbx1* expressing cells in the pharyngeal endoderm are envisaged as signaling to target cells within the branchial arches. (Photographs courtesy of Elizabeth Lindsay and Antonio Baldini.)

The regulation of *TBX1* itself is, as yet, not well characterized although progress has been made in identifying tissue-specific enhancers. In particular, it appears that *Tbx1* is regulated by the *Foxa2* and related forkhead transcription factors, and that these genes may be acting downstream of Shh (Yamagishi *et al.*, 2003b). Targeted mutagenesis of the chordin gene results in a DGS-like phenotype in those embryos surviving an early lethality. *Tbx1* and *Fgf8* expression is downregulated in these mutants (Bachiller *et al.*, 2003).

Df1 mice and behavior

Given the cognitive deficits and increased incidence of behavioral difficulty in 22q11DS attempts have been made to identify behavioral correlates in the mouse deletion model. The *Df1* mice have sensorimotor gating and learning abnormalities as detected in PPI (prepulsed inhibition) and conditioned fear tests (Paylor *et al.*, 2001). Efforts are underway to identify specific gene haploinsufficiencies that might be responsible for this phenotype. Clearly, there are limits to how far any findings can be extrapolated between the two species, but nevertheless these experiments offer a novel route into the dissection of genes underlying brain development and behavioral traits.

Other models

Mutagenesis screens in the zebrafish have been informative in the dissection of several developmental and genetic pathways. The phenotype of the *vgo* zebrafish is strongly reminiscent of that seen in *Tbx1* null mice, with a failure of pharyngeal segmentation and the presence of a single pharyngeal arch artery (Piotrowski & Nusslein-Volhard, 2000). Subsequently, it has been shown that the *vgo* phenotype is secondary to mutations of zebrafish *Tbx1*, the *vgo* mutant therefore provides another model for exploring the developmental basis of the syndrome (Piotrowski *et al.*, 2003). Work to date demonstrates reduced *Nkx2.5* expression in the secondary heart field. Interestingly, the heterozygous fish have no apparent abnormalities, emphasizing that different vertebrate species have differing dosage requirements for *Tbx1* during development.

TBX1 mutations are rare in non-deletion VCFS/DGS

Despite extensive searches (Gong *et al.*, 2001; Lindsay *et al.*, 2001; Conti *et al.*, 2003), just three unequivocal mutations of *TBX1* have been described in non-deletion cases of VCFS/DGS or conotruncal heart defect (Yagi *et al.*, 2003). The mutations described to date are predicted to be loss of function, and occur in conserved amino acids of TBX1 (Yagi *et al.*, 2003). They are all in patients from Japan, which may reflect an increased frequency of *TBX1* mutation in this ethnic group. Although one or two of the other sequence variants described may lead to some loss of function of TBX1, this remains to be proven biochemically. It is possible that, in some of the patients screened, mutations within intronic regions, transcriptional control regions or multiexon deletions have been missed. However, given the numbers of patients screened, mutations within the coding region, particularly of the T box would have been expected. Even so, it may reasonably be concluded that *TBX1* mutations are not a common cause of non-deletion VCFS and the syndrome in these patients presumably has a different etiology. There are a number of explanations for this unexpected result. Several genes are known that are haploinsufficient in humans, but not in mice. For instance, in humans, heterozygous mutations of *PAX3* cause Waardenburg syndrome which includes sensorineural deafness. In mouse, heterozygous mutations of *Pax3* cause a white belly spot, but the mice have normal auditory evoked potentials. It is therefore conceivable that the opposite pertains i.e. *Tbx1* is haploinsufficient in mice but not in man. In the context of a 3Mb deletion, however, the embryo's tolerance for *TBX1* hemizygosity would be diminished, resulting in emergence of haploinsufficiency in this scenario. If this were true then the Japanese mutations may represent predisposition alleles interacting with some additional insult. Some commentators have suggested that disruption of an important functional chromosomal architecture existing in the critical region could affect transcription of genes within 22q11 and play a role in the pathogenesis of the disorder (Novelli *et al.*, 2000). These arguments are based upon the complexity of the different deletions seen, and the fact that many of the genes from the TDR are expressed in the pharyngeal arches and/or the neural crest. Indeed, recent evidence based upon microarray data from *Drosophila melanogaster* does suggest that gene expression patterns are correlated over large chromosomal distances (Weitzman, 2002). If this is true for 22q11, and additionally reflects an underlying functional interrelationship, then the deletion of genes adjacent to *TBX1* could well exacerbate the effects of *TBX1* haploinsufficiency. However, the available data provide strong support for the hypothesis that *TBX1* deficiency is the primary cause of the predominant malformations seen in 22q11DS (Baldini 2000). Early results from array-based comparative genome hybridization suggests some patients previously diagnosed as probable 22q11DS actually have deletions elsewhere in the genome (our unpublished data).

Chromosome 10p deletion syndromes

Partial monosomy 10p has been described in association with VCFS/DGS-like abnormalities and comparison of deletions led to identification of the DGSII locus (Daw *et al.*, 1996). Later studies suggested that two regions of 10p might be involved (Gottlieb *et al.*, 1998a; Schuffenhauer *et al.*, 1998). A syndrome of hypoparathyroidism, sensorineural deafness and renal anomalies (HDR) was associated with the more distal deletions, and cardiac anomalies with thymic hypo/aplasia or T cell defect thought to be due to hemizygosity of a more proximal gene or genes (Lichtner *et al.*, 2000). HDR is now known to be due to *GATA3* loss of function mutations (Van Esch *et al.*, 2000). The partial monosomy 10p sub-spectrum of heart defect and thymus hypoplasia/aplasia still remains unexplained. The search for genes involved in heart and thymic development concentrated on a region 4Mb proximal to the *GATA3* gene. The gene *BRUNOL3* appeared a good candidate based upon positional and expression pattern but no loss of function mutations have yet been found (Lichtner *et al.*, 2002). In clinical terms, the 10p deletions are relatively infrequent with an incidence of less than 1:50 000 live births. A study of approximately 400 patients referred for deletion testing identi-fied a single 10p deletion, visible on a standard karyotype (Berend *et al.*, 2000). Routine screening for sub-microscopic deletions of 10p is not recommended unless there is clinical suspicion of HDR syndrome.

The future

TBX1 is a member of a family of transcription factors having a DNA binding domain – the "T" box – related to that seen in the prototypic member of the family, Brachyury or T. Over 20 members of the family have now been described, some of which are transcriptional activators and others are repressors. Our preliminary data suggest that TBX1 is a transcriptional activator and that the activating activity resides in the c-terminal part of the protein. This information has been used to create a dominant-negative version of TBX1, substituting the repression domain from *Drosophila* engrailed for the activation domain. When expressed in *Xenopus laevis*, this protein severely disrupts development of the pharyngeal structures, providing another system for the analysis of TBX1 activity. Dominant negative interference can be controlled by the addition of a hormone-responsive element to the protein, thus providing a molecular switch. Similar methods have been used with success to probe the function of the related TBX5 gene, which is haploinsuf-ficient in the Holt Oram syndrome (Horb & Thomsen, 1999). It is likely that inducible systems such as Cre/loxP and tetR will be used to control *Tbx1* expres-sion in the mouse, providing information regarding the times at which *Tbx1* is required during development, and the specific cell types that require its activity.

Clearly, as a transcription factor, it is important to identify the genes regulated by *TBX1*, and thus differentially regulated in mutant embryos. Progress towards this end has been achieved using oligonucleotide-based gene arrays, comparing expression in wild type and *Df1* pharyngeal arches. The hemizygosity of genes adjacent to *Tbx1* in the *Df1* deletion provide a good internal control for the sensitivity of the technique, and early work shows that these genes are indeed identified in the subset of downregulated genes within *Df1* embryos. Similar work is being conducted on *Tbx1* null embryos and on the brains of *Df1* mice. These latter experiments could identify genes important in controlling the conditioned fear and PPI responses.

Finally, for the patient and family, how does genetics improve patient care? The FISH test (and other molecular assays) can now provide an unequivocal diagnosis which enables prenatal diagnosis where requested and, importantly, an early diagnosis which can direct further investigation and appropriate therapeutic intervention. In many countries the availability of a firm syndromic diagnosis is a necessary prerequisite to facilitated access to educational support and social services. Much of the recent molecular and developmental biology is basic science whose benefits will not be felt for years and even then are likely to be applicable to general areas rather than one specific syndrome. However, it is possible that the more recent work on the behavioral and psychiatric aspects of the syndrome may identify novel drug targets that will be of benefit not only to 22q11DS patients but also more generally.

REFERENCES

Abu-Issa, R., Smyth, G., Smoak, I. *et al.* (2002) Fgf8 is required for pharyngeal arch and cardiovascular development in the mouse. *Development*, **129** (19), 4613–25.

Akhavan, S., De Cristofaro, R., Peyvandi, F. *et al.* (2002) Molecular and functional characterization of a natural homozygous Arg67His mutation in the prothrombin gene of a patient with a severe procoagulant defect contrasting with a mild hemorrhagic phenotype, *Blood*, **100** (4), 1347–53.

Amati, F., Conti, E., Novelli, A. *et al.* (1999) Atypical deletions suggest five 22q11.2 critical regions related to the DiGeorge/velo-cardio-facial syndrome, *Eur. J. Hum. Genet.*, **7** (8), 903–9.

Augusseau, S., Jouk, S., Jalbert, P. & Priur, M. (1986) DiGeorge syndrome and 22q11 rearrangements, *Hum. Genet.*, **74**, 206.

Ayuk, P. T., Sibley, C. P., Donnai, P. *et al.* (2000) Development and polarization of cationic amino acid transporters and regulators in the human placenta, *Am. J. Physiol. Cell Physiol.*, **278** (6), C1162–71.

Bachiller, D., Klingensmith, J., Shneyder, N. *et al.* (2003) The role of chordin/Bmp signals in mammalian pharyngeal development and DiGeorge syndrome. *Development*, **130** (15), 3567–78.

Baglin, T. P., Carrell, R. W., Church, F. C. *et al.* (2002) Crystal structures of native and thrombin-complexed heparin cofactor II reveal a multistep allosteric mechanism. *Proc. Natl. Acad. Sci. USA*, **99** (17), 11079–84.

Baldini, A. (2000) DiGeorge syndrome: complex pathogenesis? Maybe, maybe not. *Mol. Med. Today*, **6** (**1**), 12.

Berend, S. A., Spikes, A. S., Kashork, C. D. *et al.* (2000) Dual-probe fluorescence in situ hybridization assay for detecting deletions associated with VCFS/DiGeorge syndrome I and DiGeorge syndrome II loci [In Process Citation]. *Am. J. Med. Genet.*, **91** (**4**), 313–17.

Bergman, A. & Blennow, E. (2000) Inv dup (22), del (22) (q11) and r (22) in the father of a child with DiGeorge syndrome. *Eur. J. Hum. Genet.*, **8** (**10**), 801–4.

Berti, L., Mittler, G., Przemeck, G. K. *et al.* (2001) Isolation and characterization of a novel gene from the DiGeorge chromosomal region that encodes for a mediator subunit. *Genomics*, **74** (**3**), 320–32.

Binder, M. (1985) The teratogenic effects of a Bis (dichloroacetyl)diamine on hamster embryos. *Am. J. Pathol.*, **118**, 179–93.

Bobanovic, L. K., Royle, S. J. & Murrell-Lagnado, R. D. (2002) P2X receptor trafficking in neurons is subunit specific. *J. Neurosci.*, **22** (**12**), 4814–24.

Bockman, D. E. & Kirby, M. L. (1984) Dependence of thymus development on derivatives of the neural crest. *Science*, **223**, 498–500.

Bockman, D. E., Redmond, M. E., Waldo, K. *et al.* (1987) Effect of neural crest ablation on development of the heart and arch arteries in the chick. *Am. J. Anat.*, **180**, 332–41.

Botta, A., Lindsay, E. A., Jurecic, V. & Baldini, A. (1997) Comparative mapping of the DiGeorge syndrome region in mouse shows inconsistent gene order and diferential degree of gene conservation. *Mammalian Genome*, **8**, 890–5.

Budarf, M. L., Konkle, B. A., Ludlow, L. B. *et al.* (1995) Identification of a patient with Bernard–Soulier syndrome and a deletion in the DiGeorge/Velo-cardio-facial chromosomal region in 22q11.2., *Hum Mol Genet*, **4**, 763–6.

Caltagarone, J., Rhodes, J., Honer, W. G. & Bowser, R. (1998) Localization of a novel septin protein, hCDCrel-1, in neurons of human brain. *Neuroreport*, **9** (**12**), 2907–12.

Carey, A. H., Kelly, D., Halford, S. *et al.* (1992) Molecular genetic study of the frequency of monosomy 22q11 in DiGeorge syndrome. *Am. J. Hum. Genet.*, **51**, 964–70.

Clouthier, D. E., Williams, S. C., Yanagisawa, H. *et al.* (2000) Signaling pathways crucial for craniofacial development revealed by endothelin-A receptor-deficient mice. *Dev Biol*, **217** (**1**), 10–24.

Conti, E., Grifone, N., Sarkozy, A. *et al.* (2003) DiGeorge subtypes of nonsyndromic conotruncal defects: evidence against a major role of TBX1 Gene. *Eur. J. Hum. Genet.*, **11** (**4**), 349–51.

Conway, S. J., Henderson, D. J., Kirby, M. L. *et al.* (1997) Development of a lethal congenital heart defect in the splotch (Pax3) mutant mouse. *Cardiovasc. Res.*, **36**, 163–73.

Cote, F., Boisvert, F. M., Grondin, B. *et al.* (2001) Alternative promoter usage and splicing of ZNF74 multifinger gene produce protein isoforms with a different repressor activity and nuclear partitioning. *DNA Cell. Biol.*, **20** (**3**), 159–73.

Daw, S. C. M., Taylor, C., Kraman, M. *et al.* (1996) A common region of 10p deleted in DiGeorge and velo-cardio-facial syndrome. *Nat. Genet.*, **13**, 458–60.

De Lucia, F., Lorain, S., Scamps, C. *et al.* (2001) Subnuclear localization and mitotic phosphorylation of HIRA, the human homologue of *Saccharomyces cerevisiae* transcriptional regulators Hir1p/Hir2p. *Biochem. J.*, **358** (**2**), 447–55.

Driscoll, D. A. (2001) Prenatal diagnosis of the 22q11.2 deletion syndrome. *Genet. Med.*, **3** (**1**), 14–18.

Du Montcel, S. T., Mendizabal, H., Ayme, S. *et al.* (1996) Prevalence of 22q11 microdeletion. *J. Med. Genet.*, **33**, 719.

Dunham, I., Shimizu, N., Roe, B. A. *et al.* (1999) The DNA sequence of human chromosome 22 [see comments] [published erratum appears in Nature 2000, 404 (6780), 904], *Nature*, **402 (6761)**, 489–95.

Edelmann, L., Pandita, R., Spiteri, E. *et al.* (1999a) A common molecular basis for rearrangement disorders on chromosome 22q11. *Hum. Mol. Genet.*, **8**, 1157–67.

Edelmann, L., Pandita, R. K., & Morrow, B. E. (1999b) Low-copy repeats mediate the common 3-Mb deletion in patients with velo-cardio-facial syndrome. *Am. J. Hum. Genet.*, **64** (**4**), 1076–86.

Emanuel, B. S., Budarf, B. S. & Scambler, P. J. (1998) The genetic basis of conotruncal heart defects: the chromosome 22q11.2 deletion. In Rosenthal, N. & Harvey, R., eds., *Heart Development*. New York: Academic Press, pp. 463–78.

Farrell, M., Stadt, H., Wallis, K. *et al.* (1999) Persistent truncus arteriosus is associated with decreased expression of HIRA by cardiac neural crest cells in chick embryos. *Circulation Research*, **84**, 127–35.

Feller, S. M. (2001) Crk family adaptors-signalling complex formation and biological roles. *Oncogene*, **20** (**44**), 6348–71.

Frank, D. U., Fotheringham, L. K., Brewer, J. A. *et al.* (2002) An Fgf8 mouse mutant phenocopies human 22q11 deletion syndrome. *Development*, **129** (**19**), 4591–603.

Funke, B., Puech, A., Saint-Jore, B. *et al.* (1998) Isolation and characterization of a human gene containing a nuclear localization signal from the critical region for velo-cardio-facial syndrome on 22q11. *Genomics*, **53** (**2**), 146–54.

Galili, N., Epstein, J. A., Leconte, I. *et al.* (1998) Gscl, a gene within the minimal DiGeorge critical region, is expressed in primordial germ cells and the developing pons. *Dev Dyn*, **212**, 86–93.

Galili, N., Nayak, S., Epstein, J. A. & Buck, C. A. (2000) Rnf4, a RING protein expressed in the developing nervous and reproductive systems, interacts with Gscl, a gene within the DiGeorge critical region. *Dev Dyn*, **218**, 102–11.

Gebhardt, G. S., Devriendt, K., Thoelen, R. *et al.* (2003) No evidence for a parental inversion polymorphism predisposing to rearrangements at 22q11.2 in the DiGeorge/Velocardiofacial syndrome. *Eur. J. Hum. Genet.*, **11** (**2**), 109–11.

Gehrmann, T. & Heilmeyer, L. M., Jr. (1998) Phosphatidylinositol 4-kinases. *Eur. J. Biochem.*, **253** (**2**), 357–70.

Gogos, J. A., Morgan, M., Luine, V. *et al.* (1998) Catechol-O-methyltransferase-deficient mice exhibit sexually dimorphic changes in catecholamine levels and behavior. *Proc. Natl. Acad. Sci. USA*, **95** (**17**), 9991–6.

Gogos, J. A., Santha, M., Takacs, Z. *et al.* (1999) The gene encoding proline dehydrogenase modulates sensorimotor gating in mice. *Nat. Genet.*, **21** (**4**), 434–9.

Goldmuntz, E., Fedon, J., Roe, B. & Budarf, M. L. (1997) Molecular characterization of a serine/threonine kinase in the DiGeorge minimal critical region. *Gene*, **198**, 379–86.

Gong, L., Liu, M., Jen, J. & Yeh, E. T. (2000) GNB1L, a gene deleted in the critical region for DiGeorge syndrome on 22q11, encodes a G-protein beta-subunit-like polypeptide (1). *Biochim. Biophys. Acta*, **1494** (1–2), 185–8.

Gong, W., Emanuel, B. S., Collins, J. *et al.* (1996) A transcription map of the DiGeorge and velo-cardio-facial syndrome critical region on 22q11. *Hum. Mol. Genet.*, **5**, 789–800.

Gong, W., Gottlieb, S., Collins, J. *et al.* (2001) Mutation analysis of TBX1 in non-deleted patients with features of DGS/VCFS or isolated cardiovascular defects. *J. Med. Genet.*, **38** (12), E45.

Goodship, J., Cross, I., Scambler, P. & Burn, J. (1995) Monozygotic twins with chromosome 22q11 deletion and discordant phenotype. *J. Med. Genet.*, **32**, 746–8.

Gottlieb, S., Driscoll, D. A., Punnett, H. H. *et al.* (1998a) Characterization of 10p deletions suggests two nonoverlapping regions contribute to the DiGeorge syndrome phenotype. *Am. J. Hum. Genet.*, **62**, 495–8.

Gottlieb, S., Hanes, S. D., Golden, J. A. *et al.* (1998b) Goosecoid-like, a gene deleted in DiGeorge and velocardiofacial syndromes, recognizes DNA with a bicoid-like specificity and is expressed in the developing mouse brain. *Hum. Mol. Genet.*, **7** (9), 1497–505.

Graham, A. (2001) The development and evolution of the pharyngeal arches. *J. Anat.*, **199** (1–2), 133–41.

Grondin, B., Cote, F., Bazinet, M. *et al.* (1997) Direct interaction of the KRAB/Cys2-His2 zinc finger protein ZNF74 with a hyperphosphorylated form of the RNA polymerase II largest subunit. *J. Biol. Chem.*, **272** (44), 27877–85.

Guris, D. L., Fantes, J., Tara, D. *et al.* (2001) Mice lacking the homologue of the human 22q11.2 gene CRKL phenocopy neurocristopathies of DiGeorge syndrome. *Nat. Genet.*, **27** (3), 293–8.

Halford, S., Lindsay, E., Nayudu, M. *et al.* (1993a) Low-copy-repeat sequences flank the DiGeorge/velo-cardio-facial syndrome loci at 22q11. *Hum. Mol. Genet.*, **2**, 191–6.

Halford, S., Wilson, D. I., Daw, S. C. M. *et al.* (1993b) Isolation of a gene expressed during early embryogenesis from the region of 22q11 commonly deleted in DiGeorge syndrome. *Hum. Mol. Genet.*, **2**, 1577–82.

Hall, C., Nelson, D. M., Ye, X. *et al.* (2001) HIRA, the human homologue of yeast Hir1p and Hir2p, is a novel cyclin-cdk2 substrate whose expression blocks S-phase progression. *Mol. Cell Biol.*, **21** (5), 1854–65.

Hatchwell, E., Long, F., Wilde, J. *et al.* (1998) Molecular confirmation of germ line mosaicism for a submicroscopic deletion of chromosome 22q11. *Am. J. Med. Genet.*, **78** (2), 103–6.

Holmes, S. E., Riazi, M. A., Gong, W. *et al.* (1997) Disruption of the clathrin heavy chain-like gene (CLTCL) associated with features of DGS/VCFS: a balanced (21;22) (p12;q11) translocation. *Hum. Mol. Genet.*, **6**, 357–67.

Horb, M. E. & Thomsen, G. H. (1999) Tbx5 is essential for heart development. *Development*, **126** (8), 1739–51.

Ishii, J., Adachi, H., Aoki, J. *et al.* (2002) SREC-II, a new member of the scavenger receptor type F family, trans-interacts with SREC-I through its extracellular domain. *J. Biol. Chem.*, **277** (42), 39696–702.

Iwarsson, E., Ahrlund-Richter, L., Inzunza, J. *et al.* (1998) Preimplantation genetic diagnosis of DiGeorge syndrome. *Mol. Hum. Reprod.*, **4** (9), 871–5.

Jacquet, H., Raux, G., Thibaut, F. *et al.* (2002) PRODH mutations and hyperprolinemia in a subset of schizophrenic patients. *Hum. Mol. Genet.*, **11** (**19**), 2243–9.

Jerome, L. A. & Papaioannou, V. E. (2001) DiGeorge syndrome phenotype in mice mutant for the T-box gene. *Tbx1. Nat Genet*, **27**, 286–91.

Kajiwara, K., Nagasawa, H., Shimizu-Nishikawa, K. *et al.* (1996) Cloning of SEZ-12 encoding seizure-related and membrane bound adhesion protein. *Biochem. Biophys. Res. Com.*, **222**, 144–8.

Kimber, W., Hseih, P., Hirotsune, S. *et al.* (1999) Deletion of 150 kb in the minimal DiGeorge/velocardiofacial syndrome critical region in mouse. *Hum. Mol. Genet.*, **12**, 2229–37.

Kirby, M. L. (1999) Contribution of neural crest to heart and vessel morphology. In Harvey, R. P. & Rosenthal, N., eds., *Heart Development.* New York: Academic Press, pp. 179–94.

Kochilas, L. K., Merscher-Gomez, S., Lu, M. M. *et al.* (2002) The role of neural crest during cardiac development in a mouse model of DiGeorge syndrome. *Dev. Biol.*, **251**, 157–66.

Kurahashi, H., Akagi, K., Inazawa, J. *et al.* (1995) Isolation and characterization of a novel gene deleted in DiGeorge syndrome. *Hum. Mol. Genet.*, **4**, 541–9.

Kurahashi, H., Nakayama, T., Osugi, Y. *et al.* (1996) Deletion mapping of 22q11 in CATCH22 syndrome: identification of a second critical region. *Am. J. Hum. Genet.*, **58**, 1377–81.

Lachman, H. M., Morrow, B., Shprintzen, R. *et al.* (1996) Association of codon 108/158 catechol-O-methyltransferase gene polymorphism with the psychiatric manifestations of velocardiofacial syndrome. *Am. J. Med. Genet.*, **67**, 468–72.

Lammer, E. J., Chen, D. T., Hoar, N. D. *et al.* (1986) Retinoic acid embryopathy. A new human teratogen and a mechanistic hypothesis. *N. Engl. J. Med.*, **313**, 837–41.

Lamorte, L., Royal, I., Naujokas, M. & Park, M. (2002) Crk adapter proteins promote an epithelial-mesenchymal-like transition and are required for HGF-mediated cell spreading and breakdown of epithelial adherens junctions. *Mol. Biol. Cell.*, **13** (**5**), 1449–61.

Laura, R. P., Witt, A. S., Held, H. A. *et al.* (2002) The Erbin PDZ domain binds with high affinity and specificity to the carboxyl termini of delta-catenin and ARVCF. *J. Biol. Chem.*, **277**(**15**), 12906–14.

Levy, A., Demczuk, S., Aurias, A. *et al.* (1995) Interstitial 22q11 deletion excluding the ADU breakpoint in a patient with DGS. *Hum. Mol. Genet.*, **4**, 2417–18.

Lichtner, P., Konig, R., Hasegawa, T. *et al.* (2000) An HDR (hypoparathyroidism, deafness, renal dysplasia) syndrome locus maps distal to the DiGeorge syndrome region on 10p13/14 [In Process Citation]. *J. Med. Genet.*, **37** (**1**), 33–7.

Lichtner, P., Attie-Bitach, T., Schuffenhauer, S. *et al.* (2002) Expression and mutation analysis of BRUNOL3, a candidate gene for heart and thymus developmental defects associated with partial monosomy 10p. *J. Mol. Med.*, **80** (**7**), 431–42.

Lindsay, E. A. & Baldini, A. (1997) A mouse gene (Dgcr6) related to the *Drosophila* gonadal gene is expressed in early embryogenesis and is the homolog of a human gene deleted in DiGeorge syndrome. *Cytogenet. Cell Genet.*, **79** (**3–4**), 243–7.

(2001) Recovery from arterial growth delay reduces penetrance of cardiovascular defects in mice deleted for the DiGeorge syndrome region. *Hum. Mol. Genet.*, **10** (**9**), 997–1002.

Lindsay, E. A., Halford, S., Wadey, R. *et al.* (1993) Molecular cytogenetic characterisation of the DiGeorge syndrome region using fluorescence in situ hybridisation. *Genomics*, **17**, 403–7.

Lindsay, E. A., Harvey, E. L., Scambler, P. J. & Baldini, A. (1998) ES2, a gene deleted in DiGeorge syndrome, encodes a nuclear protein and is expressed during early mouse development, where it shares an expression domain with a Goosecoid-like gene. *Hum. Mol. Genet.*, **7**, 629–35.

Lindsay, E. A., Botta, A., Jurecic, V. *et al.* (1999) Congenital heart disease in mice deficient for the DiGeorge syndrome region. *Nature*, **401**, 379–83.

Lindsay, E. A., Vitelli, F., Su, H. *et al.* (2001) Tbx1 haploinsufficiency identified by functional scanning of the DiGeorge syndrome region is the cause of aortic arch defects in mice. *Nature*, **401**, 97–101.

Liu, H., Heath, S. C., Sobin, C. *et al.* (2002) Genetic variation at the 22q11 PRODH2/DGCR6 locus presents an unusual pattern and increases susceptibility to schizophrenia. *Proc. Natl. Acad. Sci. USA*, **99** (**6**), 3717–22.

Lorain, S., Quivy, J.-P., Monier-Gavelle, F. *et al.* (1998) Core histones and HIRIP3, a novel histone-binding protein, directly interact with the WD repeat protein HIRA. *Mol. Cell Biol.*, **18**, 5546–56.

Magnaghi, P., Roberts, C., Lorain, S. *et al.* (1998) HIRA, a mammalian homologue of *Saccharomyces cerevisiae* transcriptional co-repressors, interacts with Pax3. *Nat. Genet.*, **20**, 74–7.

Malakhov, M. P., Malakhova, O. A., Kim, K. I. *et al.* (2002) UBP43 (USP18) specifically removes ISG15 from conjugated proteins. *J. Biol. Chem.*, **277** (**12**), 9976–81.

Mangos, S., Vanderbeld, B., Krawetz, R. *et al.* (2001) Ran binding protein RanBP1 in zebrafish embryonic development. *Mol Reprod Dev*, **59** (**3**), 235–48.

Mariner, D. J., Wang, J. & Reynolds, A. B. (2000) ARVCF localizes to the nucleus and adherens junction and is mutually exclusive with p120 (ctn) in E-cadherin complexes. *J. Cell. Sci.*, **113** (**8**), 1481–90.

Maynard, T. M., Haskell, G. T., Bhasin, N. *et al.* (2002) RanBP1, a velocardiofacial/DiGeorge syndrome candidate gene, is expressed at sites of mesenchymal/epithelial induction. *Mech. Dev.*, **111** (**1–2**), 177–80.

McKerracher, L. & Winton, M. J. (2002) Nogo on the go. *Neuron*, **36** (**3**), 345–8.

McKie, J. M., Sutherland, H. F., Harvey, E. *et al.* (1998) A human gene similar to *Drosophila melanogaster* peanut maps to the DiGeorge Syndrome region of 22q11. *Hum Genet*, **101**, 6–12.

McQuade, L., Christodoulou, J., Budarf, B. *et al.* (1999) Patient with a 22q11.2 deletion with no overlap of the minimal DiGeorge syndrome critical region (MDGCR). *Am. J. Med. Genet.*, **86**, 27–33.

Merscher, S., Funke, B., Epstein, J. A. *et al.* (2001) TBX1 is responsible for the cardiovascular defects in velo-cardio-facial/DiGeorge syndrome. *Cell*, **104**, 619–29.

Meyer, H. H., Shorter, J. G., Seemann, J. *et al.* (2000) A complex of mammalian ufd1 and npl4 links the AAA-ATPase, p97, to ubiquitin and nuclear transport pathways. *EMBO J.*, **19** (**10**), 2181–92.

Miyamori, H., Takino, T., Kobayashi, Y. *et al.* (2001) Claudin promotes activation of pro-matrix metalloproteinase-2 mediated by membrane-type matrix metalloproteinases. *J. Biol. Chem.*, **276** (**30**), 28204–11.

Morita, K., Sasaki, H., Furuse, M. & Tsukita, S. (1999) Endothelial claudin: claudin-5/TMVCF constitutes tight junction strands in endothelial cells. *J. Cell Biol.*, **147** (**1**), 185–94.

Novelli, G., Amati, F. & Dallapiccola, B. (2000) Individual haploinsufficient loci and the complex phenotype of DiGeorge syndrome. *Mol. Med. Today*, **6**(1), 10–11.

O'Donnell, H., McKeown, C., Gould, C. *et al.* (1997) Detection of a deletion within 22q11 which has no overlap with the DiGeorge syndrome critical region. *Am. J. Hum. Genet.*, **60**, 1544–8.

Osborne, L. R., Li, M., Pober, B. *et al.* (2001) A 1.5 million-base pair inversion polymorphism in families with Williams-Beuren syndrome. *Nat. Genet.*, **29** (3), 321–5.

Paylor, R., McIlwain, K. L., McAninch, R. *et al.* (2001) Mice deleted for the DiGeorge/velocardiofacial syndrome region show abnormal sensorimotor gating and learning and memory impairments. *Hum. Mol. Genet.*, **10** (23), 2645–50.

Pfeifer, D., Kist, R., Dewar, K. *et al.* (1999) Campomelic dysplasia translocation breakpoints are scattered over 1 Mb proximal to SOX9: evidence for an extended control region. *Am. J. Hum. Genet.*, **65** (1), 111–24.

Piotrowski, T. & Nusslein-Volhard, C. (2000) The endoderm plays an important role in patterning the segmented pharyngeal region in zebrafish (*Danio rerio*). *Dev. Biol.*, **225** (2), 339–56.

Piotrowski, T., Ahn, D. G., Schilling, T. F. *et al.* (2003) The zebrafish van gogh mutation disrupts Tbx1, which is involved in the DiGeorge deletion syndrome in humans. *Development*, **130** (20), 5043–52.

Puech, A., Saint-Jore, B., Funke, B. *et al.* (1997) Comparative mapping of the human 22q11 chromosomal region and the orthologous region in mice reveals complex changes in gene organization. *Proc. Natl. Acad. Sci. USA*, **94**, 14608–13.

Puech, A., Saint-Jore, B., Merscher, S. *et al.* (2000) Normal cardiovascular development in mice deficient for 16 genes in 550 kb of the velocardiofacial/DiGeorge syndrome region. *Proc. Natl. Acad. Sci. USA*, **97** (18), 10090–5.

Rape, M., Hoppe, T., Gorr, I. *et al.* (2001) Mobilization of processed, membrane-tethered SPT23 transcription factor by CDC48 (UFD1/NPL4), a ubiquitin-selective chaperone. *Cell*, **107** (5), 667–77.

Ravassard, P., Cote, F., Grondin, B. *et al.* (1999) ZNF74, a gene deleted in DiGeorge syndrome, is expressed in human neural crest-derived tissues and foregut endoderm epithelia. *Genomics*, **62** (1), 82–5.

Ray-Gallet, D., Quivy, J. P., Scamps, C. *et al.* (2002) HIRA is critical for a nucleosome assembly pathway independent of DNA synthesis. *Mol. Cell*, **9** (5), 1091–100.

Roberts, C., Daw, S. C., Halford, S. & Scambler, P. J. (1997) Cloning and developmental expression analysis of chick Hira (Chira), a candidate gene for Di George Syndrome. *Hum. Mol. Genet.*, **6**, 237–45.

Roberts, C., Sutherland, H. F., Farmer, H. *et al.* (2002) Targeted mutagenesis of the Hira gene results in gastrulation defects and patterning abnormalities of mesoendodermal derivatives prior to early embryonic lethality. *Mol. Cell. Biol.*, **22**, 2318–28.

Robinson, H. B. Jr. (1975) DiGeorge's or the III-IV pharyngeal pouch syndrome. Pathology and a theory of pathogenesis. *Perspect. Ped. Path.*, **2**, 173–206.

Ryan, A. K., Goodship, J. A., Wilson, D. I. *et al.* (1997) Spectrum of clinical features associated with interstitial chromosome 22q11 deletions: a European collaborative study. *J. Med. Genet.*, **34**, 798–804.

Saint-Jore, B., Puech, A., Heyer, J. *et al.* (1998) Goosecoid-like (Gscl), a candidate gene for velocardiofacial syndrome, is not essential for normal mouse development. *Hum. Mol. Genet.,* **7** (**12**), 1841–9.

Sandrin-Garcia, P., Macedo, C., Martelli, L. R. *et al.* (2002) Recurrent 22q11.2 deletion in a sibship suggestive of parental germline mosaicism in velocardiofacial syndrome. *Clin. Genet.,* **61** (**5**), 380–3.

Scambler, P. J. (2000) The 22q11 deletion syndromes. *Hum. Mol. Genet.,* **9**, 2421–6.

Schuffenhauer, S., Lichter, P., Peykar-Derakhshandeh, P. *et al.* (1998) Deletion mapping on chromosome 10p and definition of a critical region for the second DiGeorge syndrome locus (DGS2). *Eur. J. Hum. Genet.,* **6**, 213–25.

Shaikh, T. H., Kurahashi, H., Saitta, S. C. *et al.* (2000) Chromosome 22-specific low copy repeats and the 22q11.2 deletion syndrome: genomic organization and deletion endpoint analysis. *Hum. Mol. Genet.,* **9** (**4**), 489–501.

Shaikh, T. H., Kurahashi, H. & Emanuel, B. S. (2001) Evolutionarily conserved low copy repeats (LCRs) in 22q11 mediate deletions, duplications, translocations, and genomic instability: an update and literature review. *Genet. Med.,* **3** (**1**), 6–13.

Su, Q., Mochida, S., Tian, J. H. *et al.* (2001) SNAP-29: a general SNARE protein that inhibits SNARE disassembly and is implicated in synaptic transmission. *Proc. Natl. Acad. Sci. USA,* **98** (**24**), 14038–43.

Sutherland, H. F., Wadey, R., McKie, J. M. *et al.* (1996) Identification of a novel transcript disrupted by a balanced translocation associated with DiGeorge syndrome. *Am. J. Hum. Genet.,* **59**, 23–31.

Sutherland, H. F., Kim, U. -J. & Scambler, P. J. (1998) Cloning and comparative mapping of the DiGeorge syndrome critical region in the mouse. *Genomics,* **52**, 37–43.

Taddei, I., Morishima, M., Huynh, T. & Lindsay, E. A. (2001) Genetic factors are major determinants of phenotypic variability in a mouse model of the DiGeorge/del22q11 syndromes. *Proc. Natl. Acad. Sci. USA,* **98** (**20**), 11428–31.

Takihara, Y., Tomotsune, D., Shirai, M. *et al.* (1997) Targeted disruption of the mouse homologue of the *Drosophila* polyhomeotic gene leads to altered anteroposterior patterning and neural crest defects. *Development,* **124**, 3673–82.

Taricani, L., Tejada, M. L. & Young, P. G. (2002) The fission yeast ES2 homologue, Bis1, interacts with the Ish1 stress-responsive nuclear envelope protein. *J. Biol. Chem.,* **277** (**12**), 10562–72.

Taylor, C., Wadey, R., O'Donnell, H. *et al.* (1997) Cloning and mapping of murine DGCR2 and its homology to the Sez-12 seizure-related protein. *Mamm. Genome,* **8**, 371–5.

Thomas, T., Kurihara, H., Yamagish, H. *et al.* (1998) A signaling cascade involving endothelin-1, dHAND, and Msx1 regulates development of neural-crest-derived branchial arch mesenchyme. *Development,* **125**, 3005–14.

Van Esch, H., Groenen, P., Nesbit, M. A. *et al.* (2000) GATA3 haplo-insufficiency causes human HDR syndrome. *Nature,* **406** (**6794**), 419–22.

Van Geet, C., Devriendt, K., Eyskens, B. *et al.* (1998) Velocardiofacial syndrome patients with a heterozygous chromosome 22q11 deletion have giant platelets. *Pediatr. Res.,* **44** (**4**), 607–11.

Vermot, J., Niederreither, K., Garnier, J. M. *et al.* (2003) Decreased embryonic retinoic acid synthesis results in a DiGeorge syndrome phenotype in newborn mice. *Proc. Natl. Acad. Sci. USA*, **100** (**4**), 1763–8.

Vitelli, F., Morishima, M., Taddei, I. *et al.* (2002a) Tbx1 mutation causes multiple cardiovascular defects and disrupts neural crest and cranial nerve migratory pathways. *Hum. Mol. Genet.*, **11** (**8**), 915–22.

Vitelli, F., Taddei, I., Morishima, M. *et al.* (2002b) A genetic link between Tbx1 and fibroblast growth factor signaling. *Development*, **129** (**19**), 4605–11.

Waibler, Z., Schafer, A. & Starzinski-Powitz, A. (2001) mARVCF cellular localisation and binding to cadherins is influenced by the cellular context but not by alternative splicing. *J. Cell. Sci.*, **114** (**21**), 3873–84.

Wakamiya, M., Lindsay, E. A., Rivera-Perez, J. A. *et al.* (1998) Functional analysis of Gscl in the pathogenesis of the DiGeorge and velocardiofacial syndromes. *Hum. Mol. Genet.*, **7** (**12**), 1835–40.

Weitzman, J. B. (2002) Transcriptional territories in the genome. *J. Biol.*, **1** (**1**), 2.

Wilming, L. G., Snoeren, C. A. S., van Rijswijk, A. *et al.* (1997) The murine homologue of HIRA, a DiGeorge syndrome candidate gene, is expressed in embryonic structures affected in CATCH22 patients. *Hum. Mol. Genet.*, **6**, 247–58.

Wilson, D. I., Cross, I. E., Wren, C. *et al.* (1994) Minimum prevalence of chromosome 22q11 deletions. *Am. J. Hum. Genet.* **55**, A169.

Wilson, T. A., Blethen, S. L., Vallone, A. *et al.* (1993) DiGeorge anomaly with renal agenesis in infants of mothers with diabetes. *Am. J. Med. Genet.*, **1078**, 1082.

Yagi, H., Furutani, Y., Hamada, H. *et al.* (2003) Role of TBX1 in human del22q11.2 syndrome. *Lancet*, **362** (**9393**), 1366–73.

Yamagishi, H., Garg, V., Matsuoka, R. *et al.* (1999) A molecular pathway revealing a genetic basis for human cardiac and craniofacial defects. *Science*, **283**, 1158–61.

Yamagishi, C., Hierck, B. P., Gittenberger-de Groot, A. C. *et al.* (2003a) Functional attenuation of Ufd1l, a 22q11.2 deletion syndrome candidate gene, leads to cardiac outflow septation defects in chicken embryos. *Pediatr. Res.*, **53** (**4**), 546–53.

Yamagishi, H., Maeda, J., Hu, T. *et al.* (2003b) Tbx1 is regulated by tissue-specific forkhead proteins through a common Sonic hedgehog-responsive enhancer. *Genes Dev.*, **17** (**2**), 269–81.

Ye, Y., Meyer, H. H. & Rapoport, T. A. (2001) The AAA ATPase Cdc48/p97 and its partners transport proteins from the ER into the cytosol. *Nature*, **414** (**6864**), 652–6.

Yoshida, K., Kuo, F., George, E. L. *et al.* (2001) Requirement of CDC45 for postimplantation mouse development. *Mol. Cell. Biol.*, **21** (**14**), 4598–603.

Congenital cardiovascular disease and velo-cardio-facial syndrome

Bruno Marino[1], Federica Mileto[1], Maria Cristina Digilio[2], Adriano Carotti[3] and Roberto Di Donato[3]

[1] Department of Pediatrics, University of Rome "La Sapienza", Italy
[2] Department of Clinical Genetics, Bambino Gesù Hospital, Rome, Italy
[3] Department of Pediatic Cardiac Surgery, Bambino Gesù Hospital, Rome, Italy

Cardiovascular defects (CVD) are an important feature in children with DiGeorge/velo-cardio-facial/conotruncal anomaly face syndrome (DGS/VCFS/CTAF) associated with a chromosome 22q11 deletion (del 22q11). In a landmark paper, Freedom *et al.* (1972) reported a series of ten patients with conotruncal anomalies and aortic arch anomalies associated with DiGeorge syndrome (Freedom *et al.*, 1972). In the last 20 years, many papers have documented various types of congenital heart defects in this condition (Kinouchi *et al.*, 1976; Young *et al.*, 1980; Conley *et al.*, 1979; Moerman *et al.*, 1980; Marmon *et al.*, 1984; Van Mierop & Kutsche, 1986; Goldmuntz *et al.*, 1993, 1998; Takahashi *et al.*, 1995; Lewin *et al.*, 1996; Webber *et al.*, 1996; Momma *et al.*, 1996a; Marino *et al.*, 1997a, 1999b, 2001; Mehraein *et al.*, 1997; Fokstuen *et al.*, 1998; Iserin *et al.*, 1998; Borgmann *et al.*, 1999; Young *et al.*, 1999; Frohn-Mulder *et al.*, 1999).

Cardiovascular defects affect 75% of VCFS individuals and are the major cause of mortality (about 90% of all deaths) in this syndrome (Ryan *et al.*, 1997; Matsuoka *et al.*, 1998). Thus, VCFS represents a very important syndrome in pediatric cardiology and, after Down syndrome, is the most frequent genetic condition associated with CVD (Goodship *et al.*, 1998).

It is interesting to note that the first description of a congenital heart defect in a patient *probably* affected by a del 22q11 was made in 1671 by Nicolai Stensen. He wrote:

There was a cleft palate and hare-lip on the right side, and the mother attributed this anomaly to the fact that she was fond of rabbit stew … the unusual form of the arteries arising from the heart attracted the chief attention and called for admiration. In particular, the pulmonary artery was much narrower than the aorta …. when I opened the right ventricle, the probe that was passed forward and upward along the interventricular septum entered directly into the aorta just as readily as the probe passed from the left ventricle into the aorta (Raskind, 1972, 1979).

Velo-Cardial-Facial Syndrome: A Model for Understanding Microdeletion Disorders, ed. Kieran C. Murphy and Peter J. Scambler. Published by Cambridge University Press. © Cambridge University Press, 2005.

Goldmuntz *et al.* (1993) reported that a substantial proportion (29%) of patients with a "non-syndromic" conotruncal defect were found to have a chromosome 22q11 deletion. This data, if confirmed, would have completely changed the genetic counseling of congenital heart disease. Nowadays, it is widely accepted that one or more additional extracardiac features of this syndrome are associated in virtually all patients with CVD and VCFS (Takahashi *et al.*, 1995; Webber *et al.*, 1996; Momma *et al.*, 1996a; Marino *et al.*, 1997a, 2001; Mehraein *et al.*, 1997; Fokstuen *et al.*, 1998; Ryan *et al.*, 1997; Matsuoka *et al.*, 1998; Goodship *et al.*, 1998; Amati *et al.*, 1995; Digilio *et al.*, 1996a, 1997, 1999b). Moreover, non syndromic children with isolated conotruncal anomalies are at very low risk for del 22q11 (Webber *et al.*, 1996; Marino *et al.*, 1997a; Digilio *et al.*, 2003a). Notably, not all patients with CVD and del 22q11 present with all the diagnostic criteria for DGS/ VCFS/CTAF syndrome (Ryan *et al.*, 1997; Matsuoka *et al.*, 1998 Marino *et al.*, 2001). Many children, particularly neonates, have a subtle phenotype with only one or two additional extracardiac features (Amati *et al.*, 1995; Digilio *et al.*, 1996a, 1997a, 1999a), so the diagnosis of the syndrome can be difficult at a young age and the guidelines for routine genetic tests are still controversial (Amati *et al.*, 1995; Digilio *et al.*, 1996a, 1997a, 1999b, 2003a-b; Johnson *et al.*, 1996; Bristow & Bernstein, 1998; Goldmuntz *et al.*, 1998; Goodship *et al.*, 1998).

The characteristic CVD occurring in VCFS individuals are conotruncal defects consisting in anomalies of the outflow tract of the heart (Freedom *et al.*, 1972; Kinouchi *et al.*, 1976; Young *et al.*, 1980; Conley *et al.*, 1979; Moerman *et al.*, 1980; Marmon *et al.*, 1984; Van Mierop & Kutsche, 1986; Goldmuntz *et al.*, 1993; Takahashi *et al.*, 1995; Lewin *et al.*, 1996; Webber *et al.*, 1996; Momma *et al.*, 1996a; Marino *et al.*, 1997a). These malformations include tetralogy of Fallot (TF), pulmonary atresia with ventricular septal defect (PA-VSD), truncus arteriosus (PTA), interrupted aortic arch (IAA), ventricular septal defect (VSD) and isolated anomalies of the aortic arch (AAA). Furthermore, in patients with this syndrome other cardiac defects have been occasionally reported including: atrial septal defect (Ryan *et al.*, 1997; Marino *et al.*, 2001), atrioventricular canal (Marino *et al.*, 1991; Kumar *et al.*, 1996; Ryan *et al.*, 1997), tricuspid atresia (Marino *et al.*, 1997b), transposition of great arteries (Melchionda *et al.*, 1995; Ryan *et al.*, 1997; Marino *et al.*, 2001), hypoplastic left ventricle (Consevage *et al.*, 1996), heterotaxy (Marino *et al.*, 1996a; Penman Splitt *et al.*, 1996; Yates *et al.*, 1996), aortic coarctation and persistent ductus arteriosus (Ryan *et al.*, 1997; Matsuoka *et al.*, 1998).

The prevalence and types of CVD are different at the various ages of presentation of patients with this syndrome. In neonates and infants presenting with the full VCFS phenotype, the presence of CVD is more frequent and the cardiac anomalies are usually more severe including, in particular, IAA-B, PTA and PA-VSD (Conley *et al.*, 1979; Moerman *et al.*, 1980; Takahashi *et al.*, 1995; Marino *et al.*, 1997a;

Goldmuntz *et al.*, 1998; Matsuoka *et al.*, 1998). In VCFS children and adolescents, the CVD tend to be less severe and include VSD and isolated AAA (Takahashi *et al.*, 1995; Momma, K. *et al.*, 1996a; McElhinney *et al.*, 2001a; Toscano *et al.*, 2002). Tetralogy of Fallot is present in similar proportions in all age groups.

Specific patterns of cardiac anatomy have been described in subjects with various genetic syndromes (Marino & Digilio, 2000). Children with Down syndrome (Marino *et al.*, 1990a), Noonan syndrome (Marino *et al.*, 1999c), Holt–Oram syndrome (Bennhagen & Menahem, 1998), and Ellis–van Creveld syndrome (Digilio *et al.*, 1999a) present distinctive types and subtypes of CVD differing, in some aspects, from those observed in patients without genetic anomalies. Many recent contributions also show that in VCFS individuals the CVD are characterized by some anatomic aspects resulting in specific cardiac phenotypes. It is interesting to note that the human spectrum of CVD associated with del 22q11 is different from and larger than that obtained with various proposed experimental animal models. For instance, in the chick embryo, after cardiac neural crest ablation, PTA and dextroposed aorta are the prevalent cardiac defects and IAA is extremely rare (Nishibatake *et al.*, 1987; Waldo *et al.*, 1999). On the contrary, mice heterozygously deleted for part of the chromosome 16 including *UFD1L* (Lindsay *et al.*, 1999) present with an aberrant subclavian artery and/or VSD, but also IAA, and those null for *Tbx1* (Vitelli *et al.*, 2002) have PTA and VSD. Thus, no single animal experiment produces the entire spectrum of CVD observed in VCFS individuals.

In this chapter we describe the cardiac anatomy of CVD associated with VCFS and its diagnostic and surgical implications.

Types of cardiac defects

Tetralogy of Fallot

This heart malformation consists of a large subaortic VSD with overriding of the aorta and pulmonary stenosis at infundibular and valvular levels. Tetralogy of Fallot is the single most common type of cardiac anomaly seen in children with del 22q11, and this holds true even excluding cases with pulmonary atresia (Momma *et al.*, 1995, 1996a; Marino *et al.*, 1996b, 1997a, 2001; Mehraein *et al.*, 1997; Ryan *et al.*, 1997; Fokstuen *et al.*, 1998; Goldmuntz *et al.*, 1998; Matsuoka *et al.*, 1998; Frohn-Mulder *et al.*, 1999; Maeda *et al.*, 2000; Lu *et al.*, 2001a).

Genetic syndromes and extracardiac anomalies are quite frequent in patients with TF, accounting for about 20–30% of the cases (Marino *et al.*, 1996b). Tetralogy of Fallot is found in 20–45% of patients with VCFS and CVD (Ryan *et al.*, 1997; Matsuoka *et al.*, 1998; Marino *et al.*, 2001) and 10–15% of patients with TF are found to have a 22q11 deletion (Amati *et al.*, 1995; Marino *et al.*, 1997a; Goodship *et al.*, 1998; Maeda *et al.*, 2000).

Table 3.1. Additional cardiovascular defects in children with Tetralogy of Fallot and del 22q11

Heart defects		Hypoplasia/absence of the infundibular septum
		Dysplasia/absence of the pulmonary valve
		(Absence of the ductus arteriosus)
Great arteries defects	Aorta	Right aortic arch
		Cervical aortic arch
		Aberrant subclavian artery
		Isolation of subclavian artery
	Pulmonary arteries	Major aorto-pulmonary collateral arteries
		Diffuse hypoplasia of the pulmonary arteries
		Discontinuity of the pulmonary arteries
		Absence of the left pulmonary artery

Additional CVD defects are common in patients with TF and VCFS, occurring in about half of the patients with this syndrome (Momma *et al.*, 1995, 1996a; Marino *et al.*, 1996b, 1997a; Frohn-Mulder *et al.*, 1999; Maeda *et al.*, 2000; Lu *et al.*, 2001a). These additional anomalies are peculiar and can involve the heart and/or the great arteries (Table 3.1). The associated cardiac defects are hypoplasia or absence of the infundibular septum (TF with "double committed" VSD) (Momma *et al.*, 1995; Marino *et al.*, 1996b) and absence of the pulmonary valve with huge dilatation of the pulmonary arteries and bronchial compression (Figure. 3.1 A, B) (Johnson *et al.*, 1995a). Absence of the infundibular septum was also reported in other patients with TF and genetic syndromes such as trisomy 18 and 13 (Marino *et al.*, 1996; Van Praagh *et al.*.). Tetralogy of Fallot with absent pulmonary valve has been described with an absence of the ductus arteriosus. The associated vascular defects involve systemic and pulmonary circulations and include right or cervical aortic arch, aberrant subclavian artery, isolation of subclavian artery (perfused by the vertebral artery), major aorto-pulmonary collateral arteries (MAPCA) with absent ductus arteriosus, and anomalies of the pulmonary arteries, such as diffuse hypoplasia and small central pulmonary arteries. Furthermore the pulmonary arteries can be discontinuous with the left pulmonary artery arising from the ductus arteriosus. Absence of the left pulmonary artery has been also reported, probably due to discontinuity of the pulmonary arteries and to early closure of the ductus (Figure 3.2).

Pulmonary atresia with ventricular septal defect

This malformation presents an intracardiac anatomy similar to that observed in children with TF but the pulmonary infundibulum and/or the pulmonary valve are atretic. Since the prevalence of VCFS is different between patients with classic

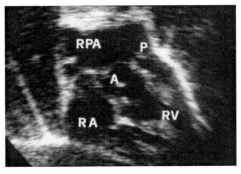

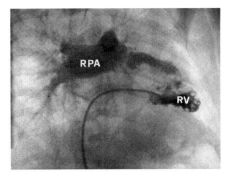

A   B

Figure 3.1   Tetralogy of Fallot with absent pulmonary valve. (A) Echocardiography in subcostal right oblique
view; (B) Angiocardiography in right oblique projection. Note the huge dilatation of the right
pulmonary artery (RPA). RA = right atrium; RV = right ventricle; A = aorta; P = pulmonary artery.

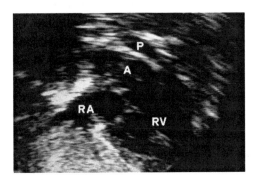

Figure 3.2   Tetralogy of Fallot with absent left pulmonary artery. Echocardiography in subcostal right
oblique view. Note the single right pulmonary artery (P).

TF and those with PA-VSD (Digilio *et al.*, 1996b; Anaclerio *et al.*, 2001), it is better
to describe these two malformations separately. In this cardiac defect various types
of genetic syndromes are frequent, accounting for about 25–50% of patients
(Jadele *et al.*, 1992; Digilio *et al.*, 1996b; Momma *et al.*, 1996b; Chessa *et al.*,
1998; Hofbeck *et al.*, 1998; Marino & Digilio, *et al.*, 2000; Anaclerio *et al.*, 2001).
PA-VSD occurs in 15–30% of children with del 22q11 (Ryan *et al.*, 1997; Goodship
et al., 1998; Matsuoka *et al.*, 1998; Marino *et al.*, 2001) and in a population of
patients with PA-VSD the prevalence of del 22q11 ranges between 20–50%
(Digilio *et al.*, 1996b; Anaclerio *et al.*, 2001).

From the anatomical point of view two main groups of PA-VSD can be
recognized: in the first group the pulmonary blood is supplied by a patent ductus

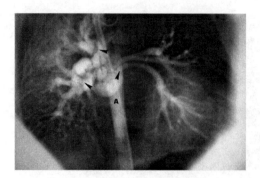

Figure 3.3   Pulmonary atresia with ventricular septal defect and major aorto-pulmonary collateral arteries. Angiocardiography in antero-posterior projection. Note the right-sided descending aorta (A) and the collateral arteries (arrows).

arteriosus and the pulmonary arteries are confluent and usually good sized. This group can be correctly defined "Tetralogy of Fallot with pulmonary atresia." In the second group the pulmonary blood is predominantly supplied by MAPCAs, the pulmonary arteries can be nonconfluent and/or hypoplastic and the ductus arteriosus is usually absent. These cases can be better defined as PA-VSD with MAPCAs (Figure 3.3). In VCFS children the second pattern is more common (Momma *et al.*, 1996b; Chessa *et al.*, 1998; Hofbeck *et al.*, 1998; Anaclerio *et al.*, 2001). Moreover, VCFS is reported to be associated with complex loop morphology of the pulmonary arteries and the connections between central and peripheral pulmonary arteries are impaired (Chessa *et al.*, 1998; Hofbeck *et al.*, 1998). This anatomic pattern is probably due to an early embryological defect involving the IV and VI primitive aortic arches (Vitelli *et al.*, 2002). This complex nature of the pulmonary vascular tree is associated with increased bronchial circulation and, in some occasions, with arterial bronchial compression causing bronchomalacia. These aspects frequently produce persistent airway hyper-responsiveness with broncho-spasm in the pre- and post-operative periods in these patients (Jadele *et al.*, 1992; Ackerman *et al.*, 2001). Primary bronchomalacia related to del 22q11 is unlikely. These respiratory symptoms are quite frequent in patients with PA-VSD (Jadele *et al.*, 1992) but are not unique to children with VCFS (Ackerman *et al.*, 2001).

In these patients, as well as in children with TF, the presence of del 22q11 can be associated with additional anomalies of the aorta including right and/or cervical aortic arch and aberrant or cervical subclavian artery (Table 3.2). Due to anatomical and genetic differences PA-VSD with MAPCA could be considered a separate entity from PA-VSD with a single left-sided patent ductus arteriosus and confluent pulmonary arteries that can be classified in the spectrum of TF (Anaclerio *et al.*, 2001).

Table 3.2. Additional cardiovascular defects in children with pulmonary atresia with ventricular septal defect (PA-VSD) and del 22q11

Aorta	Right aortic arch
	Cervical aortic arch
	Aberrant subclavian artery
Pulmonary arteries	MAPCA (with complex loop)
	(absent ductus arteriosus)
	Hypoplasia/discontinuity of the pulmonary artery
	Absence of the left pulmonary artery

MAPCA = major aorto-pulmonary collateral arteries

Velo-cardio-facial syndrome is exceptionally rare in patients with PA with intact ventricular septum (Li *et al.*, 2003) as well as in cases of PA with complex intracardiac anomalies such as l-loop ventricle and/or double inlet left ventricle (Anaclerio *et al.*, 2001).

Persistent truncus arteriosus

This cardiac defect consists in a single outlet from the heart supplying the systemic, the coronary, and the pulmonary circulations. Genetic syndromes and extracardiac anomalies are very frequent in this cardiac defect representing about 30–40% of all the cases (Raatikka *et al.*, 1981; Radford *et al.*, 1988). Since the first clinical and pathological reports on cardiac defects associated with VCFS were published, PTA was described as one of the most frequent heart malformations (Freedom *et al.*, 1972; Conley *et al.*, 1979; Moerman *et al.*, 1980; Marmon *et al.*, 1984; Van Mierop & Kutsche, 1986) and subsequent studies have confirmed these findings (Raatikka *et al.*, 1981; Radford *et al.*, 1988; Dallapiccola *et al.*, 1989). The prevalence of PTA in the largest series of VCFS children ranges between 5–10% (Ryan *et al.*, 1997; Goodship *et al.*, 1998; Matsuoka *et al.*, 1998; Frohn-Mulder *et al.*, 1999; Marino *et al.*, 2001) whereas the prevalence of VCFS is about 30–35% in individuals with PTA (Momma *et al.*, 1997; Marino *et al.*, 1998; Matsuoka *et al.*, 1998).

Additional CVDs affecting the great arteries including systemic and pulmonary circulations have also been described in VCFS (Marmon *et al.*, 1984; Van Mierop, L.H.S. *et al.*, 1986; Momma *et al.*, 1997; Marino *et al.*, 1998, 2001, 2002) (Table 3.3). Discontinuity of the pulmonary arteries with the left pulmonary artery arising from the ductus arteriosus (Figure 3.4A) (also described as PTA type A3), ostial stenosis with diffuse hypoplasia (Figure 3.4B), crossing of the pulmonary arteries, presence of MAPCA, and unilateral absence of one pulmonary artery (usually the left after an early closure of the ductus) were frequently found in children with

Table 3.3. Additional cardiovascular defects in children with Persistent truncus arteriosus and del 22q11

Heart defects		Dysplasia/stenosis truncal valve
		Muscular subtruncal conus
		Truncal origin from the right ventricle
Great arteries defects	Aorta	Right aortic arch
		Cervical aortic arch
		Interrupted aortic arch type B
	Pulmonary arteries	Discontinuity (type A3)
		Stenosis/hypoplasia
		Crossing
		Major aorto-pulmonary collateral arteries

PTA and VCFS (Momma *et al.*, 1997; Marino *et al.*, 1998, 2002). These variants of pulmonary artery morphology are quite rare in patients with PTA without VCFS and can be cervical or interrupted between the left subclavian and the left carotid arteries (Type B). Additional malformations may involve the heart, for instance, severe dysplasia with stenosis of the truncal valve (Marino *et al.*, 1998; Borgmann *et al.*, 1999) (Figure 3.4A) and origin of the PTA from the right ventricle surrounded by a complete muscular infundibulum (Figure 3.4B). It is interesting to note that many of these additional cardiac features were previously reported in children with PTA associated with multiple extracardiac dysmorphic features resembling VCFS (Perez Martinez *et al.*, 1975; Patel *et al.*, 1978; Vairo *et al.*, 1989).

In model systems, PTA can be caused by a reduced number of neural crest cells reaching the outflow tract of the heart, causing a complete defect of the aorto-pulmonary, truncal, and infundibular septa (Momma *et al.*, 1997; Marino *et al.*, 2002). This situation is also found in *Tbx1* -/- embryos (see Chapter 2). However, genetic (Vitelli *et al.*, 2002) and other defects can cause the abnormal development of pharyngeal arch endoderm and secondary disruption of aortico-pulmonary, truncal and conal septation, as well as conal alignment and absorption. Finally, the additional CVDs could be a consequence of specific defects of the primitive branchial arch arteries.

Interrupted aortic arch

In this malformation the aortic arch is interrupted with discontinuity between the ascending and descending aorta. The distal aorta is supplied by the pulmonary artery and by the ductus arteriosus. Extracardiac anomalies and/or genetic

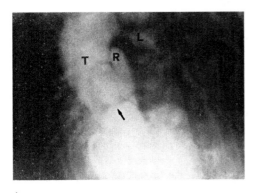

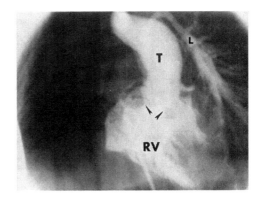

A   B

C

Figure 3.4   Truncus arteriosus. (A) Angiocardiography showing stenosis with dysplasia of the truncal valve (arrow) and discontinuity of the pulmonary arteries with origin of the left pulmonary artery (L) from the left-sided ductus arteriosus while the right pulmonary artery (R) rises from the truncus (T). Truncus arteriosus type A3.

(B) Angiocardiography showing diffuse hypoplasia of the left pulmonary artery (L). Note the origin of the truncus (T) exclusively from the right ventricle (RV) surrounded by a complete muscular infundibulum (arrows).

(C) Angiocardiography showing truncus arteriosus with right aortic arch (A).

syndromes are very common in this cardiac defect ranging between 40–80% of cases (Moerman *et al.*, 1987; Lewin *et al.*, 1997; Rauch *et al.*, 1998; Marino *et al.*, 1999a; Momma *et al.*, 1999a; Loffredo *et al.*, 2000; Marino & Digilio, 2000). In neonates with VCFS, IAA is one of the most frequent cardiac defects (Moerman *et al.*, 1987; Lewin *et al.*, 1997; Ryan *et al.*, 1997; Matsuoka *et al.*, 1998; Rauch *et al.*, 1998; Marino *et al.*, 1999a, 2001; Momma *et al.*, 1999a; Loffredo *et al.*, 2000). Interrupted aortic arch is found in 5–20% of patients with VCFS and CVD (Ryan *et al.*, 1997; Matsuoka *et al.*,

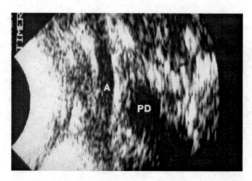

Figure 3.5   Interrupted aortic arch. Echocardiography in suprasternal view showing interrupted aortic arch type C. A = ascending aorta; PD = pulmonary artery.

1998; Marino *et al.*, 2001) while 45–50% of all patients with IAA are found to have VCFS, increasing to 60–80% of those with IAA type B.

According to the classic anatomic categorization based on the site of interruption (Celoria & Patton *et al.*, 1959) patients with IAA are classified into three groups: type A when the IAA is distal to the left subclavian artery; type B when the IAA is between the left carotid and the left subclavian arteries; and type C when the IAA is proximal to the left carotid artery.

In VCFS children, IAA type B is highly prevalent while IAA type A is quite rare (Moerman *et al.*, 1987; Lewin *et al.*, 1997; Rauch *et al.*, 1998; Marino *et al.*, 1999a; Momma *et al.*, 1999a; Loffredo *et al.*, 2000). In our experience, VCFS is also associated with the rare IAA type C (Figure 3.5). Due to its frequent association with VCFS (60–80%), IAA type B is one of the conotruncal phenotypes more strongly related to genetic syndromes as well as TF with absent PV, PA-VSD and MAPCA PTA with discontinuity of the pulmonary arteries and atrioventricular canal with TF.

In this malformation, a right aortic arch and abnormalities of the subclavian artery opposite to the aortic arch are frequently reported (Moerman *et al.*, 1987; Lewin *et al.*, 1997; Rauch *et al.*, 1998; Marino *et al.*, 1999a; Momma *et al.*, 1999a). The anomalies of the subclavian artery include: cervical origin, thoracic origin (aberrant), and isolation (Table 3.4). Other unusual and complex anomalies of the great arteries have been occasionally reported (Agnoletti *et al.*, 2001; Sett *et al.*, 2001).

It is interesting to note that in patients with IAA type B and VCFS, a hypoplasia of the posteriorly deviated infundibular septum has been described (Marino *et al.*, 1999a; Momma *et al.*, 1999a). This aspect is reminiscent of the hypoplasia of the anteriorly deviated infundibular septum observed in some children with TF and VCFS and could be considered the "mirror image" of that infundibular morphology (Momma *et al.*, 1995; Marino *et al.*, 1996b). Likewise, a doubly

Table 3.4. Interrupted aortic arch and del 22q11

Types
   Interruption between left carotid and left subclavian artery (type B)
   Interruption proximal to the left carotid artery (type C)
Additional anomalies
   Truncus arteriosus
   Right aortic arch
   Cervical origin
   Anomalies of the subclavian artery
   Thoracic origin
   Isolation
   Hypoplasia/absence of the infundibular septum

committed VSD is seen in association with IAA as well as with TF in children with VCFS.

Pathogenetic differences between IAA type A and type B were previously suggested on the basis of the different prevalence of associated cardiac anomalies (Braunlin *et al.*, 1982; Oppenheimer-Dekker *et al.*, 1982; Van Mierop & Kutsche, 1984). In fact, double inlet ventricle, transposition of great arteries and aorto-pulmonary window are less common in IAA type B than in type A while the right aortic arch and the anomalies of the subclavian artery are commonly associated with IAA type B but are rare in type A (Braunlin *et al.*, 1982; Oppenheimer-Dekker *et al.*, 1982; Van Mierop & Kutsche, 1984). Moreover, VCFS is quite rare in children where the IAA is in the setting of double inlet ventricle, ventricular inversion (l-loop of the ventricle), transposition of the great arteries and aorto-pulmonary window (Marino *et al.*, 1999a). In contrast, VCFS is quite frequent in individuals presenting with both IAA and PTA.

In summary, IAA type A is a cardiac malformation pathogenetically related to aortic coarctation and usually due to alteration of cardiac hemodynamics, whereas IAA type B is secondary to abnormal cellular interactions during development (Van Mierop & Kutsche, 1984; Marino *et al.*, 1999a). In particular, the aortic arch proximal to the left carotid artery and between left carotid and the left subclavian arteries is a specific developmental weak point directly affected by del 22q11. In the setting of VCFS, IAA type B and C are probably not due to intracardiac subaortic stenosis, as usually suggested. These malformations are caused by a neural crest defect expressed at aortic arch level and at infundibular septum level (Marino *et al.*, 1999a; Momma *et al.*, 1999) or by the effect of a specific deleted gene involved in the development of pharyngeal arches and cardiac infundibulum (Vitelli *et al.*, 2002).

Isolated aortic arch anomalies

Anomalies of aortic arch position and branching include a large spectrum of congenital vascular defects. Genetic syndromes are quite rare in these malformations. In VCFS children with conotruncal defects, the AAA are significantly more common than in non-deleted individuals (Freedom *et al.*, 1972; Young *et al.*, 1980; Momma *et al.*, 1996a; Marino *et al.*, 1997a, 2001; Goldmuntz *et al.*, 1998; Matsuoka *et al.*, 1998; Ryan *et al.*, 1997). In addition, isolated AAA without intracardiac defects are frequently associated with VCFS (Kazuma *et al.*, 1997; Kumar *et al.*, 1997; Momma *et al.*, 1999; Wang *et al.*, 1999; Lee *et al.*, 2001; McElhinney *et al.*, 2001a,b). These malformations can result in a vascular ring with symptomatic airway compression.

The exact prevalence of isolated AAA in VCFS individuals is unknown. Several studies have reported that approximately 5–10% of children with VCFS have isolated AAA (Momma *et al.*, 1996a, 1999b) while 24% of individuals with isolated AAA are found to have a 22q11 deletion (McElhinney *et al.*, 2001a). In addition, it is possible that among the 25% of VCFS individuals without CVD reported by Ryan *et al.* (1997), there are some patients with asymptomatic and undiagnosed isolated AAA.

The most frequent AAA associated with VCFS are: right aortic arch (Figure 3.6), double aortic arch (with a dominant right arch) (Figure 3.7), cervical aortic arch, persistent fifth aortic arch and aberrant or isolated subclavian artery (Figure 3.6) (Momma *et al.*, 1996a, 1999; Ryan *et al.*, 1997; Kazuma *et al.*, 1997; Kumar *et al.*, 1997; Wang *et al.*, 1999; Lee *et al.*, 2001; McElhinney *et al.*, 2001b). All these anomalies can be associated with many anatomic vascular variants that can cause vascular ring (Table 3.5). In children with AAA the association with abnormalities of the proximal branch of the pulmonary arteries and the ductus arteriosus is an indication for del 22q11 screening (Momma *et al.*, 1999; McElhinney *et al.*, 2001a). It is interesting to note that in some cases the AAA is associated with aortic root dilatation. These various and complex anomalies of position and of branching of the aortic arch and brachiocephalic arteries can be explained on the basis of defects during embryogenesis causing anomalous regression and/or persistence of the primitive branchial arches (Figure 3.8) (Momma *et al.*, 1999b).

Ventricular septal defect

This malformation consists of a communication between the two ventricles. As a single cardiac anomaly the VSD is the most frequent form of CVD (Lewis *et al.*, 1996). Extracardiac anomalies are not frequent in these children and are more common in infants with large VSD than in individuals with small defects (Lewis *et al.*, 1996). There are no data on the prevalence of VCFS in children with VSD but

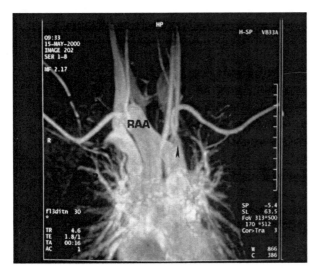

Figure 3.6   Right aortic arch with aberrant left subclavian artery. Magnetic resonance imaging in sagittal plane showing the right aortic arch (RAA) and the anomalous left subclavian artery (arrow).

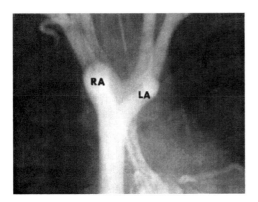

Figure 3.7   Double aortic arch. Angiocardiography showing the dominant right aortic arch (RA) and the left aortic arch (LA).

several studies have reported that 10–50% of VCFS individuals have VSD (Young *et al.*, 1980; Van Mierop & Kutsche, 1986; Momma *et al.*, 1996a; Ryan *et al.*, 1997; Matsuoka *et al.*, 1998; Goodship *et al.*, 1998; Marino *et al.*, 1999b, 2001). Analyzing VCFS individuals with an older mean age, including children and adolescents, the prevalence of VSD is higher (Young *et al.*, 1980; Momma *et al.*, 1996a; Matsuoka *et al.*, 1998).

     The VSD observed in VCFS individuals is usually perimembranous (with or without malalignment) or doubly committed subarterial (Yamagishy *et al.*, 2000; Toscano *et al.*, 2002) (Figure 3.9). Ventricular septal defect with posterior

Table 3.5. Isolated aortic arch anomalies in children with del 22q11

Right Aortic Arch
    with aberrant left subclavian artery (ring)
    with right or bilateral ductus arteriosus
    with stenosis or hypoplasia of the left pulmonary artery
    with mirror-image brachiocephalic arteries
    with isolated left subclavian artery
Double aortic arch
    with right arch dominant (ring)
Left aortic arch
Aberrant right subclavian artery

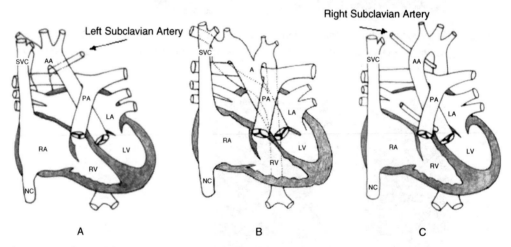

Figure 3.8   Three of the most frequent patterns of Isolated AAA founded in children with del 22q11.
(A) Right Aortic arch with aberrant left subclavian artery (vascular ring). (B) Double Aortic arch
with right arch dominant (vascular ring). (C) Left Aortic arch with aberrant right subclavian
artery (no vascular ring).

deviation of the infundibular septum has also been described (Goldmuntz *et al.*,
1998; Mc Elhinney *et al.*, 2003). On the contrary, a large muscular VSD is very
rare in VCFS children (Toscano *et al.*, 2002). The size of the perimembranous
and subarterial VSD associated with VCFS can be either large or restrictive
(Young *et al.*, 1980; Momma *et al.*, 1996a; Yamagishy *et al.*, 2000; Marino *et
al.*, 2001; Toscano *et al.*, 2002). Prolapses of the aortic cusps have been described
in association with subarterial VSD (Young *et al.*, 1980). Doubly committed
subarterial VSD is due to deficiency of the infundibular septum and is quite rare
in the Caucasian population (1.5% of all VSD), but is more common in the

Table 3.6. Ventricular septal defect and del 22q11

Types
  Perimembranous
  Doubly committed subarterial
Additional vascular anomalies
  Right aortic arch (with or without aberrant subclavian artery)
  Cervical aortic arch
  Double aortic arch

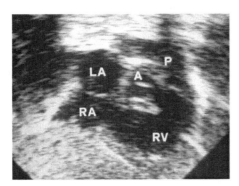

Figure 3.9   Double committed subarterial ventricular septal defect. Echocardiography in right oblique subcostal view showing the absence of the infundibular septum and the doubly committed ventricular septal defect.

Oriental population (10–15% of all VSD). It is interesting to note that in series of Caucasian patients with VSD and VCFS there is a predominance of double committed VSD (Ferencz *et al.*, 1997; Toscano *et al.*, 2002).

Moreover, in patients with VSD and VCFS additional anomalies of the position and branching of the aortic arch (Figure 3.7) are present more commonly compared with nondeleted individuals with VSD (Toscano *et al.*, 2002). These additional anomalies of the aortic arch include right aortic arch (with or without aberrant left subclavian artery) (Figure 3.10), cervical aortic arch and double aortic arch (Table 3.6). In patients with VSD and VCFS it is possible to observe additional anomalies of the pulmonary arteries such as discrete stenosis or diffuse hypoplasia. These vascular malformations, like those observed in association with all types of conotruncal defect and VCFS, are probably due to the anomalous migration and/or distribution of neural crest cells affecting the embryonic aortic arches (Momma *et al.*, 1999), or to the direct effect of a defective gene on conal septation (Vitelli *et al.*, 2002).

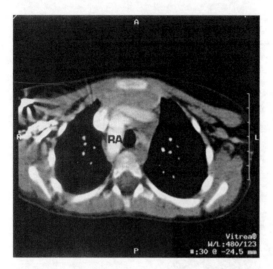

Figure 3.10   Right aortic arch associated with ventricular septal defect. Computed tomography scan in coronal plane showing the right aortic arch (RA).

Other cardiovascular defects

Among the other conotruncal anomalies Transposition of Great Arteries and "Double Outlet Right Ventricle" have occasionally been described in patients with VCFS (Freedom *et al.*, 1972; Conley *et al.*, 1979; Moerman *et al.*, 1980; Van Mierop & Kutsche, 1986; Melchionda *et al.*, 1995; Ryan *et al.*, 1997; Matsuoka *et al.*, 1998; Marino *et al.*, 2001). Due to their lesser association with genetic syndromes (Ferencz *et al.*, 1997) and with familial recurrence (Digilio *et al.*, 2001) these cardiac malformations are currently classified separately from the "classic" conotruncal defects. In some instances transposition of the great arteries and double outlet right ventricle could be related to anomalies of ventricular looping (Digilio *et al.*, 2001). Transposition of great arteries when associated with VCFS can have either intact ventricular septum or VSD with or without pulmonary stenosis or atresia (Freedom *et al.*, 1972; Conley *et al.*, 1979; Moerman *et al.*, 1980; Van Mierop & Kutsche, 1986; Melchionda *et al.*, 1995; Ryan *et al.*, 1997; Matsuoka *et al.*, 1998; Marino *et al.*, 2001). When associated with VCFS, double outlet right ventricle is usually found with a subaortic VSD and normally related great arteries.

Atrial septal defect (ostium II type) has been reported in a small proportion of VCFS individuals (Ryan *et al.*, 1997; Marino *et al.*, 2001). Usually the patients with this heart malformation are "non syndromic" (Ferencz *et al.*, 1997) but a subgroup is associated with Holt–Oram syndrome (Bennhagen & Menahem, 1998) and some patients have been described in association with conduction abnormalities and mutation of the gene NKX2–5 (Schott *et al.*, 1998) or mutation of the gene GATA4 (Garg *et al.*, 2003; Sarkozy *et al.*, 2005).

Atrioventricular canal (also known as atrioventricular septal defect) is the classic heart malformation of children with Down syndrome (Marino *et al.*, 1990) but has been reported also in individuals with other syndromes including Noonan syndrome (Marino *et al.*, 1999c), Ellis–Van Creveld syndrome (Digilio *et al.*, 1999a) and Heterotaxy (Francalanci *et al.*, 1996). In the rare cases described in VCFS individuals, the atrioventricular septal defect was of the complete type (Marino *et al.*, 1991; Kumar *et al.*, 1996; Ryan *et al.*, 1997).

Tricuspid atresia can occur in families with recurrence of conotruncal defects (Bonnet *et al.*, 1999) and has been rarely reported in association with VCFS (Marino *et al.*, 1997b). It is noteworthy that tricuspid atresia can result after experimental ablation of neural crest, probably by an indirect mechanism as a consequence of an abnormality of intracardiac flow (Besson *et al.*, 1986).

Hypoplastic left heart syndrome has been reported in a few neonates with VCFS (Wilson *et al.*, 1993), one of them having a mosaic deletion (Consevage *et al.*, 1996).

Aortic coarctation has also occasionally been reported (Wilson *et al.*, 1991) as well as patent ductus arteriosus (Ryan *et al.*, 1997; Matsuoka *et al.*, 1998).

Defects of lateralization are very rare in VCFS (Marino *et al.*, 1996) although sporadic cases have been reported (Penman Splitt *et al.*, 1996), one of them presenting with heterotaxy, polysplenia, and left isomerism (Yates *et al.*, 1996).

Recently, a very uncommon pattern of conotruncal defect, namely Isolated infundibuloarterial inversion has been described in a patient in association with persistence of the fifth aortic arch and del 22q11 (Lee *et al.*, 1999).

Anomalous origin of one pulmonary artery is a rare vascular malformation, usually associated with normal intracardiac anatomy. Anomalous origin of the right pulmonary artery from the ascending aorta commonly occurs in nonsyndromic children but has been reported in a patient with VCFS (Johnson *et al.*, 1995b). The more rare anomalous origin of the left pulmonary artery from the ascending aorta has been described in two VCFS individuals in association with right aortic arch and right-sided ductus arteriosus (Dodo *et al.*, 1995). This pattern is probably due to a persistence of the fifth aortic arch (Dodo *et al.*, 1995) and is similar to that described in some individuals with isolated AAA (Momma *et al.*, 1999; McElhinney *et al.*, 2001a, b). Unilateral pulmonary agenesis with absent left pulmonary artery and vein has been reported in a child with VCFS (Conway *et al.*, 2002).

Common findings

Children with CVD and VCFS usually have laevocardia, viscero-atrial situs solitus with d-loop of the ventricle, and atrioventricular concordance. Both atrioventricular valves are usually well formed and the ventricles are balanced. The great

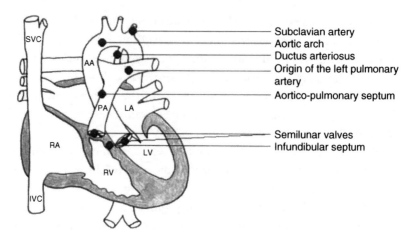

Figure 3.11 Cardiac sites at major risk of malformation in patients with del 22q11.

arteries (if both present) are normally related to each other and frequently there is a large subaortic (or doubly committed) VSD with dextroposed aorta. The infundibular septum is very frequently affected: it can be hypoplastic/absent (TF, PA, PTA, IAA type B, VSD), anteriorly deviated causing subpulmonary obstruction (TF, PA) or posteriorly deviated causing subaortic obstruction (IAA type B VSD). In addition, the aorto-pulmonary septation is frequently involved in the cardiac defect as well as the aortic arch showing many anomalies of the position and branching, including anomalies of the subclavian and carotid arteries (Rauch *et al.*, 2002) (Tables 3.1–3.6).

The pulmonary arteries are another sector characteristically affected in VCFS: they can be discontinuous (with the left pulmonary artery arising from the ductus arteriosus), or show diffuse hypoplasia, ostial stenosis, crossing (Recto *et al.*, 1997), defects of arborization and MACPAs. The origin of the left pulmonary artery seems to be a crucial point. The ductus arteriosus can be anomalous in shape, in position (Lee *et al.*, 2001) or even absent. Moreover, the semilunar valves can be dysplastic; the pulmonary valve can be bicuspid, stenotic, or absent (TF with absent PV); the truncal valve can be stenotic or severely insufficient, but also the aortic valve can be absent (Weintraub *et al.*, 1989), quadricuspid (Nakagawa *et al.*, 2000), or stenotic. All these anatomic characteristics constitute quite specific patterns of CVD in children with VCFS (Figure 3.11). These cardiac phenotypes should alert the pediatric cardiologist to the possible presence of this genetic syndrome. However, it should be kept in mind that not all patients with CVD and VCFS present with such a specific cardiac phenotype. Moreover, these peculiar cardiac malformations can be present in a subgroup of children with nonsyndromic CVD (Conti *et al.*, 2003). These patterns of malformations are therefore specific but not exclusive to VCFS.

No specific data are available about the myocardial structure and function in VCFS individuals but this aspect deserves consideration, since neural crest cells can also influence myocardial development (Waldo, et al., 1999).

Clinical implications

There is limited information available on the natural history and the clinical course of children with CVD and VCFS. Prenatal diagnosis of this association, by means of fetal echocardiography and amniocentesis is possible nowadays. The prevalence of del 22q11 in fetuses with conotruncal defects is quite high (Boudjemline et al., 2000, 2001). Some of the additional cardiac and extracardiac anomalies can be prenatally diagnosed, and although the expected risks for cardiac surgery are quite low, the possibility of developmental delay associated with this syndrome, may influence the prenatal counseling (Boudjemline et al., 2001) (see Chapter 11 for more details).

Neonates with VCFS and CVD may present with low birth weight and growth retardation. Calcium levels need careful monitoring and neonatal hypocalcemia can be a sign of this syndrome. Although hypocalcemia is usually transitory, it needs to be treated in the neonatal period. Humoral immunodeficiency is generally subclinical but in some neonates and infants it can be significant (Franklin et al., 1996; Rhoden et al., 1996; Pierdominici et al., 2000, 2003). Among children with conotruncal defects, the increased mortality for subjects with a lower percentage of blood lymphocytes (Rhoden et al., 1996) has not been confirmed. However, from the immunologic point of view, some preventive measures (Leana-Cox et al., 1996, Rhoden et al., 1996) could be taken into account including: (1) analysis of lymphocyte populations prior to blood transfusion; (2) administration of irradiated blood products; (3) aggressive and immediate treatment of infection; (4) use of killed viral vaccines (see Chapter 6 for more details).

Familial recurrence of VCFS can include concordant or discordant types of CVD (Leana-Cox et al., 1996; Digilio et al., 1997b, 2003a; Iascone et al., 2002). Discordant cardiac phenotypes have also been reported in monozygotic twins (Goodship et al., 1995; Lu et al., 2001b; Iascone et al., 2002). The majority of deleted parents of a child with CVD and VCFS have an apparently normal cardiovascular system (Digilio et al., 1997b).

Currently, two-dimensional and Color-Doppler echocardiography is the definitive tool for the diagnosis of conotruncal defects. Echocardiographic identification of thymic tissue can help in the diagnosis of this syndrome (Yeager & Sanders, 1995; Moran et al., 1999) and this measure deserves attention in all children with CVD and VCFS. Intracardiac and vascular anatomy can be accurately shown by echocardiography and the majority of children with CVD may safely undergo primary repair guided only by the ultrasound diagnosis (Hutha *et al.*, 1987; Marino *et al.*, 1990b; Santoro *et al.*, 1994; Carotti *et al.*, 1997; Tworetzky *et al.*, 1999). However, in VCFS individuals, since the CVD can be frequently complicated by additional cardiac and vascular defects, the preoperative diagnostic use of cardiac catheterization and angiocardiography should be carefully considered (Marino *et al.*, 1996b) and is mandatory in some complex cases. Magnetic resonance imaging can improve the diagnostic possibilities in particular for the vascular malformations, including positional and branching anomalies of the aortic arch and anomalies of the pulmonary arteries (Toscano *et al.*, 2002).

The guidelines for del 22q11 screening of neonates and infants with conotruncal defects are still controversial (see Chapter 11). Goldmuntz *et al.* (1998), due to the difficult clinical recognition of the extracardiac features in the neonatal age, suggested extending 22q11 deletion screening to all individuals with IAA, TA and TF irrespective of their clinical phenotype. Other authors (Bristow & Bernstein, 1998; Goodship *et al.*, 1998; Digilio *et al.*, 1999b; Marino *et al.*, 2001) suggest a more selective screening based on: (1) the prevalence of del 22q11 in each specific cardiac defect; (2) the presence of extracardiac features of VCFS; (3) the presence of additional CVD characteristic of this syndrome.

Following these suggestions, deletion screening is indicated in all patients with IAA type B and C, PA with VSD and MAPCA and PTA as there is a high prevalence of VCFS associated with these cardiac defects. For patients with TF without extracardiac signs and without any of the specific additional CVDs associated with VCFS, genetic screening is probably not indicated. Conversely, deletion screening is indicated in all children with congenital heart disease and phenotypic signs of VCFS and/or specific additional CVD of this syndrome. Little information is available on adult VCFS individuals with sporadic or familiar CVD (Kieran *et al.*, 1999; Hokanson *et al.*, 2001; Momma *et al.*, 2001).

Surgical implications

Advances in pediatric cardiac surgery have made it possible to treat the majority of patients with CVD with a very low operative risk and excellent long-term outlook. Technical achievements and especially a shift in surgical timing towards younger ages are chiefly responsible for this encouraging trend in the management of isolated congenital heart malformations (Castaneda, A. R. *et al.*, 1989; Maharasingam & Ostam-Smith, 2003).

Intuitively, though not clearly demonstrated, the coexistence of a genetic syndrome with a CVD may add to the complexity of the clinical picture, both at the cardiac and the extracardiac level (McElhinney *et al.*, 2002; Shashi *et al.*, 2003). In VCFS, there are as yet no definitive data showing increased mortality and morbidity for all patients following congenital heart surgery. Nevertheless, for specific defects the increasing awareness of the additional features and pitfalls of the syndrome imposes adjustments to the standard management of children with similar nonsyndromic CVD.

General issues

Surgical repair of conotruncal defects associated with VCFS must deal, as described above, with additional anomalies in four areas of the cardiovascular system: (1) the aortic arch; (2) the pulmonary arteries; (3) the infundibular septum and the under-lying doubly committed VSD; and (4) the semilunar valves. These additional cardi-ovascular malformations can influence the treatment and the surgical results of children with VCFS. In a recent review of our experience, the overall early surgical mortality of children with VCFS is significantly higher than that of patients without genetic syndromes (unpublished data). However these data could be biased by the different severity of cardiac defects in the two groups of patients. Analyzing separately each cardiac defect in patients with TF, PTA, AAA, and in those with VSD, the presence of del 22q11 and related additional cardiovascular anomalies were not a risk factor for heart surgery (Anaclerio *et al.*, 2004; Michielon *et al.*, 2004). Conversely, additional cardiovascular anomalies and perhaps immunological complication in patients with PA with VSD and MAPCAs and of those with IAA can complicate the surgical result, and in these groups of children the immediate surgical mortality was higher in our series of patients (Anaclerio *et al.*, 2004).

Tetralogy of Fallot

In our experience, del 22q11 does not affect the hospital survival in this cardiac defect (Anaclerio *et al.*, 2004; Michielon *et al.*, 2004). This information, however, is not sufficient to rule out an impact of the syndrome on the degree of surgical complexity and on postoperative morbidity. As previously described, the key feature of hypoplasia or absence of the infundibular septum with the associated feature of "doubly committed" or "subarterial" VSD, typical of VCFS, possibly introduces the need for relevant modifications of the "classical" surgical technique. (1) The VSD closure, in the subarterial quadrant, requires anchoring of the patch to a deficient infundibular septum or even, when the septum is lacking, to the corresponding segment of pulmonary valve annulus. Both semilunar valves may be damaged by this suture with ensuing pulmonary or, more bothersome, aortic regurgitation (Vargas *et al.*, 1986; Marino & Digilio, 2003). (2) The release of the septal and parietal insertions of the infundibular septum is often either impossible or simply ineffective, and most of the subpulmonary resection relies on the division of redundant muscle bundles in the underlying trabecular portion of the right ventricle. (3) The right ventricular outflow tract reconstruction is most often accomplished by a transannular patch because the subarterial extension of the VSD patch produces a narrowing beneath the pulmonary ring which indicates an extensive outflow patch enlargement across the pulmonary annulus (Neirotti *et al.*, 1978), even if this is frequently of adequate size (Okita *et al.*, 1995). Some of these patients do not tolerate long-standing pulmonary insufficiency and require late revision of the right ventricular outflow tract for insertion of a valved conduit.

The intracardiac repair of tetralogy of Fallot with "absent pulmonary valve syndrome," and VCFS, is similar to that of TF with doubly committed, or subarterial, VSD. However, as a result of the propensity toward progressive pulmonary arterial dilatation and secondary bronchial compression, the pulmonary arteries must be often trimmed down and the right ventricular outflow reconstruction is preferably accomplished by valved conduit interposition (Stellin *et al.*, 1983; Ilbawi *et al.*, 1986; Carotti *et al.*, 2003).

Surgical repair of patients with TF and "unilateral absence of pulmonary artery" (more often the left pulmonary artery) faces the problem of a much lesser peripheral arterial bed compared with normal. Early timing of surgery is considered beneficial in these patients to optimize the chances of pulmonary arterial growth and maturation and to prevent pulmonary thrombosis. Furthermore, it is crucial both to completely eliminate any cause of right ventricular outflow tract obstruction and to avoid postoperative pulmonary regurgitation by inserting a valve (monocusp outflow patch or valved conduit). Mortality, in this anatomical setting, has ranged between 8%–48% (Zhang *et al.*, 1997).

Pulmonary atresia with ventricular septal defect

For a long time, the bizarre anatomy of the pulmonary vascular supply has been a major stumbling block for the complete repair of this anomaly. Several, often controversial, staged surgical approaches have been proposed (Sawatari *et al.*, 1989; Iyer & Mee, 1991) revolving around two main strategies: (1) palliative right ventricular outflow patch reconstruction to promote the growth of the pulmonary arteries; (2) "unifocalization" of as many MAPCA as possible, with or without involvement of the native pulmonary arteries and with or without interposition of prosthetic material. In general, successful definitive repair has been deemed possible when at least 70% of the whole pulmonary vascular supply was recruited. In 1995, Hanley and colleagues made an historical contribution by introducing the revolutionary technique of single-stage unifocalization and repair of PA-VSD and MAPCA (Reddy *et al.*, 1995). Since then, this approach has further evolved, with the establishment of new indices, both pre- (Carotti *et al.*, 1998) and intra-operative (Reddy *et al.*, 1997) and with some modifications of the original technique (Lucani & Starnes, 1996; Tchervenkov *et al.*, 1997). Children with VCFS have been described as having smaller central pulmonary arteries and higher degrees of pulmonary arterial arborization anomalies (Hofbeck *et al.*, 1998). In contrast, in our surgical series, the presence of del 22q11 did not relate to any peculiar anatomic phenotype of pulmonary vascular supply or side of the aortic arch (Carotti et al., 1998; Mahle et al., 2003). On the other hand, in our series, an increased occurrence of "unfavourable" anatomical associations did characterize the subgroup of people with VCFS, PA-VSD-MAPCA, and absent right pulmonary artery. These patients mainly have a right aortic arch and an unstable left-sided arterial duct originating from the left subclavian artery. Interestingly, the same pulmonary arterial anatomy in otherwise normal patients occurs with left aortic arch and a usually stable left-sided arterial duct directly arising from the aorta (unpublished data). We speculate that the different physiology of the duct may contribute to the surgical risk associated with an earlier surgical approach in patients with VCFS. In our center, a so-called "integrated approach" is adopted based on: (a) the preoperative measurement of the pulmonary arterial bed size (using the so-called "total neo-pulmonary artery index") and (b) on the intraoperative use of the so-called "flow study" to judge the effective repair feasibility once the unifocalization has been carried out. Essentially, cases with dominant MAPCA are managed with single-stage unifocalization and repair whereas those with dominant, though hypoplastic, pulmonary arteries are treated by a preliminary right ventricular outflow patch reconstruction followed by a secondary single-stage unifocalization and repair (Carotti et al., 1998). Results are excellent with hospital survival of about 90% and good hemodynamic performance at intermediate follow-up. A recent re-examination of our series of 37 patients operated on for PA-VSD-MAPCA shows a 40% prevalence of del 22q11. Among them, 20% developed life-threatening postoperative fungal infections, which likely related to a decreased count of CD_4 lymphocytes in peripheral blood samples in two-thirds of the cases (Albanese et al., 2000). In summary, in our experience, del 22q11 was significantly linked with poor outcome ($P < 0.005$), mostly caused by infections and airway bleeding episodes.

Truncus arteriosus

Since the first successful repair by McGoon et al. (1968), surgical management of truncus arteriosus has markedly evolved to include earlier surgical timing. Most centres now successfully perform PTA repair in the neonatal age, excluding the severe morbidity produced by accelerated pulmonary vascular obstructive disease (Thompson et al., 2001). Standard repair includes patch closure of the VSD connecting the left ventricle with the aorta and right ventricle-to-pulmonary artery valved conduit reconstruction. Interestingly, repair of truncus arteriosus in the neonatal period can be performed routinely with excellent survival, even in patients with major associated abnormalities and, most likely, with a genetic syndrome, e.g. VCFS (Schreiber et al., 2000). Major associated anomalies possibly related to del 22q11 and requiring surgical management at an increased risk include: moderate or severe truncal valve regurgitation (and/or stenosis) (30%) (Rajasinghe *et al.*, 1997), interrupted aortic arch (10–20%) (Sano *et al.*, 1990), coronary artery abnormalities (18%) (de la Cruz *et al.*, 1990), and nonconfluent pulmonary arteries (10–15%) (Brizard *et al.*, 1997). In our experience these additional cardiovascular defects do not cause a higher surgical mortality in infants with VCFS (Anaclerio *et al.*, 2004).

Interrupted aortic arch

Additional cardiovascular anomalies characteristic of VCFS may have an impact on the results of reparative surgery. In fact, the more proximal location of the interruption, typical of VCFS, can be a risk factor for surgery. The rare IAA type C is a highly lethal lesion, whereas only a surprisingly minor difference is found between type B and type A (Sell *et al.*, 1998). Characteristically, the caliber of the ascending aorta is less than normal in IAA type B, and definitely diminutive in IAA type C, reflecting a more limited territory of distribution than in the case of normal ascending aorta or even of IAA type A. This observation may suggest two mechanisms potentially affecting the repair of IAA type B and C: (1) a chronically volume unloaded left ventricle resulting in a mild to moderate degree of hypoplastic left heart syndrome, with a restricted suitability to handle the whole cardiac output; (2) a considerable size discrepancy between the ascending and the descending aorta, which may complicate the anastomosis and, even with the most extensive proximal reconstruction, imply the persistence of a tapered and possibly inadequate aortic root.

Another relevant, though controversial, issue is the management of subaortic stenosis in cases of IAA. Resection of the infundibular septum at the primary operation has been suggested by some (Bove *et al.*, 1993), while others adopt a more conservative approach (Sell *et al.*, 1998). Considering in particular VCFS individuals with IAA type B or C, the typical hypoplasia of the posteriorly deviated infundibular septum generally provides a limited substrate for subaortic resection. Furthermore, surgical closure of the so-called doubly committed VSD, also typical of IAA with del 22q11, is frequently (40% of the cases) associated with secondary development of left ventricular outflow obstruction suggesting that the anatomical basis for the obstruction is already present at birth. It is noteworthy that, in these cases with deficient infundibular septum, both VSD closure and subaortic resection are best accomplished via a transpulmonary approach (Serraf *et al.*, 1996). In our surgical experience del 22q11 is a risk factor for immediate surgical mortality (Anaclerio *et al.*, 2004).

Isolated aortic arch anomalies

The variability of isolated aortic arch anomalies, with or without a vascular ring, demands a full preoperative anatomical delineation followed by an individualized surgical approach. Furthermore, while performing arch surgery in these cases, it should be appreciated that the potential for recurrent obstruction may be different from cases with a normal left aortic arch (McElhinney *et al.*, 2000).

Ventricular septal defect

Surgical closure of the perimembranous VSD is feasible by a transatrial approach while in children with doubly committed subarterial VSD, the best surgical approach is through the pulmonary artery (Schmidt *et al.*, 1988).

Prolapse of an aortic cusp is frequently (about 40% of the cases) associated with doubly committed subarterial VSD (Tohyama *et al.*, 1997; Sim *et al.*, 1999). The anatomical substrate for this aortic valve deformity comprises a deficiency in the infundibular musculature and a congenital defect of the lower margin of the aortic sinus and underdevelopment of the valve commissures (Van Praagh & McNamara, 1968; Tatsuno *et al.*, 1973). Furthermore, smaller VSDs are more frequently associated with aortic valve prolapse and regurgitation by generating greater shunt velocity through the communication and, hence, a greater Venturi effect pulling down the aortic cusp into the VSD (Tatsuno *et al.*, 1973). Others, however, have observed a higher prevalence of aortic cusp prolapse and regurgitation in patients with higher pulmonary flow (Tohyama *et al.*, 1997).

A timely VSD closure may suffice to prevent the evolution from an early stage of aortic cusp deformity to a severe degree of valve prolapse and regurgitation (Schmidt *et al.*, 1988). However, once the aortic lesion becomes full-blown, sophisticated valve reconstruction procedures must be considered (Bonhoeffer *et al.*, 1992; Yacoub *et al.*, 1997).

Perioperative policy

Before cardiac surgery, all children with cardiac defects and VCFS need an accurate clinical investigation to exclude the presence of additional, extracardiac anomalies. In fact, laryngotracheal (Mc Elhinney *et al.*, 2003) and esophageal anomalies, gastrointestinal or renal defects can influence the postoperative period. According to the possible immunologic depression observed in VCFS individuals, the following perioperative preventive measures should be always taken into account:

(1) Transfusion of irradiated blood products, to avoid the risk of fatal graft-versus-host disease (Franklin, R. C. G. *et al.*, 1996).

(2) Administration of a modified perioperative antimicrobial prophylaxis, including a glycopeptide (i.e. vancomycin) and an aminoglycoside (i.e. amikacin) antibiotic.

(3) Addition of a perioperative anti-fungal prophylaxis in patients with a decreased count of CD_4 lymphocytes undergoing very complex surgical

procedures (i.e. one-stage total unifocalization with or without repair of pulmonary atresia with ventricular septal defect and major aorto-pulmonary collateral arteries) (Albanese *et al.*, 2000).

REFERENCES

Ackerman, M. J., Wylam, M. E., Feldt, R. H. *et al.* (2001) Pulmonary atresia with ventricular septal defect and persistent airway hyperresponsiveness. *J. Thorac. Cardiovasc. Surg.* **122** (1), 169–77.

Agnoletti, G., Borghi, A. & Annecchino, F. (2001) A rare form of interrupted aortic arch. *Ital. Heart J.*, **2** (3), 228–30.

Albanese, S. B., Carotti, A., D'Argenio, P. *et al.* (2000) Is 22q11 microdeletion a risk factor for perioperative fungal infections in patients operated on for PA-VSD-MAPCAs? *Proceedings, Third International Meeting of the Therapy of Infectious Disease.* Florence.

Amati, F., Mari, A., Digilio, M. C. *et al.* (1995) 22q11 deletions in isolated and syndromic patients with tetralogy of Fallot. *Hum. Genet.*, **95**, 479–82.

Anaclerio, S., Marino, B., Carotti, A. *et al.* (2001) Pulmonary atresia with ventricular septal defect: prevalence of deletion 22q11 in the different anatomic patterns. *Ital. Heart J.*, **2** (5), 384–7.

Anaclerio, S., Di Ciompo, V., Michielon, G. *et al.* (2004) Conotruncal heart defects: impact of genetic syndromes on immediate operative mortality. *Ital. Heart J.*, **5** (8), 624–628.

Bennhagen, R. G. & Menahem, S. (1998) Holt–Oram syndrome and multiple ventricular septal defects: an association suggesting a possible genetic marker? *Cardiol. Young.* **8**, 128–30.

Besson, W. T., Kirby, M. L., Van Mierop, L. H. S. *et al.* (1986) Effects of the size of lesions of the cardiac neural crest at various embryonic ages on incidence and type of cardiac defects. *Circulation* **73**, 360–4.

Bonhoeffer, P., Fabbrocini, M., Lecompte, Y. *et al.* (1992) Infundibular septal defect with severe aortic regurgitation: a new surgical approach. *Ann. Thorac. Surg.*, **53** (5), 851–3.

Bonnet, D., Fermont, L., Kachaner, J. *et al.* (1999) Tricuspid atresia and conotruncal malformations in five families. *J. Med. Genet.*, **36**, 349–50.

Borgmann, S., Luhmer, I., Arslan-Kirchner, M. *et al.* (1999) A search for chromosome 22q11.2 deletions in a series of 176 consecutively catheterized patients with congenital heart disease: no evidence for deletions in non-syndromic patients. *Eur. J. Pediatr.*, **158**, 958–63.

Boudjemline, Y., Fermont, L., Le Bidois, J. *et al.* (2000) Prenatal diagnosis of conotruncal heart diseases. Result in 337 cases. *Arch. Mal. Coeur. Vaiss.*, **93** (5), 583–6.

(2001) Prevalence of 22q11 deletion in fetuses with conotruncal cardiac defects: a 6-years prospective study. *J. Pediatr.*, **138**, 520–4.

Bove, E. L., Minich, L. L., Pridjian, A. K. *et al.* (1993) The management of severe subaortic stenosis, ventricular septal defect, and aortic arch obstruction in the neonate. *J. Thorac. Cardiovasc. Surg.*, **105** (2), 289–96.

Braunlin, E., Peoples, W. M., Freedom, R. M. *et al.* (1982) Interruption of the aortic arch with aorticopulmonary septal defect. *Ped. Cardiol.*, **3**, 329–35.

Bristow, J. D. & Bernstein, H. S. (1998) Counseling families with chromosome 22q11 deletions: the catch in CATCH-22. *J. Am. Coll. Cardiol.* **32** (2), 499–501.

Brizard, C. P., Cochrane, A., Austin, C. *et al.* (1997) Management strategy and long-term outcome for truncus arteriosus. *Eur. J. Cardiothorac. Surg.* **11** (4), 687–96.

Carotti, A., Marino, B., Bevilacqua, M. *et al.* (1997) Primary repair of isolated ventricular septal defect in infancy guided by echocardiography. *Am. J. Cardiol.*, **79**, 1498–501.

Carotti, A., Di Donato, R. M., Squitieri, C. *et al.* (1998) Total repair of pulmonary atresia with ventricular septal defect and major aortopulmonary collaterals: an integrated approach. *J. Thorac. Cardiovasc. Surg.*, **116** (6), 914–23.

Carotti, A., Marino, B. & Di Donato, R. M. (2003) Influence of chromosome 22q11.2 microdeletion on surgical outcome after treatment of tetralogy of Fallot with pulmonary atresia. *J. Thorac. Cardiovasc. Surg.*, **126** (4), 1666–7.

Castaneda, A. R., Mayer, J. E. Jr., Jonas, R. A. *et al.* (1989) The neonate with critical congenital heart disease: repair – a surgical challenge. *J. Thorac. Cardiovasc. Surg.* **98** (5), 869–75.

Celoria, C. G. & Patton, R. B. (1959) Congenital absence of the aortic arch. *Am. Heart J.*, **58**, 407–13.

Chessa, M., Butera, G., Bonhoeffer, P. *et al.* (1998). Relation of genotype 22q11 deletion to phenotype of pulmonary vessels in tetralogy of Fallot and pulmonary atresia-ventricular septal defect. *Heart*, **79**, 186–90.

Conley, M. E., Beckwith, J. B., Mancer, J. F. K. *et al.* (1979) The spectrum of the DiGeorge syndrome. *J. Pediatr.*, **94**, 883–90.

Consevage, M. W., Seip, J. R., Belchis, D. A. *et al.* (1996) Association of a mosaic chromosomal 22q11 deletion with hypoplastic left heart syndrome. *Am. J. Cardiol.*, **77**, 1023–5.

Conti, E., Grifone, N., Sarkozy, A. *et al.* (2003) DiGeorge subtypes of non syndromic conotruncal defects: evidence against a major role of TBX1 gene. *Eur. J. Hum. Genet.*, **11**, 349–51.

Conway, K., Gibson, R. L., Perkins, J. *et al.* (2002) Pulmonary agenesis: expansion of the VCFS phenotype. *Am. J. Med. Genet.*, **113**, 89–92.

Dallapiccola, B., Marino, B., Giannotti, A. *et al.* (1989) DiGeorge anomaly associated with partial deletion of chromosome 22. Report of a case with X/22 translocation and review of the literature. *Ann. Genet.*, **32** (2), 92–6.

de la Cruz, M. V., Cayre, R., Angelici, P. *et al.* (1990) Coronary arteries in truncus arteriosus. *Am. J. Cardiol.*, **66** (20), 1482–6.

Digilio, M. C., Marino, B., Giannotti, A. *et al.* (1996a) Search for 22q11 deletion in non-syndromic conotruncal cardiac defects. *Eur. J. Pediatr.*, **155**, 619–24.

Digilio, M. C., Marino, B., Grazioli, S. *et al.* (1996b) Comparison of occurrence of genetic syndromes in ventricular septal defect with pulmonic stenosis (classic tetralogy of Fallot) versus ventricular septal defect with pulmonic atresia. *Am. J. Cardiol.*, **77**, 1375–6.

Digilio, M. C., Marino, B., Giannotti, A. *et al.* (1997a) Conotruncal heart defects and chromosome 22q11 microdeletion. *J. Pediatr.*, **130**, 675–7.

(1997b) Familial deletions of chromosome 22q11. *Am. J. Med. Genet.*, **73**, 95–6.

Digilio, M. C., Marino, B., Ammirati, A. *et al.* (1999a) Cardiac malformations in patients with oral-facial-skeletal syndrome: clinical similarities with heterotaxia. *Am. J. Genet.*, **84**, 350–6.

Digilio, M. C., Marino, B., Giannotti, A. *et al.* (1999b). Guidelines for 22q11 deletion screening of patients with conotruncal defects. *J. Am. Coll. Cardiol.*, **33** (6), 1746–7.

Digilio, M. C., Casey, B., Toscano, A. *et al.* (2001) Complete transposition of the great arteries. Patterns of congenital heart disease in familial precurrence. *Circulation*, **104**, 2809–14.

Digilio, M. C., Angioni, A., De Santis, M. *et al.* (2003a) Spectrum of clinical variability in familial deletion 22q11.2: from full manifestation to extremely mild clinical anomalies. *Clin. Genet.*, **63**, 1–6.

Digilio, M. C., Marino, B. & Dallapiccola, B. (2003b) Screening for celiac disease in patients with deletion 22q11.2 (DiGeorge/velo-cardio-facial syndrome). *Am. J. Med. Genet.*, **121**, 286–8.

Dodo, H., Alejos, J. C., Perlof, J. K. *et al.* (1995) Anomalous origin of the left main pulmonary artery from the ascending aorta associated with DiGeorge syndrome. *Am. J. Cardiol.*, **75**, 1294–5.

Ferencz, C., Loffredo, C. A. & Correa-Villasenor, A. (1997) Genetic and enviromental risk factors of major cardiovascular malformations: the Baltimore–Washington Infant Study 1981–1989. *Armonk, Futura*, New York.

Fokstuen, S., Arbenz, U., Artan, S. *et al.* (1998) 22q11.2 deletions in a series of patients with non-selective congenital heart defects: incidence, type of defects and parental origin. *Clin. Genet.*, **53**, 63–9.

Francalanci, P., Marino, B., Boldrini, R. *et al.* (1996) Morphology of the atrioventricular valve in asplenia syndrome: a peculiar type of atrioventricular canal defect. *Cardiovasc. Pathol.*, **5**, 145–51.

Franklin, R. C. G., Onuzo, O., Miller, P. A. *et al.* (1996) Transfusion associated graft-versus-host disease in DiGeorge syndrome – index case report with survey of screening procedures and use of irradiated blood components. *Cardiol. Young.*, **6**, 222–7.

Freedom, R. M., Rosen, F. S. & Nadas, A. S. (1972) Congenital cardiovascular disease and anomalies of the third and fourth pharyngeal pouch. *Circulation*, **46**, 165–72.

Frohn-Mulder, I. M. E., Wesby, V., Swaay, E. *et al.* (1999) Chromosome 22q11 deletions in patients with selected outflow tract malformations. *Genet. Counsel.*, **10** (1), 35–41.

Garg, V., Kathiriya, I. S., Barnes, R. *et al.* (2003) GATA4 mutations cause human congenital heart defects and reveal an interaction with TBX5. *Nature*, **424**, 443–7.

Goldmuntz, E., Driscoll, D., Budarf, M. L. *et al.* (1993) Microdeletions of chromosomal region 22q11 in patients with congenital conotruncal cardiac defects. *J. Med. Genet.*, **30**, 807–12.

Goldmuntz, E., Clark, B. J., Mitchell, L. E. *et al.* (1998) Frequency of 22q11 deletions in patients with conotruncal defects. *J. Am. Coll. Cardiol.*, **32** (2), 492–8.

Goodship, J., Gross, I., Scambler, P. *et al.* (1995). Monozygotic twins with chromosome 22q11 deletion and discordant phenotype. *J. Med. Genet.*, **32**, 746–8.

Goodship, J., Cross, I., LiLing, J. *et al.* (1998) A population study of chromosome 22q11 deletions in infancy. *Arch. Dis. Child.*, **79**, 348–51.

Hofbeck, M., Rauch, A., Buheitel, G. *et al.* (1998). Monosomy 22q11 in patients with pulmonary atresia, ventricular septal defect, and major aortopulmonary collateral arteries. *Heart*, **79** (2), 180–5.

Hokanson, J. S., Pierpont, M. E., Hirsch, B. *et al.* (2001) 22q11.2 microdeletions in adults with familial tetralogy of Fallot. *Genet. Med.*, **3** (1), 61–4.

Hutha, J. C., Glasow, P., Murphy D. J., Jr. *et al.* (1987) Surgery without catheterization for congenital heart defects: management of 100 patients. *J. Am. Coll. Cardiol.*, **9**, 823–9.

Iascone, M. R., Vittorini, S., Sacchelli, M. *et al.* (2002) Molecular characterization of 22q11 deletion in a three-generation family with maternal transmission. *Am. J. Med. Genet.*, **108**, 319–21.

Ilbawi, M. N., Fedorchik, J., Muster, A. J. *et al.* (1986) Surgical approach to severely symptomatic newborn infants with tetralogy of Fallot and absent pulmonary valve. *J. Thorac. Cardiovasc. Surg.*, **91** (4), 584–9.

Iserin, L., de Lonlay, P., Viot, G. *et al.* (1998) Prevalence of the microdeletion 22q11 in newborn infants with congenital conotruncal cardiac anomalies. *Eur. J. Pediatr.*, **157**, 881–4.

Iyer, K. S. & Mee, R. B. (1991) Staged repair of pulmonary atresia with ventricular septal defect and major systemic to pulmonary artery collaterals. *Ann. Thorac. Surg.*, **51** (1), 65–72.

Jadele, K. B., Michels, V. V., Puga, F. J. *et al.* (1992) Velo-cardio-facial syndrome associated with ventricular septal defect, pulmonary atresia, and hypoplastic pulmonary arteries. *Pediatrics*, **89** (5), 915–19.

Johnson, M. C., Strauss, A. W., Dowton, S. B. *et al.* (1995a) Deletion within chromosome 22 is common in patients with absent pulmonary valve syndrome. *Am. J. Cardiol.*, **76**, 66–9.

Johnson, M. C., Watson, M. S., Strauss, A. W. *et al.* (1995b) Anomalous origin of the right pulmonary artery from the aorta and CATCH 22 syndrome. *Ann. Thorac. Surg.*, **60**, 681–3.

Johnson, M. C., Watson, M. S. & Strauss, A. W. (1996) Chromosome 22q11 monosomy and the genetic basis of congenital heart disease. *J. Pediatr.*, **129** (1), 1–3.

Kazuma, N., Murakami, M., Suzuki, Y. *et al.* (1997). Cervical aortic arch associated with 22q11.2 deletion. *Pediatr. Cardiol.*, **18** (2), 149–51.

Kieran, M., Thompson, P. W., Davies, S. J. *et al.* (1999) The prevalence of chromosome 22q11 deletions in an adult congenital heart disease population. *J. Med. Genet.*, **36** (1), S59.

Kinouchi, A., Mori, K., Ando, M. *et al.* (1976) Facial appearance with conotruncal anomalies. *Pediatr. Jpn.*, **17**, 84–9.

Kumar, A., Sapire, D. W., Lockhart, L. H. *et al.* (1996) Atrioventricular septal defect with pulmonary atresia in DiGeorge anomaly: expansion of the cardiac phenotype. *Am. J. Med. Genet.*, **61**, 89–91.

Kumar, A., McCombs, J. L. & Sapire, D. W. (1997) Deletions in chromosome 22q11 region in cervical aortic arch. *Am. J. Cardiol.*, **79**, 388–90.

Leana-Cox, J., Pangkanon, S., Eanet, K. R. *et al.* (1996) Familial DiGeorge/velocardiofacial syndrome with deletions of chromosome area 22q11: report of five families with a review of the literature. *Am. J. Med. Genet.*, **65**, 309–16.

Lee, M. G., Chiu, I. S., Fang, W. *et al.* (1999) Isolated infundibuloarterial inversion and fifth aortic arch in an infant: a newly recognized cardiovascular phenotype with chromosome 22q11 deletion. *Int. J. Cardiol.*, **71**, 89–91.

Lee, M. L., Chaou, W. T., Wang, Y. M. *et al.* (2001) A new embryologic linkage between chromosome 22 deletion and a right ductus from a right aortic arch in a neonate with DiGeorge syndrome. *Int. J. Cardiol.*, **79**, 315–16.

Lewin, M. B., Lindsay, E. A. & Baldini, A. (1996) 22q11 deletions and cardiac disease. *Progr. Pediatr. Cardiol.*, **6**, 19–28.

Lewin, M. B., Lindsay, E. A., Jurecic, V. *et al.* (1997) A genetic etiology for interruption of the aortic arch type B. *Am. J. Cardiol.*, **80**, 493–7.

Lewis, D. A., Loffredo, C. A. and Correa-Villasenor, A. (1996) Descriptive epidemiology of perimembranous and muscular ventricular septal defect in the Baltimore-Washington Infant Study. *Cardiol. Young.*, **6**, 281–90.

Li, C., Chudley, A. E., Soni, R. *et al.* (2003) Pulmonary atresia with intact ventricular septum and major aortopulmonary collaterals: associations with deletion 22q11.2. *Pediatr. Cardiol.*, **24**, 585–7.

Lindsay, E. A., Botta, A., Jurecic, V. *et al.* (1999) Congenital heart disease in mice deficient for the DiGeorge syndrome region. *Nature*, **401**, 379–83.

Loffredo, C. A., Ferencz, C., Wilson, P. D. *et al.* (2000) Interrupted aortic arch: an epidemiologic study. *Teratology*, **61**, 368–75.

Lu, H. J., Chung, M. Y., Betau, H. *et al.* (2001a) Molecular characterization of tetralogy of Fallot within DiGeorge critical region of the chromosome 22. *Ped. Cardiol.*, **22** (**4**), 279–84.

Lu, J. H., Chung, M. Y., Hwang, B. *et al.* (2001b) Monozygotic twins with chromosome 22q11 microdeletion and discordant phenotypes in cardiovascular patterning. *Pediatr. Cardiol.*, **22**, 260–3.

Lucani, G. B. & Starnes, V. A. (1996). Clamshell for pulmonary atresia, ventricular septal defect, and aortopulmonary collaterals. *Ann. Thorac. Surg.*, **62** (**4**), 1247–8.

Maeda, J., Yamagishi, H., Matsuoka, R. *et al.* (2000) Frequent association of 22q11.2 deletion with tetralogy of Fallot. *Am. J. Med. Genet.*, **92**, 269–72.

Maharasingam, M. & Ostam-Smith, I. (2003) A cohort study of neurodevelopmental outcome in children with DiGeorge syndrome following cardiac surgery. *Arch. Dis. Child.*, **88**, 61–4.

Mahle, W. T., Crisalli, J., Coleman, K. *et al.* (2003) Deletion of chromosome 22q11.2 and outcome in patients with pulmonary atresia and ventricular septal defect. *Ann. Thorac. Surg.*, **76** (**2**), 567–71.

Marino, B., Vairo, U., Corno, A. *et al.* (1990a) Atrioventricular canal in Down syndrome: prevalence of associated cardiac malformations compared with patients without Down syndrome. *Am. J. Dis. Child.*, **144**, 1120–2.

Marino, B., Corno, A., Carotti, A. *et al.* (1990b) Pediatric cardiac surgery guided by echocardiography. *Scand. J. Cardiovasc. Surg.*, **24**, 197–201.

Marino, B., Marcelletti, C., Giannotti, A. *et al.* (1991) DiGeorge anomaly with atrio-ventricular canal. *Chest*, **99**, 242–3.

Marino, B., Digilio, M. C., Giannotti, A. *et al.* (1996a) Heterotaxia syndromes and 22q11 deletion. *J. Med. Genet.*, **33** (**12**), 1052.

Marino, B., Digilio, M. C., Grazioli, S., *et al.* (1996b) Associated cardiac anomalies in isolated and syndromic patients with patients with tetralogy of Fallot. *Am. J. Cardiol.*, **77**, 505–8.

(1997a) Cardiac defect and deletion 22q11. *J. Med. Genet.*, **34**, 20.

Marino, B., Digilio, M. C., Novelli, G. *et al.* (1997b) Tricuspid atresia and 22q11 deletion. *Am. J. Med. Genet.*, **72**, 40–2.

Marino, B., Digilio, M. C. & Dallapiccola, B. (1998) Severe truncal valve displasia: association with DiGeorge syndrome? *Ann. Thorac. Surg.*, **66**, 980.

Marino, B., Digilio, M. C., Persiani, M. *et al.* (1999a) Deletion 22q11 in patients with interrupted aortic arch. *Am. J. Cardiol.*, **84**, 360–1.

Marino, B., Digilio, M. C., Toscano, A. *et al.* (1999b) Congenital heart defects in patients with DiGeorge/velocardiofacial syndrome and del 22q11. *Genet. Counsel.*, **10** (**1**), 25–33.

(1999c) Congenital heart diseases in children with Noonan syndrome: an expanded cardiac spectrum with high prevalence of atrioventricular canal. *J. Pediatr.*, **136**, 703–6.

Marino, B. & Digilio, M. C. (2000) Congenital heart disease and genetic syndromes: specific correlation between cardiac phenotype and genotype. *Cardiovasc. Pathol.*, **9** (**6**), 303–15.

Marino, B., Digilio, M. C., Toscano, A. *et al.* (2001) Anatomic patterns of conotruncal defects associated with deletion 22q11. *Genet. Med.*, **3** (**1**), 45–8.

Marino, B., Digilio, M. C. & Toscano, A. (2002) Common arterial trunk, DiGeorge syndrome and microdeletion 22q11. *Prog. Ped. Cardiol.*, **15**, 9–17.

Marino, B. & Digilio, M. C. (2003) Tetralogy of Fallot with aortic valvular stenosis and deletion 22q11. *Ann. Thorac. Surg.*, **75**, 2007–12.

Marmon, L. M., Balsara, R. K., Chen, R. *et al.* (1984) Congenital cardiac anomalies associated with DiGeorge syndrome: a neonatal experience. *Ann. Thorac. Surg.*, **38** (**2**), 146–50.

Matsuoka, R., Kimura, M., Scambler, P. J. *et al.* (1998). Molecular and clinical study of 183 patients with conotruncal anomaly face syndrome. *Hum Genet.* **103**, 70–80.

McElhinney, D. B., Thompson, L. D., Weinberg, P. M. *et al.* (2000) Surgical approach to complicated cervical aortic arch: anatomic, developmental, and surgical considerations. *Cardiol. Young.*, **10** (**3**), 212–19.

McElhinney, D. B., Clark, B. J., Weinberg, P. M. *et al.* (2001a) Association of chromosome 22q11 deletion with isolated anomalies of aortic arch laterality and branching. *J. Am. Coll. Cardiol.*, **37** (**8**), 2114–19.

McElhinney, D. B., Hoydu, A. K., Gaynor, J. W. *et al.* (2001b) Patterns of right aortic arch and mirror-image branching of the brachiocefalic vessels without associated anomalies. *Pediatr. Cardiol.*, **22**, 285–91.

McElhinney, D. B., Jacobs, I., McDonald-McGinn, D. M. *et al.* (2002) Chromosomal and cardiovascular anomalies associated with congenital laryngeal web. *Int. J. Pediatr. Otorhinolaryngol.*, **66**, 23–7.

McElhinney, D. B., Driscoll, D. A., Levin, E. R. *et al.* (2003) Chromosome 22q11 deletion in patients with ventricular septal defect: frequency and associated cardiovascular anomalies. *Pediatrics*, **112** (**6**), 472–6.

McGoon, D. C., Rastelli, G. C. & Ongley, P. A. (1968) An operation for the correction of truncus arteriosus. *J. Am. Med. Assoc.*, **205** (**2**), 69–73.

Mehraein, Y., Wippermann, C. F., Michel-Behnke, I. *et al.* (1997) Microdeletion 22q11 in complex cardiovascular malformations. *Hum. Genet.*, **99**, 433–42.

Melchionda, S., Digilio, M. C., Mingarelli, R. *et al.* (1995) Transposition of the great arteries associated with deletion of chromosome 22q11. *Am. J. Cardiol.*, **75**, 95–8.

Michielon, G., Marino, B., Formigari, R. *et al.* (2004) Impact of genetic syndromes on surgical correction of tetralogy of Fallot. *Circulation*, Abstract Book, Am Heart Association.

Moerman, P., Goddeeris, P., Lauwerijns, J. *et al.* (1980) Cardiovascular malformations in DiGeorge syndrome (congenital absence or hypoplasia of the thymus). *Br. Heart J.*, **44**, 452–9.

Moerman, P., Dumoulin, M., Lauweryns, J. *et al.* (1987) Interrupted right aortic arch in DiGeorge syndrome. *Br. Heart J.*, **58**, 274–8.

Momma, K., Kondo, C., Ando, M. *et al.* (1995) Tetralogy of Fallot associated with chromosome 22q11 deletion. *Am. J. Cardiol.*, **76**, 618–21.

Momma, K., Kondo, C., Matsuoka, R. *et al.* (1996a) Cardiac anomalies associated with a chromosome 22q11 deletion in patients with conotruncal anomaly face syndrome. *Am. J. Cardiol.*, **78**, 591–4.

Momma, K., Kondo, C. & Matsuoka, R. (1996b) Tetralogy of Fallot with pulmonary atresia associated with chromosome 22q11 deletion. *J. Am. Coll. Cardiol.*, **27** (1), 198–202.

Momma, K., Ando, M. & Matsuoka, R. (1997) Truncus arteriosus communis associated with chromosome 22q11 deletion. *J. Am. Coll. Cardiol.*, **30** (4), 1067–71.

Momma, K., Ando, M., Matsuoka, R. *et al.* (1999a) Interruption of the aortic arch associated with deletion of chromosome 22q11 is associated with a subarterial and doubly committed ventricular septal defect in Japanese patients. *Cardiol. Young.*, **9** (5), 451–7.

Momma, K., Matsuoka, R. & Takao, A. (1999b) Aortic arch anomalies associated with chromosome 22q11 deletion (CATCH 22). *Pediatr. Cardiol.*, **20**, 97–102.

Momma, K., Takao, A., Matsuoka, R. *et al.* (2001) Tetralogy of Fallot associated with chromosome 22q11.2 deletion in adolescents and young adults. *Genet. Med.*, **3** (1), 56–60.

Moran, A. M., Colan, S. D., Mayer, J. E. *et al.* (1999) Echocardiographic identification of thymic hypoplasia in tetralogy of Fallot/tetralogy pulmonary atresia. *Am. J. Cardiol.*, **84**, 1268–71.

Nakagawa, M., Okamoto, N., Fujino, H. *et al.* (2000). Tetracuspid aortic valve in a patient with 22q11.2 microdeletion. *Am. J. Med. Genet.*, **93**, 74–5.

Neirotti, R., Galindez, E., Kreutzer, G. *et al.* (1978) Tetralogy of Fallot with subpulmonary ventricular septal defect. *Ann. Thorac. Surg.*, **25** (1), 51–6.

Nishibatake, M., Kirby, M. L. & Van Mierop, L. H. S. (1987) Pathogenesis of persistent truncus arteriosus and dextroposed aorta in the chick embryo after neural crest ablation. *Circulation*, **75** (1), 255–64.

Okita, Y., Miki, S., Ueda, Y. *et al.* (1995) Early and late results of repair of tetralogy of Fallot with subarterial ventricular septal defect. A comparative evaluation of tetralogy with perimembranous ventricular septal defect. *J. Thorac. Cardiovasc. Surg.*, **110** (1), 180–5.

Oppenheimer-Dekker, A., Gittenberger-de Groot, A. C. & Roozendaal, H. (1982) The ductus arteriosus and associated cardiac anomalies in interruption of the aortic arch. *Ped. Cardiol.*, **2**, 185–93.

Patel, R. G., Freedom, R. M., Bloom, K. R. *et al.* (1978) Truncal or aortic valve stenosis in functionally single arterial trunk. *Am. J. Cardiol.*, **42**, 800–9.

Penman Splitt, M., Burn, J. & Goodship, J. (1996) Defects in the determination of left-right asymmetry. *J. Med. Genet.*, **33**, 498–503.

Perez Martinez, V. M., Diaz Gongola, G., Calabrò, R. *et al.* (1975) Tronco arterial comun con interrupcion del istmo aortico. Peculiaridades anatomicas e implicaciones quirurgicas en relacion al tronco arterial comun habitual. *Revista Latina de Cardiologia*, 6 (4), 291–6.

Pierdominici, M., Marziali, M., Giovanetti, A. *et al.* (2000) T cell receptor repertoire and function in patients with DiGeorge and velocardiofacial syndromes. *Clin. Exp. Immunol.*, 121, 127–32.

Pierdominici, M., Mazzetta, F., Caprini, E. *et al.* (2003) Biased T-cell receptor repertoires in patients with chromosome 22q11.2 deletion syndrome (DiGeorge syndrome/velocardiofacial syndrome). *Clin. Exp. Immunol.*, 132, 323–31.

Raatikka, M., Rapola, J., Tuuteri, L. *et al.* (1981) Familial third and fourth pharyngeal pouch syndrome with truncus arteriosus: DiGeorge syndrome. *Pediatrics*, 67 (2), 173–5.

Radford, D. J., Perkins, L., Lachman, R. *et al.* (1988) Spectrum of Di George syndrome in patients with truncus arteriosus: expanded Di George syndrome. *Pediatr. Cardiol.*, 9 (2), 95–101.

Rajasinghe, H. A., McElhinney, D. B., Reddy, V. M. *et al.* (1997) Long-term follow-up of truncus arteriosus repaired in infancy: a twenty-year experience. *J. Thorac. Cardiovasc. Surg.*, 113 (5), 869–79.

Raskind, W. J. (1972) Historic aspect of congenital heart disease. *Birth Defects: Orig. Article Ser.*, 8 (1), 2–8.

(1979) Pediatric cardiology: A brief report perspective. *Ped. Cardiol.*, 1, 63–71.

Rauch, A., Hofbeck, M., Leipold, G. *et al.* (1998) Incidence and significance of 22q11.2 hemizygosity in patients with interrupted aortic arch. *Am. J. Med. Genet.*, 78, 322–31.

Rauch, R., Rauch, A., Koch, A. *et al.* (2002) Cervical origin of the subclavian artery as a specific marker for monosomy 22q11. *Am. J. Cardiol.*, 89, 481–4.

Recto, M. R., Parness, I. A., Gelb, B. D. *et al.* (1997) Clinical implications and possible association of malposition of the branch pulmonary arteries with DiGeorge syndrome and microdeletion of chromosomal region 22q11. *Am. J. Cardiol.*, 80, 1624–7.

Reddy, V. M., Liddicoat, J. R. & Hanley, F. L. (1995) Midline one-stage complete unifocalization and repair of pulmonary atresia with ventricular septal defect and major aortopulmonary collaterals. *J. Thorac. Cardiovasc. Surg.*, 109 (5), 832–45.

Reddy, V. M., Petrossian, E., McElhinney, D. B. *et al.* (1997) One-stage complete unifocalization in infants: when should the ventricular septal defect be closed? *J. Thorac. Cardiovasc. Surg.*, 113 (5), 858–68.

Rhoden, D. K., Leatherbury, L., Helman, S. *et al.* (1996) Abnormalities in lymphocyte populationsin infants with neural crest cardiovascular defects. *Pediatr. Cardiol.*, 17, 143–9.

Rubay, J. F., Macartney, F. J. & Anderson, R. H. (1987) A rare variant of common arterial trunk. *Br. Heart J.*, 57 (2), 202–4.

Ryan, A. K., Goodship, J. A., Wilson, D. I. *et al.* (1997) Spectrum of clinical features associated with interstitial chromosome 22q11 deletions: a European collaborative study. *J. Med. Genet.*, 34, 798–804.

Sano, S., Brawn, W. J. & Mee, R. B. (1990) Repair of truncus arteriosus and interrupted aortic arch. *J. Cardiovasc. Surg.*, 5 (3), 157–62.

Santoro, G., Marino, B., Di Carlo, D. *et al.* (1994) Echocardiographically guided repair of tetralogy of Fallot. *Am. J. Cardiol.*, **73**, 808–11.

Sarkozy, A., Conti, E., Neri, C. *et al.* (2005) Spectrum of atrial septal defects associated with mutations of NKK 2.5 and GATA 4 transcription factors. *J. Med. Genet.*, **42**, 16–21.

Sawatari, K., Imai, Y., Kurosawa, H. *et al.* (1989) Staged operation for pulmonary atresia and ventricular septal defect with major aortopulmonary collateral arteries. New technique for complete unifocalization. *J. Thorac. Cardiovasc. Surg.*, **98** (5), 738–50.

Schmidt, K. G., Cassidy, S. C., Silverman, N. H. *et al.* (1988) Doubly committed subarterial ventricular septal defects: echocardiographic features and surgical implications. *J. Am. Coll. Cardiol.*, **12** (6), 1538–46.

Schott, J. J., Benson, D. W., Basson, C. T. *et al.* (1998) Congenital heart disease caused by mutations in the transcription factor NKX2-5. *Science*, **281**, 108–11.

Schreiber, C., Eicken, A., Balling, G. *et al.* (2000) Single centre experience on primary correction of common arterial trunk: overall survival and freedom from reoperation after more than 15 years. *Eur. J. Cardiothorac. Surg.*, **18** (1), 68–73.

Sell, J. E., Jonas, R. A., Mayer, J. E. *et al.* (1998) The results of a surgical program for interrupted aortic arch. *J. Thorac. Cardiovasc. Surg.*, **115** (6), 864–77.

Serraf, A., Lacour-Gayet, F., Robotin, M. *et al.* (1996) Repair of interrupted aortic arch: a ten-year experience. *J. Thorac. Cardiovasc. Surg.*, **112** (5), 1150–60.

Sett, S. S., Sandor, G. G. S. & Mawson, J. B. (2001) Interrupted right aortic arch and origin of the left pulmonary artery from the aorta in DiGeorge syndrome. *Cardiol. Young.*, **11** (6), 676–9.

Shashi, V., Berry, M. N. & Hines, M. H. (2003) Vasomotor instability in neonates with chromosome 22q11 deletion syndrome. *Am. J. Med. Genet.*, **121**, 231–4.

Sim, E. K., Grignani, R. T., Wong, M. L. *et al.* (1999) Influence of surgery on aortic valve prolapse and aortic regurgitation in doubly committed subarterial ventricular septal defect. *Am. J. Cardiol.*, **84** (12), 1445–8, A8.

Stellin, G., Jonas, R. A., Goh, T. H. *et al.* (1983) Surgical treatment of absent pulmonary valve syndrome in infants: relief of bronchial obstruction. *Ann. Thorac. Surg.*, **36** (4), 468–75.

Takahashi, K., Kido, S., Hoshino, K. *et al.* (1995) Frequency of a 22q11 deletion in patients with conotruncal cardiac malformations: a prospective study. *Eur. J. Pediatr.*, **154**, 878–81.

Tatsuno, K., Konno, S., Ando, M. *et al.* (1973) Pathogenetic mechanisms of prolapsing aortic valve and aortic regurgitation associated with ventricular septal defect. Anatomical, angiographic, and surgical considerations. *Circulation*, **48** (5), 1028–37.

Tchervenkov, C. I., Salasidis, G., Cecere, R. *et al.* (1997) One-stage midline unifocalization and complete repair in infancy versus multiple-stage unifocalization followed by repair for complex heart disease with major aortopulmonary collaterals. *J. Thorac. Cardiovasc. Surg.*, **114** (5), 727–37.

Thompson, L. D., McElhinney, D. B., Reddy, M. *et al.* (2001) Neonatal repair of truncus arteriosus: continuing improvement in outcomes. *Ann. Thorac. Surg.*, **72** (2), 391–5.

Tohyama, K., Satomi, G. & Momma, K. (1997) Aortic valve prolapse and aortic regurgitation associated with subpulmonic ventricular septal defect. *Am. J. Cardiol.*, **79** (9), 1285–9.

Toscano, A., Anaclerio, S., Digilio, M. C. *et al.* (2002) Ventricular septal defect and deletion of chromosome 22q11: anatomical types and aortic arch anomalies. *Eur. J. Pediatr.,* **161**, 116–17.

Tworetzky, W., McElhinney, D. B., Brook, M. M. *et al.* (1999) Echocardiographic diagnosis alone for the complete repair of major congenital heart defects. *J. Am. Coll. Cardiol.,* **33** (1), 228–33.

Vairo, U., Marino, B., Gagliardi, M. G. *et al.* (1989) Truncus arteriosus con discontinuitá delle arterie polmonari: studio ecocardiografico e angiocardiografico. *Cardiovasc. Imag.,* **1** (3), 44–8.

Van Mierop, L. H. S. & Kutsche, L. M. (1984) Interruption of the aortic arch and coarctation of the aorta: pathogenetic relations. *Am. J. Cardiol.,* **54**, 829–34.

(1986) Cardiovascular anomalies in DiGeorge syndrome and importance of neural crest as a possible pathogenetic factor. *Am. J. Cardiol.,* **58**, 133–7.

Van Praagh, R. & McNamara, J. J. (1968) Anatomic types of ventricular septal defect with aortic insufficiency. Diagnostic and surgical considerations. *Am. Heart J.,* **75** (5), 604–19.

Van Praagh, S., Truman, T., Firpo, A., Bano-Rodrigo, A. *et al.* (1989) Cardiac malformations in trisomy-18: a study of 41 postmortem cases. *J. Am. Coll. Cardiol.,* **13**, 1586–97.

Vargas, F. J., Kreutzer, G. O., Pedrini, M. *et al.* (1986) Tetralogy of Fallot with subarterial ventricular septal defect. Diagnostic and surgical considerations. *J. Thorac. Cardiovasc. Surg.,* **92** (5), 908–12.

Vitelli, F., Morishima, M., Taddei, I. *et al.* (2002) Tbx1 mutation causes multiple cardiovascular defects and disrupts neural crest and cranial nerve migratory pathways. *Hum. Mol. Genet.,* **11** (8), 915–22.

Waldo, K., Zdanowicz, M., Burch, J. *et al.* (1999) A novel role for cardiac neural crest in heart development. *J. Clin. Invest.,* **103**, 1499–507.

Wang, J. N., Wu, J. M. & Yang, Y. J. (1999) Double-lumen aortic arch with anomalous left pulmonary artery origin from the main pulmonary artery-bilateral persistent fifth aortic arch – a case report. *Int. J. Cardiol.,* **69**, 105–8.

Webber, S. A., Hatchwell, E., Barber, J. C. K. *et al.* (1996) Importance of microdeletions of chromosomal region 22q11 as a cause of selected malformations of the ventricular outflow tracts and aortic arch: a three-year prospective study. *J. Pediatr.,* **129**, 26–32.

Weintraub, R. G., Chow, C. W. & Gow, R. M. (1989) Absence of the leaflets of the aortic valve in DiGeorge syndrome. *Int. J. Cardiol.,* **23**, 255–7.

Wilson, D. I., Cross, I. E., Goodship, J. A. *et al.* (1991) DiGeorge syndrome with isolated aortic coarctation and isolated ventricular septal defect in three sibs with a 22q11 deletion of maternal origin. *Br. Heart J.,* **66**, 308–12.

Wilson, D. I., Burn, J., Scambler, P. *et al.* (1993) DiGeorge syndrome: part of CATCH 22. *J. Med. Genet.,* **30**, 852–6.

Yacoub, M. H., Khan, H., Stavri, G. *et al.* (1997) Anatomic correction of the syndrome of prolapsing right coronary aortic cusp, dilatation of the sinus of Valsalva, and ventricular septal defect. *J. Thorac. Cardiovasc. Surg.,* **113** (2), 253–61.

Yamagishy, H., Maeda, J., Tokumura, M. *et al.* (2000). Ventricular septal defect associated with microdeletions of chromosome 22q11.2. *Clin. Genet.,* **58**, 493–6.

Yates, R. W. M., Raymond, F. L., Cook, A. *et al.* (1996) Isomerism of the atrial appendages associated with 22q11 deletion in a fetus. *Heart,* **76**, 548–9.

Yeager, S. B. & Sanders, S. P. (1995) Echocardiographic identification of thymic tissue in neonates with congenital heart disease. *Am. Heart J.*, **129**, 837–9.

Young, D., Shprintzen, F. R. J. & Golderb, R. B. (1980) Cardiac malformations in the velocardiofacial syndrome. *Am. J. Cardiol.*, **46**, 643–8.

Young, D. E. J., Booth, P., Barumi, J. *et al.* (1999) Chromosome 22q11 microdeletion and congenital heart disease – a survey in a pediatric population. *Eur. J. Pediatr.*, **158**, 566–70.

Zhang, G. C., Wang, Z. W., Zhang, R. F. *et al.* (1997) Surgical repair of patients with tetralogy of Fallot and unilateral absence of pulmonary artery. *Ann. Thorac. Surg.*, **64** (4), 1150–3.

4

Palatal anomalies and velopharyngeal dysfunction associated with velo-cardio-facial syndrome

Richard E. Kirschner

Division of Plastic and Reconstructive Surgery, The Children's Hospital of Philadelphia, PA, USA

Structural and functional palatal anomalies are among the most common manifestations in VCFS, with cleft lip, cleft palate, and velopharyngeal dysfunction reported as features of affected patients. Up to 8% of patients with isolated palatal clefts, including submucosal clefts, may have an underlying 22q11 deletion, making this the most common genetic syndrome associated with palatal clefts. Moreover, 22q11 deletions have been identified as the most common genetic basis of congenital velopharyngeal dysfunction.

The high incidence of cleft palate and velopharyngeal dysfunction associated with VCFS makes many affected children candidates for palatal or velopharyngeal surgery. This chapter describes the spectrum of palatal phenotypes associated with VCFS and presents guidelines for their diagnosis and surgical management.

Cleft palate and VCFS

Defining the palatal phenotype in VCFS

Palatal anomalies are frequently associated with other congenital malformations and may be seen as features of numerous genetic syndromes. Occasionally, cleft palate or velopharyngeal dysfunction may be the first and most conspicuous presenting sign of a genetic disorder, whereas the associated features and the underlying syndrome remain undiagnosed for many years. In other instances, more severe or life-threatening anomalies may command the clinicians' immediate attention, leaving more subtle palatal abnormalities unrecognized. Since early syndrome recognition is essential to provide for appropriate early intervention and for appropriate family genetic counseling, clinicians caring for children with syndromic disorders should possess a thorough understanding of the phenotypic features of these diagnoses.

It is now well recognized that VCFS may be associated with a wide range of palatal phenotypes, including cleft palate, submucosal cleft palate, bifid uvula, and absence

Velo-Cardial-Facial Syndrome: A Model for Understanding Microdeletion Disorders, ed. Kieran C. Murphy and Peter J. Scambler. Published by Cambridge University Press. © Cambridge University Press, 2005.

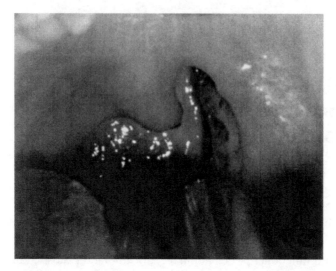

Figure 4.1   Absence of the left palatopharyngeus muscle in a child with a 22q11 deletion, a rare finding.

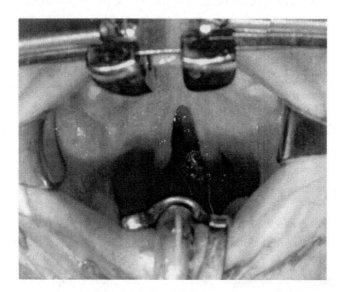

Figure 4.2   Velar cleft associated with a 22q11 deletion.

or hypoplasia of the musculus uvulae or other palatal muscles (Shprintzen *et al.*, 1981; Goldberg *et al.*, 1993; McDonald-McGinn *et al.*, 1999) (Figure 4.1). Clefts of both the primary (anterior to the incisive foramen) and the secondary (posterior to the incisive foramen) palate have been documented in affected patients (McDonald-McGinn *et al.*, 1999). The vast majority of clefts associated with a 22q11 deletion, however, involve the secondary palate alone. Palatal clefts in affected patients may completely divide the soft palate or both the soft and hard palate (Figure 4.2). These

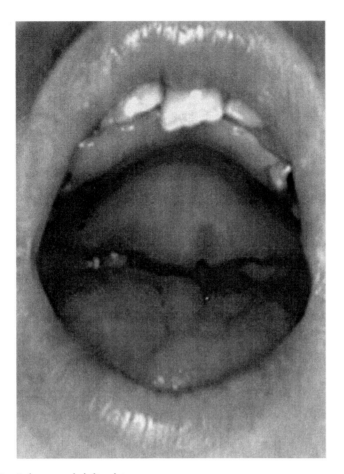

Figure 4.3   Submucosal cleft palate.

overt clefts are invariably associated with alterations in the anatomy of the muscles responsible for velopharyngeal closure, most notably the levator veli palatini. The paired levator muscles normally take their origin from the inferior surface of the temporal bone and descend to the posterior soft palate where they course transversely to form a muscular sling. In the cleft palate, the levator and the palatopharyngeal muscles of each side fuse to form a common muscle that courses parallel to the cleft margin, inserting into the posterior edge of the hard palate. Thus, only isometric contraction of the levators is possible, providing ineffective velar motion.

More frequently, VCFS individuals present with a submucosal cleft palate. In its classic form, submucosal cleft palate may be readily diagnosed by intraoral examination. The triad of bifid uvula, central velar translucency (or *zona pellucidum*), and notching of the posterior hard palate is pathognomonic for the presence of a submucosal cleft (Figure 4.3). The bony notch can usually be seen or palpated at the posterior margin of the hard palate (where the posterior nasal spine is normally

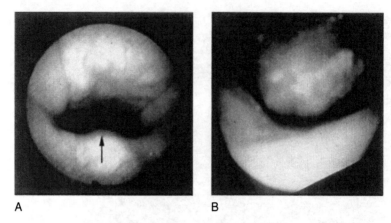

A   B

Figure 4.4   (A) The musculus uvulae is seen as a small bulge (arrow) in the posterior velum on nasendoscopy. (B) Occult submucosal cleft associated with a 22q11 deletion. The musculus uvulae is absent.

present) but may be difficult to appreciate in young infants. The principal abnormality in submucosal clefts is a diastasis of the velar muscles within an intact mucosal envelope. Rather than forming a transverse sling across the posterior soft palate, the paired levator veli palatini muscles insert aberrantly into the posterior edge of the hard palate. Dissection of the soft palate in patients with submucosal clefts has revealed a continuum of muscular abnormalities ranging from partial decussation to complete diastasis of the levator muscles. Contraction of the abnormally oriented velar muscles in submucosal clefts can often be visualized as an abnormal V-shaped ridge upon intraoral examination.

Submucosal clefts of the palate may occur in the absence of the classic triad of overt signs, a condition termed "occult submucosal cleft palate" (Kaplan, 1975; Croft *et al.*, 1978). Affected patients may demonstrate normal palatal morphology on intraoral examination or may present with a bifid uvula in the absence of a zona pellucidum or a bony notch. The majority of cases of isolated bifid uvula likely represent occult submucosal clefts (Shprintzen *et al.*, 1985). Nasendoscopic evaluation of occult submucosal cleft palate reveals a midline V-shaped defect and absence of the normal midline bulge of the musculus uvulae (Figure 4.4). Since the diagnosis cannot be made based upon intraoral examination alone, the presence of an occult submucosal cleft is frequently unnoticed until later evaluation of velopharyngeal dysfunction.

The incidence of cleft palate among VCFS individuals has been reported to range from 9% to as high as 98% (Lipson *et al.*, 1991; Finkelstein *et al.*, 1993; Goldberg *et al.*, 1993; Ryan *et al.*, 1997; Cohen *et al.*, 1999; McDonald-McGinn *et al.*, 1999). This wide variation primarily reflects a difference in reporting technique, with some centers reporting open clefts and submucosal clefts separately. Moreover, the incidence of occult clefts is dependent upon the diligence with which the diagnosis is sought. The true incidence of cleft palate in VCFS remains uncertain, since the figure reported by any single center may reflect some degree of ascertainment bias. The incidence of cleft palate reported by centers in which the majority of patients are ascertained at a younger age (i.e., those presenting with cardiac anomalies) may be artificially low. In such centers, submucosal clefts may remain unrecognized until careful palatal examination and diagnostic testing are performed for the evaluation of velopharyngeal insufficiency. Since language delays are common in affected children, so too may be perceptual evidence of velopharyngeal insufficiency.

In a recent European collaborative study, Ryan et al. (1997) noted clefts of the secondary palate, including submucosal clefts, in 14% of 496 patients with a 22q11 deletion. In a review of 181 patients, mostly children under 5 years of age, McDonald-McGinn et al. (1999) reported a diagnosis of overt cleft palate in 11%, submucosal cleft palate in 16%, bifid uvula in 5%, and cleft lip with or without cleft palate in 2%. Cohen et al. (1999) documented the incidence of palatal anomalies among 126 adults with a 22q11 to be significantly higher, with cleft palate noted in 41% of patients. As noted above, the higher rate of palatal findings seen in adults may be the result of ascertainment bias.

The prevalence of 22q11 deletions among patients referred for evaluation of clefts of the secondary palate has been reported to be approximately 8%. However, when 50 patients with isolated palatal clefts were screened for a 22q11 deletion at the Children's Hospital of Philadelphia Cleft Palate Clinic, none were found to be deleted (Driscoll et al., 1995). Similarly, Mingarelli et al. (1996) did not discover a single deletion among 38 patients screened with isolated clefts of the secondary palate. Thus, although patients with a 22q11 deletion may comprise a significant percentage of the cleft palate population, it is unlikely that 22q11 deletions are responsible for a significant number of apparently nonsyndromic clefts.

Surgical management of cleft palate: timing

The primary goal of cleft palate surgery is the establishment of a normal velopharyngeal valving system that will separate the oral and nasal cavities during speech. Most studies carried out to date support the belief that speech outcome after cleft palate repair is better when the palate is repaired before the development of meaningful, connected speech (Dorf & Curtin, 1982, 1990; Kirschner et al., 2000). While the available data suggest that earlier closure of the palate is associated with better velopharyngeal function and better articulation skills, design flaws make most published studies difficult to interpret. Consequently, there is little consensus regarding the optimal timing of cleft palate repair, particularly in patients with VCFS, in whom language delays are common. The current recommendations for palatal closure by 12–18 months of age are based upon cleft palate treatment protocols that have been established on the basis of outcome studies involving nondeleted patients (Kirschner & LaRossa, 2000). Although early closure is more likely to yield better results than later surgery, the timing of cleft palate repair in patients with a 22q11 deletion must be balanced against other abnormalities (i.e., cardiac) that may take priority over the palate.

Surgical management of cleft palate: technique

The technique described by von Langenbeck (1861) is perhaps the oldest method of palatal repair utilizing mucoperiosteal flaps. The medial cleft margins are pared, bilateral incisions are made medial to the alveolar ridges, and bipedicled mucoperiosteal flaps are elevated. The margins of the cleft are then sutured to one another, a maneuver aided by relaxation of the soft tissues at the lateral incisions.

Modifications of the von Langenbeck technique are still employed in some centers today. A significant drawback of the technique, however, is its inability to provide for significant palatal lengthening. In the early twentieth century, Ganzer (1920) first proposed the idea of lengthening the palate at the time of repair by V–Y retropositioning. This concept was promoted by Veau & Ruppe (1922) and later modified by Wardill (1937) and Kilner (1937). The technique involves elevation of bilateral unipedicled mucoperioteal flaps that are elevated from the hard palate, retropositioned, and sutured to one another, thereby closing the cleft defect while lengthening the palate. In practice, the actual gain in palatal length may be limited due to contraction of the longitudinal scar. Moreover, the repair leaves relatively large areas of denuded bone to heal by secondary intention, theoretically predisposing to inhibition of normal maxillary growth. Nevertheless, variations of the Veau–Wardill–Kilner technique are still widely used worldwide.

Kriens (1969) proposed dissection and anatomic repositioning of the levator veli palatini muscles to reconstruct the levator sling at the time of cleft palate repair. Although several authors have since documented the efficacy of intravelar veloplasty in reducing the incidence of velopharyngeal dysfunction after palate repair, shortcomings in study design have made it difficult to reliably determine if the procedure offers significant benefit. In the only prospective, randomized study of intravelar veloplasty reported to date, Marsh et al. (1989) concluded that the procedure failed to provide a measurable improvement in speech outcome. Others have noted, however, that the variability in outcomes reported after intravelar veloplasty may reflect differences in surgical technique and have reported significantly better velopharyngeal function after extensive release and retropositioning of the abnormally oriented levators (Cutting et al., 1995).

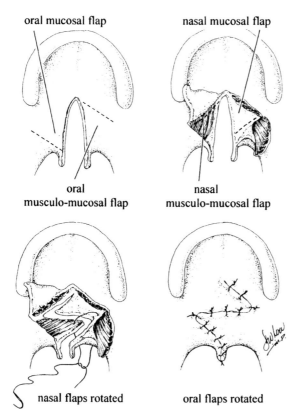

oral mucosal flap

nasal mucosal flap

oral
musculo-mucosal flap

nasal
musculo-mucosal flap

nasal flaps rotated

oral flaps rotated

Figure 4.5   Furlow double-opposing Z-plasty.

The double-opposing Z-plasty technique for velar repair was introduced by Furlow (1978). By incorporating mirror-image Z-plasty incisions of the oral and nasal mucosa, Furlow's method lengthens the soft palate while preventing longitudinal scar contracture. Transposition of the posteriorly based musculomucosal flaps re-orients the levator veli palatini muscles and reconstructs the levator sling (Figure 4.5). By separating the muscle from mucosa on only one surface, the dissection is rendered somewhat simpler than that of the standard intravelar veloplasty and theoretically produces less intravelar scarring. A 20-year experience with the double-opposing Z-palatoplasty at The Children's Hospital of Philadelphia has demonstrated significantly improved speech results in non-deleted cleft palate patients over historical controls, resulting in reduced rates of secondary surgery for the management of velopharyngeal dysfunction (Kirschner et al., 1999). Although this and other studies suggest that the Furlow method results in better velopharyngeal function than straight-line techniques of cleft palate repair, definitive assertion of the technique's superiority awaits the completion of well-controlled, prospective trials.

There are currently few studies documenting long-term speech outcome after cleft palate repair in VCFS individuals. Available data suggest, however, that cleft palate repair is rarely sufficient to prevent velopharyngeal insufficiency in such patients (D'Antonio *et al.*, 2001; Kirschner *et al.*, 2001; Lykins & Sie, 2001). This is likely a reflection of the fact that cleft palate in VCFS is frequently associated with other anomalies, such as velopharyngeal disproportion and velar hypotonia, that may contribute to velopharyngeal dysfunction and that may be inadequately addressed by palate repair alone. Accordingly, parents of affected infants should be counseled about the likely need for secondary management of velopharyngeal dysfunction after cleft palate repair.

The only indication for surgical management of submucosal cleft palate in patients with VCFS is the presence of velopharyngeal dysfunction, and the goal of management is provision of adequate velopharyngeal closure (Gosain *et al.*, 1996). There are no data to support the use of "prophylactic" surgical intervention in children diagnosed with a submucosal cleft palate prior to the age at which a definitive diagnosis of velopharyngeal dysfunction is possible. As is the case for overt clefts, there has been little information published regarding the optimal surgical approach to submucosal cleft palate associated with velopharyngeal dysfunction in patients with a 22q11 deletion. Indeed, there is little consensus with respect to the optimal surgical management of submucosal cleft palate in the general population. Numerous surgical approaches for the management of submucosal cleft palate in nondeleted patients have been described, including palatal lengthening by pushback techniques (with or without intravelar veloplasty), Furlow Z-plasty, and pharyngeal flap surgery (Gosain *et al.*, 1996). Some authors have reported using a combination of two or more techniques. Poor study design and small sample size in most reported series preclude definitive assessment of the superiority of one technique over another. Of all techniques, the pharyngeal flap has most consistently been associated with improved velopharyngeal function, although Furlow Z-plasty may also yield acceptable results in selected patients.

The limited data available suggest that palatal repair alone may be inadequate to treat velopharyngeal dysfunction in patients with submucosal clefts associated with a 22q11 deletion. As described later in this chapter, velopharyngeal dysfunction in VCFS individuals is often of multifactorial etiology and may occur in the presence or absence of submucosal clefting. Since palatal procedures alone often fail to address co-existing abnormalities that may play a significant role in faulty velopharyngeal valving in this group of patients, it is understandable that the results of such procedures are usually poor. Certainly, there is a small group of VCFS patients with submucosal clefts in whom velar motion is quite good and the size of the gap is small. Such patients may be adequately treated by Furlow Z-plasty. Effective management of velopharyngeal dysfunction in most patients, however, requires pharyngoplasty, either a pharyngeal flap or a sphincter pharyngoplasty. Although some have suggested treatment of such patients by combined palate repair and pharyngoplasty, there is no evidence to support the use of adjunctive palatal procedures when pharyngoplasty is employed as the primary means of surgical management.

Velopharyngeal insufficiency and VCFS

Deletion of 22q11 is currently the most common genetic cause of velopharyngeal dysfunction. Abnormalities of velopharyngeal valving are among the most common clinical features of VCFS and may occur both in the presence or absence of cleft palate. Clinical experience at several centers has revealed that up to 75% of patients with a 22q11 deletion will ultimately exhibit some degree of velopharyngeal insufficiency (Brondum-Nielson & Christensen, 1996; Cohen *et al.*, 1999; McDonald-McGinn *et al.*, 1999; Vantrappen *et al.*, 1999). Moreover, a recent report by Zori *et al.* (1998) notes that more than one-third of all patients who present for evaluation of apparently isolated velopharyngeal insufficiency may have an undiagnosed 22q11 deletion. Since velopharyngeal dysfunction may significantly impair a child's speech intelligibility and communication skills, early multidisciplinary evaluation and management of the velopharynx is an important part of the overall management of VCFS children.

Anatomy and physiology of the velopharyngeal valve

The primary abnormality in patients with velopharyngeal dysfunction is inadequacy of the velopharyngeal valving mechanism. Velopharyngeal valving is a complex process that relies on the coordinated interaction of many variables. Closure of the velopharyngeal valve during speech requires not only the proper velopharyngeal anatomy but also precise programming in the central nervous system for coordinated neuromuscular function. Affected individuals are unable to appropriately separate the oral and nasal cavities during speech, sucking, and swallowing. All unrepaired overt clefts, and some submucosal clefts, are associated with velopharyngeal dysfunction. As commonly seen in patients with VCFS, impaired velopharyngeal valving may also occur in the absence of palatal clefting.

The soft palate and pharyngeal walls form the velopharyngeal valve, the functional integrity of which is dependent upon the structure and function of the soft palate, the velopharyngeal musculature, and the supporting skeletal structures. During velopharyngeal closure, the velum is displaced superiorly and posteriorly, forming a genu at its posterior aspect that is easily appreciated on lateral radiographs. This genu, formed just above the level of contact or attempted contact between the velum and the posterior pharyngeal wall, has been termed the velar eminence. The paired levator veli palatini muscles function as the primary elevators of the soft palate. These muscles originate from the petrous portion of the temporal bone and travel inferiorly and anteromedially, inserting into the palatal aponeurosis in the middle third of the soft palate. Contraction of the levators lifts the soft palate upward and backward and contributes to formation of the velar eminence. The musculus uvulae, a small intrinsic muscle located on the dorsum of the soft palate, originates from the palatal aponeurosis and extends posteriorly into the uvula. Contraction of the musculus uvulae may also contribute to formation of the velar eminence, and its absence is a hallmark of occult submucosal clefts. The superior constrictor takes its origin from the soft palate, the medial pterygoid plate and hamulus, the pterygomandibular raphe, and the mandible. Its fibers course posteromedially to insert on the median pharyngeal raphe. The exact contribution of the superior constrictor remains debatable. While contraction of the superior constrictor may displace the lateral pharyngeal walls medially and the posterior pharyngeal wall anteriorly, electromyographic evidence suggests that this muscle may play little role in velopharyngeal closure during speech. The paired palatopharyngeus muscles arise from the lateral and posterior pharyngeal walls and insert into the velum. Although there is some evidence that these muscles may narrow the velopharyngeal orifice and may lower the velum, it is unlikely that they play a significant role in velopharyngeal valving.

In normal individuals, displacement of the soft palate upward and backward is the primary event that results in closure of the velopharyngeal valve. Resting velar length does not necessarily correlate with pharyngeal depth because the velum is longer during function than at rest. This lengthening of the soft palate during speech, termed "velar stretch," plays an important role in achieving velopharyngeal closure (McWilliams et al., 1990). Medial displacement of the lateral pharyngeal walls contributes to velopharyngeal valving as well, although the extent of lateral pharyngeal wall movement may differ between individuals. Occasionally, a dynamic, localized projection of the posterior pharyngeal wall, a so-called Passavant's ridge, may contribute to velopharyngeal closure. Although apparent as a compensatory mechanism in some individuals with faulty velopharyngeal valving, a Passavant's ridge may also be present in some normal individuals (McWilliams et al., 1990). In summary, the velum and the pharyngeal walls work in concert with one another to achieve velopharyngeal closure. Closure of the velopharyngeal valve during speech is a complex and highly coordinated activity that requires proper anatomical relationships, precise neurological programming, and adequate muscular function (see Chapter 10 for more details). Even minor alterations in a single variable may result in velopharyngeal dysfunction.

Table 4.1. Variables that may contribute to velopharyngeal dysfunction in patients with a 22q11 microdeletion

Palatopharyngeal disproportion
Palatal and/or pharyngeal hypotonia
Overt or submucosal cleft palate
Hypoplastic adenoid pad

Nature of velopharyngeal dysfunction in VCFS

The etiology of velopharyngeal dysfunction in patients with a 22q11 deletion is multifactorial (Table 4.1). In the majority of patients, inability to achieve velopharyngeal closure appears to be due primarily to palatopharyngeal disproportion. Cephalometric studies have demonstrated that an abnormally obtuse basicranium (platybasia) in affected patients results in an increased ratio between pharyngeal depth and palatal length, the so-called "need ratio," thereby predisposing to inadequate velopharyngeal valving (Shprintzen, 1982; Arvystas & Shprintzen, 1984; Riski *et al.*, 2000). Three-dimensional volumetric magnetic resonance analysis has confirmed that cranial base abnormalities associated with VCFS result in significant increases in pharyngeal dimensions that may contribute to velopharyngeal insufficiency on the basis of palatopharyngeal disproportion (Ruotolo *et al.*, 2003).

Adenoid hypoplasia may also contribute to velopharyngeal insufficiency in some VCFS individuals (Williams *et al.*, 1987). The adenoid pad is usually located in the nasopharyngeal concavity, the most frequent site of contact between the soft palate and posterior pharynx during velopharyngeal closure. In the setting of velopharyngeal dysfunction due to palatopharyngeal disproportion, adenoid volume may play a critical role in achieving velopharyngeal closure. Adenoid hypoplasia has been documented as a common feature in VCFS and may play a significant role in the development of speech disorders in affected patients (Havkin *et al.*, 2000). Moreover, the increase in pharyngeal depth resulting from removal of the adenoids in patients with a 22q11 deletion may lead to severe hypernasality. Chronic otitis media and upper respiratory tract infections are common in VCFS individuals and are more likely related to immune dysfunction than to adenoid abnormalities (see Chapter 6 for more details). Early diagnosis is therefore essential in order to prevent velopharyngeal dysfunction after adenoidectomy. Although velopharyngeal insufficiency is considered to be an uncommon complication of adenoidectomy in the general population, Perkins *et al.* (2000) have recently reported that 64.3% of patients with post-adenoidectomy velopharyngeal insufficiency who were tested for a 22q11 deletion were found to be deleted. Thus, the presence of velopharyngeal insufficiency after adenoidectomy should alert the clinician to the possibility of a previously undiagnosed VCFS.

Hypotonia of the velopharyngeal musculature is an inconstant feature in VCFS. Often severe, the resulting hypodynamism of the soft palate and pharyngeal walls may contribute significantly to velopharyngeal dysfunction. Since all surgical procedures for the management of velopharyngeal dysfunction rely upon some degree of velopharyngeal motion to achieve adequate valving, the results of standard pharyngoplasty techniques in VCFS individuals may be disappointing. Optimization of outcome after surgical intervention is therefore critically dependent upon a thorough preoperative assessment of velopharyngeal function and individualization of treatment.

Assessment of velopharyngeal function

Accurate velopharyngeal evaluation in VCFS individuals requires a coordinated team approach, a cooperative effort between a qualified speech pathologist and an experienced plastic surgeon or otolaryngologist. The purpose of such multidisciplinary assessment is to gather information on the anatomical and functional status of the velopharyngeal mechanism and to formulate an appropriate therapeutic strategy. It cannot be over-emphasized that assessment of velopharyngeal function in VCFS individuals must be carried out in a thoughtful and reliable fashion with careful attention to the timing and techniques of the evaluation. The potential ramifications of errors in diagnosis are significant. Misguided surgical intervention, both in timing and in technique, is as serious an error as is the recommendation for continued speech therapy in cases where there can be little expectation of further improvement. Both errors should be avoided at all costs.

Evaluation of velopharyngeal function is usually performed using a variety of methods, as there is currently no single technique for assessment of the velopharynx that provides definitive and complete information. The first step in evaluating the VCFS individual is the performance of a careful perceptual speech assessment (see Chapter 10 for more details). In the end, it is this perceptual evaluation that is most important in determining whether a recommendation should be made for surgical management of velopharyngeal dysfunction. Assessment of nasal air emission, resonance, phonation, and articulation provides important information regarding competency of the velopharyngeal valving mechanism, and any perceptual evidence of velopharyngeal dysfunction should prompt further evaluation. The use of rating scales, such as that described by McWilliams & Philips (1979), may be useful for summarizing perceptual speech data and for making preliminary judgments regarding velopharyngeal function.

Nasal air emission may be audible or may be evidenced by condensation on a mirror placed beneath the nose during speech. Velopharyngeal dysfunction is characterized by the abnormal escape of air through the nose during speech and, in most cases, by increased nasal resonance. Facial grimacing and alar flaring during speech may also be observed in children with velopharyngeal dysfunction. Children with velopharyngeal dysfunction may attempt to compensate for their inability to achieve complete velopharyngeal closure by increasing their vocal effort, resulting in hoarseness, whereas others may have difficulty creating a voice that is sufficiently loud because of air wastage through an incompetent velopharynx. Some affected patients may deliberately speak softly in an attempt to limit abnormal nasal air escape.

Articulation is the process whereby the structures responsible for speech production (i.e., the lips, tongue, teeth, etc.) come into contact with one another in order to modify the breath stream and sounds generated by the vocal cords. In order to compensate for the inability to produce pressure consonant sounds, many children with velopharyngeal dysfunction develop alterations in the typical patterns of contact or eliminate such contact altogether. Accurate assessment of velopharyngeal function requires ability of the patient to properly articulate at least some of the phonemes that require velopharyngeal closure, and the presence of compensatory articulation errors may make accurate assessment of velopharyngeal function difficult. Velopharyngeal evaluation performed in the presence of multiple glottal stops, nasal substitutions, and omission errors may lead to improper or unnecessary recommendations for surgical intervention (see Chapter 10 for more details). When compensatory articulation errors preclude proper evaluation, presurgical speech therapy is warranted in order to correct compensatory misarticulation and to allow valid assessment of velopharyngeal function.

In addition to perceptual speech evaluation, intraoral examination is an important part of velopharyngeal screening. A thorough examination should be performed to rule out a diagnosis of submucosal cleft palate and to assess tonsillar size. As discussed below, presence of significant tonsillar hypertrophy should alert the clinician to the need for tonsillectomy prior to pharyngeal flap surgery. Simple inspection of the oral cavity and oropharynx, however, provides no useful information regarding the functional status of the velopharyngeal valve. When perceptual assessment suggests the diagnosis of velopharyngeal dysfunction, definitive evaluation requires visualization of the velopharyngeal mechanism during speech. The most direct means of visualization is through flexible fiberoptic nasendoscopy. By viewing the velopharynx from above during speech production, the examiner can obtain valuable information regarding the structure of the palate (i.e., the presence or absence of a submucosal cleft), the extent and symmetry of velar and pharyngeal wall motion, and on the pattern of velopharyngeal closure. A persistent opening in the velopharyngeal valve during speech is considered definitive evidence of velopharyngeal insufficiency.

Multiview videofluoroscopy can also provide useful information on velopharyngeal function. The examination, which requires the expertise of both a

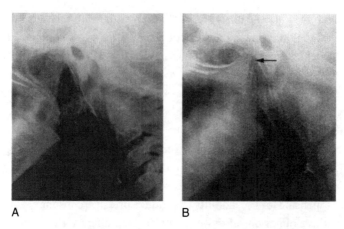

A   B

Figure 4.6   (A) Lateral videofluoroscopic image taken at rest. (B) Persistent velopharyngeal gap (arrow) during phonation confirms the diagnosis of velopharyngeal dysfunction.

radiologist and a speech pathologist, allows for radiographic visualization of the soft palate and the pharynx during speech production. Use of frontal, lateral, and basal or modified Towne views provides complementary information on velar and lateral pharyngeal wall motion and allows for three-dimensional visualization of the velopharynx. A small amount of barium may be instilled through the nose in order to better visualize the velopharyngeal structures. As with nasendoscopy, a persistent gap between the soft palate and the posterior pharynx during speech is diagnostic evidence of velopharyngeal insufficiency (Figure 4.6).

Nasendoscopy and videofluoroscopy provide complementary information on velopharyngeal function. While nasendoscopy provides the better direct view of the velopharyngeal valve during speech and allows for assessment of occult sub-mucosal clefts, the nasal airway, and the larynx, lateral view videofluoroscopy provides information not available by endoscopy, such as the level of attempted velar contact with the posterior pharynx and position of the tongue during phoneme production. It is often neither practical nor necessary to perform two studies of velopharyngeal function, and nasendoscopy alone is currently the best single examination. Videofluoroscopy remains an excellent technique for young children who are unable to cooperate with endoscopy. Both studies provide information on the size, shape, and location of the velopharyngeal gap and demonstrate the relative contributions of velar, lateral pharyngeal wall, and poster-ior pharyngeal wall movement to velopharyngeal closure. An International Working Group has proposed standards for the measurement and reporting of nasendoscopy and multiview videofluoroscopy that may serve as objective guidelines for the diagnosis and management of velopharyngeal dysfunction (Golding-Kushner *et al.*, 1990).

Nonsurgical management of velopharyngeal insufficiency

The information gathered by perceptual, instrumental, and radiological assessment provides the basis for therapeutic decisions for velopharyngeal insufficiency. Although there is some evidence that mild velopharyngeal dysfunction may respond to speech therapy that improves articulation and strengthens closure patterns, there are currently no data to document the efficacy of articulation therapy and behavioral modification techniques in the management of velopharyngeal insufficiency associated with VCFS. Prosthetic devices may be prescribed for the management of patients with velopharyngeal insufficiency who cannot undergo surgery or who demonstrate persistent velopharyngeal insufficiency despite attempts at surgical correction. An obturator typically consists of an anterior portion with clasps that secure the obturator to the teeth and a posterior portion – the speech bulb – that extends into the velopharyngeal space. Closure of the velopharyngeal valve requires the inward movement of the pharyngeal walls, bringing them into contact with the appliance. The palatal lift is another type of prosthesis that is designed to lift the soft palate into a position in which the velum comes in close proximity to the pharyngeal walls. It may be a useful device for patients in whom the length of the palate is adequate, but palatal motion is not. While prosthetic devices have the advantage of requiring neither anesthesia nor surgery; these appliances require patient cooperation, prolonged compliance, and good dental hygiene. Multiple sessions with a prosthodontist may be needed in order to properly fit the device. Moreover, the prosthesis may be uncomfortable and may be readily damaged or lost. For these reasons, prosthetic devices have proved to be of limited utility in the management of velopharyngeal dysfunction in VCFS individuals.

Surgical management of velopharyngeal insufficiency

Surgical management of the velopharynx is indicated for the majority of patients with velopharyngeal dysfunction associated with VCFS. A recommendation for surgery should be made only after a definitive diagnosis of velopharyngeal insufficiency has been established, and this, in turn, must await acquisition of sufficient expressive language and proper articulation of at least some of the sounds that require velopharyngeal closure. At most centers, therefore, velopharyngeal surgery is typically not performed until after the age of 4 or 5 years.

The goal of surgical intervention is to correct abnormal leakage of air through the velopharyngeal valve during speech, thereby diminishing nasal air escape and hypernasality. Several reports have indicated that surgical outcome in VCFS individuals with velopharyngeal dysfunction may be poorer that that achieved in patients with nonsyndromic palatal anomalies. The constellation of anatomic and functional abnormalities associated with VCFS may therefore impair velopharyngeal valving despite surgical management. Since all operative procedures for the management of velopharyngeal dysfunction rely on at least some intrinsic velopharyngeal muscle activity in order to achieve valve closure, patients with a hypodynamic velopharynx frequently demonstrate persistent hypernasality despite surgical narrowing of the velopharyngeal orifice. Moreover, many patients with velopharyngeal dysfunction associated with VCFS are diagnosed and treated at a later age than nonsyndromic cleft palate patients, perhaps contributing to poorer overall results after speech surgery.

There is currently no consensus regarding the optimal surgical technique for management of velopharyngeal dysfunction in VCFS individuals. Nevertheless, the spectrum of anatomic and physiologic abnormalities associated with the syndrome, and the resulting spectrum of velopharyngeal valving abnormalities, dictates that the surgical approach to each patient be individualized. Historically, posterior pharyngeal flap procedures have been employed most frequently for the treatment of velopharyngeal dysfunction in this and other groups of patients. Although there are several techniques for performing pharyngeal flap surgery, all involve the creation of a flap of muscle and mucosa from the posterior pharyngeal wall and the attachment of this flap to the posterior velum (Millard, 1980). The flap remains as a permanent obturator of the velopharynx. Small ports on either side of the flap allow air to move through the nose during respiration and during the production of nasal sounds. Closure of the velopharyngeal valve during speech requires medial movement of the lateral pharyngeal walls, bringing them into apposition with the pharyngeal flap. The size of the ports is determined by the width of the flap and by the width of flap inset into the posterior velum (Argamaso, 1995; Figure 4.7). The decision regarding how wide the flap must be is made using the information obtained in preoperative studies. Since many VCFS patients with velopharyngeal dysfunction have absent or limited lateral pharyngeal wall movement during speech, pharyngeal flaps in such patients must often be made very wide.

Although not performed as commonly as pharyngeal flap surgery in patients with VCFS, the sphincter pharyngoplasty is another procedure that may be utilized for the management of velopharyngeal dysfunction. As in pharyngeal flap surgery, several techniques for this procedure have been described (Hynes, 1967; Orticochea, 1970; Jackson & Silverton, 1977). Fundamentally, however, each method requires the creation of bilateral, superiorly based flaps consisting of the mucosa of the posterior tonsillar pillars together with the underlying palatopharyngeus muscles. The flaps are transposed medially and inset into a transverse incision in the posterior pharyngeal wall, thus creating a velopharyngeal sphincter with a central port (Figure 4.8).

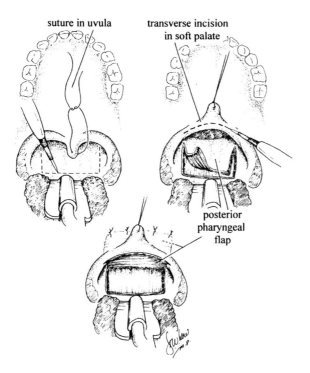

suture in uvula

transverse incision
in soft palate

posterior
pharyngeal
flap

Figure 4.7   Posterior pharyngeal flap.

Anomalies of the internal carotid arteries have been described as a frequent feature in VCFS. In as many as 25% of patients, one or both of the internal carotid arteries may be medially displaced at the level of the posterior pharynx, placing them at risk for injury at the time of pharyngoplasty (Goldberg *et al.*, 1993; Figure 4.9). Preoperative imaging studies, such as magnetic resonance angiography or computed tomography, can define the vascular anatomy in relation to potential flap donor sites, thereby allowing for precise surgical planning to minimize the risk of intra-operative vascular injury (MacKenzie-Stepner *et al.*, 1987; Mitnick *et al.*, 1996; Ross *et al.*, 1996).

Reported complications of pharyngeal flap surgery include hemorrhage, dehiscence, oronasal fistula formation, pneumonia, and cardiac arrest (Albery *et al.*, 1982; Valnicek *et al.*, 1994). Post-operatively, most patients who have undergone pharyngeal flap surgery experience some degree of nasal airway obstruction, although obstructive symptoms frequently improve as edema subsides. Snoring is common, and some patients may become obligate mouth breathers. Although hyponasal speech is frequently noted in the immediate postoperative period, a small number of patients will demonstrate persistent hyponasality after resolution of edema. Although uncommon, obstructive sleep apnea is perhaps the most feared complication of pharyngeal flap surgery. Patients with a prior history of

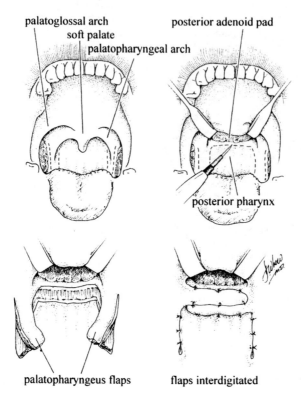

Figure 4.8   Sphincter pharyngoplasty.

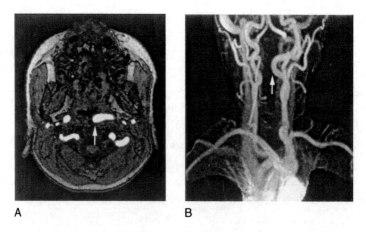

Figure 4.9   Medial deviation of the left internal carotid artery at the level of the posterior pharynx
demonstrated in (A) axial and (B) coronal magnetic resonance images.

obstructive apnea and those with significant tonsillar hyperplasia are at greater risk for obstructive complications after pharyngeal flap surgery. When the tonsils are enlarged, tonsillectomy should be performed preoperatively and velopharyngeal function reassessed prior to speech surgery. Loud snoring, nocturnal arousals, and excessive daytime somnolence after surgery may indicate the presence of obstructive apnea. Patients who manifest persistence of such signs should be referred for diagnostic evaluation, as significant obstructive apnea mandates pharyngoplasty revision.

At the present time, there are few data to support the superiority of one surgical technique over another in the management of velopharyngeal dysfunction associated with VCFS. Although the greatest experience to date has been with pharyngeal flap surgery, recent data suggest that sphincter pharyngoplasty may be an effective alternative in some patients (Witt et al., 1999). Since the anatomy and function of the velopharynx differs between patients, optimization of surgical outcome requires that the surgical technique be tailored to the individual deficiencies of each patient. Careful attention to the diagnostic information gathered during preoperative assessment and tailoring of operation interventions to the specific needs of each patient can improve surgical outcome and diminish the need for revisional procedures. Nevertheless, velopharyngeal dysfunction in patients with VCFS is a complex phenomenon that remains incompletely understood. Optimization of the management of velopharyngeal insufficiency in affected patients will ultimately require the completion of carefully designed, well-controlled prospective trials.

Summary

Early recognition of palatal clefts or velopharyngeal dysfunction in VCFS individuals is essential for early and appropriate medical intervention and for genetic counseling. Since the most common palatal manifestations in VCFS are submucosal cleft palate and velopharyngeal dysfunction, problems that may otherwise remain undetected until later in childhood, all patients identified with a 22q11 deletion should undergo early evaluation by a cleft palate team.

REFERENCES

Albery, E. H., Bennett, J. A., Pigott, R. W. & Simmons, R. M. (1982) The results of 100 operations for velopharyngeal incompetence – selected on the findings of endoscopic and radiological examination. *Br. J. Plast. Surg.*, **30**, 118–26.

Argamaso, R. V. (1995) Pharyngeal flap surgery for velopharyngeal insufficiency. *Oper. Tech. Plast. Surg.*, **2**, 233–8.

Arvystas, M. & Shprintzen, R. J. (1984) Craniofacial morphology in the velo-cardio-facial syndrome. *J. Craniofac. Genet. Dev. Biol.*, **4**, 39–45.

Brondum-Nielson, K. & Christensen, K. (1996) Chromosome 22q11 deletion and other chromosome aberrations in cases with cleft palate, congenital heart defects, and/or mental disability: A survey based on the Danish Facial Cleft Registrar. *Clin. Genet.* **50**, 116–20.

Cohen, E., Chow, E. W., Weksberg, R. & Bassett, A. S. (1999) Phenotype of adults with the 22q11 deletion syndrome: A review. *Am. J. Med. Genet.*, **86**, 359–65.

Croft, C. B., Shprintzen, R. J., Daniller, A. & Lewin, M. L. (1978) The occult submucous cleft palate and the musculus uvulae. *Cleft Palate J.*, **15**, 150–4.

Cutting, C. B., Rosenbaum, J. & Rovati, L. (1995) The technique of muscle repair in the cleft soft palate. *Oper. Tech. Plast. Reconst. Surg.*, **2**, 215–22.

D'Antonio, L. L., Davio, M., Zoller, K. *et al.* (2001) Results of Furlow Z-plasty in patients with velocardiofacial syndrome. *Plast. Reconstr. Surg.*, **107**, 1077–9.

Dorf, D. S. & Curtin, J. W. (1982) Early cleft palate repair and speech outcome. *Plast. Reconstr. Surg.* **70**, 74–9.

   (1990) Early cleft palate repair and speech outcome: A ten-year experience. In Bardach, J. & Morris, H. L., eds., *Multidisciplinary Management of Cleft Lip and Palate*. Philadelphia: W. B. Saunders, pp. 341–8.

Driscoll, D., Randall, P., McDonald-McGinn, D. M. *et al.* (1995). Are 22q11 deletions a major cause of isolated cleft palate? Presented at the 52nd annual meeting of the American Cleft Palate-Craniofacial Association, Tampa, FL.

Finkelstein, Y., Zohar, Y., Nachmani, A. *et al.* (1993) The otolaryngologist and the patient with velocardiofacial syndrome. *Arch. Otolaryngol. Head Neck Surg.*, **119**, 563–9.

Furlow, L. T., Jr. (1978) Cleft palate repair: preliminary report on lengthening and muscle transportation by Z-plasty. Presented at the annual meeting of the Southeastern Society of Plastic and Reconstructive Surgeons, Boca Raton, Florida.

Ganzer, H. (1920) Wolfsrachenplastik mit Ausnutzung des gesamten Schleimhautmaterials zur Vermeidung des Verkuerzung des Gaumensegels. *Berl. Klin. Wochenschr.*, **57**, 619.

Goldberg, R., Motzkin, B., Marion, R. *et al.* (1993) Velo-cardio-facial syndrome: A review of 120 patients. *Am. J. Med. Genet.*, **45**, 313–19.

Golding-Kushner, K. J., Argamaso, R. V., Cotton, R. T. *et al.* (1990) Standardization for the reporting of nasopharyngoscopy and multiview videofluoroscopy: a report from an international working group. *Cleft Palate J.*, **27**, 337–47.

Gosain, A. K., Conley, S. F., Marks, S. & Larson, D. L. (1996) Submucous cleft palate: Diagnostic methods and outcomes of surgical treatment. *Plast. Reconstr. Surg.*, **97**, 1497–509.

Havkin, N., Tatum, S. A., III, & Shprintzen R. J. (2000) Velopharyngeal insufficiency and articulation impairment in velocardiofacial syndrome: the influence of adenoids on phonemic development. *Int. J. Ped. Otorhinolaryngol.*, **54**, 103–10.

Hynes, W. (1967) Observations in pharyngoplasty. *Br. J. Plast. Surg.*, **20**, 244–56.

Jackson, I. T. & Silverton, J. S. (1977) The sphincter pharyngoplasty as a secondary procedure in cleft palates. *Plast. Reconstr. Surg.*, **59**, 518–24.

Kaplan, E. N. (1975). The occult submucous cleft palate. *Cleft Palate J.*, **12**, 356–68.

Kilner, T. P. (1937) Cleft lip and palate repair technique. *St. Thomas Hosp. Rep.*, **2**, 127.

Kirschner, R. E. & LaRossa, D. (2000) Cleft lip and palate. *Otolaryngol. Clin. NA*, **33**, 1191–215.

Kirschner, R. E., Wang, P., Jawad, A. F. *et al.* (1999) Cleft palate repair by modified Furlow double opposing Z-plasty: the Children's Hospital of Philadelphia experience. *Plast. Reconstr. Surg.*, **104**, 1998–2010.

Kirschner, R. E., Randall, P., Wang, P. *et al.* (2000) Cleft palate repair at 3 to 7 months of age. *Plast. Reconstr. Surg.*, **105**, 2127–32.

Kirschner, R. E., Solot, C. B., McDonald-McGinn, D. M. *et al.* (2001) Speech outcome after cleft palate repair in patients with a chromosome 22q11 deletion. Presented at the 58th Annual Meeting of the American Cleft Palate-Craniofacial Association in Minneapolis, MN.

Kriens, O. (1969) An anatomical approach to veloplasty. *Plast. Reconstr. Surg.*, **43**, 29–41.

Lipson, A. H., Yiulle, M., Angel, P. G., *et al.* (1991) Velocardiofacial (Shprintzen) syndrome: an important syndrome for the dysmorphologist to recognize. *J. Med. Genet.*, **28**, 596–604.

Lykins, C. & Sie, K. (2001) Speech surgery and velocardiofacial syndrome. Presented at the 58th Annual Meeting of the American Cleft Palate-Craniofacial Association in Minneapolis, MN.

MacKenzie-Stepner, K., Witzel, M. A., Stringer, D. A. *et al.* (1987) Abnormal carotid arteries in the velocardiofacial syndrome: a report of three cases. *Plast. Reconstr. Surg.*, **80**, 347–51.

Marsh, J., Grames, L. & Holtman, B. (1989) Intravelar veloplasty: a prospective study. *Cleft Palate J.*, **26**, 46–50.

McDonald-McGinn, D. M., Kirschner, R., Goldmuntz, E. *et al.* (1999) The Philadelphia story: The 22q11 deletion: Report on 250 patients. *Genetic Counseling*, **10**, 11–24.

McWilliams, B. J. & Philips, B. J. (1979) *Velopharyngeal Incompetence: Audio Seminars in Speech Pathology*. Philadelphia: WB Saunders.

McWilliams, B. J., Morris, H. L. & Shelton, R. L. (1990) Cleft palate speech. Philadelphia: B. C. Decker, pp. 168–206.

Millard, D. R., Jr. (1980) *Cleft Craft: The Evolution of Its Surgery. Vol. III.* Boston: Little, Brown, and Company.

Mingarelli, R., Digilio, M. C., Mari, A. *et al.* (1996) The search for hemizygosity at 22q11 in patients with isolated cleft palate. *J. Craniofac. Genet. Dev. Biol.*, **16**, 118–21.

Mitnick, R. J., Bello, J. A., Golding-Kushner, K. J. *et al.* (1996) The use of magnetic resonance angiography prior to pharyngeal flap surgery in patients with velocardiofacial syndrome. *Plast. Reconstr. Surg.*, **97**, 908–19.

Orticochea, M. (1970) Results of the dynamic muscle sphincter operation in cleft palates. *Br. J. Plast. Surg.*, **23**, 108–14.

Perkins, J. A., Sie, K. & Gray, S. (2000) Presence of 22q11 deletion in postadenoidectomy velopharyngeal insufficiency. *Arch. Otolaryngol. Head Neck Surg.*, **126**, 645–8.

Riski, J. E., Burstein, F. D., Cohen, S. R. *et al.* (2000) Cephalometric comparison of velopharyngeal dimensions in velo-cardio-facial syndrome, cleft palate, and noncleft children. Presented at the 57th annual meeting of the American Cleft Palate-Craniofacial Association in Atlanta, GA.

Ross, D. A., Witzel, M. A., Armstrong, D. C. & Thomson, H. G. (1996) Is pharyngoplasty a risk in velocardiofacial syndrome? An assessment of medially displaced carotid arteries. *Plast. Reconstr. Surg.*, **98**, 1182–90.

Ruotolo, R. A., Veitia, N., Corbin, A. *et al.* (2003) Velopharyngeal anatomy in 22q11 deletion syndrome: A three-dimensional cephalometric analysis. Presented at the 60th annual meeting of the American Cleft Palate-Craniofacial Association in Asheville, NC.

Ryan, A. K., Goodship, J. A., Wilson, D. I. *et al.* (1997) Spectrum of clinical features associated with interstitial chromosome 22q11 deletions: a European collaborative study. *J. Med. Genet.*, **34**, 798–804.

Shprintzen, R. J. (1982) Palatal and pharyngeal anomalies in craniofacial syndromes. *Birth Defects*, **28**, 53–78.

Shprintzen, R. J., Goldberg, R. B., Young, D. & Wolford, L. (1981) The velocardiofacial syndrome: a clinical and genetic analysis. *Pediatrics*, **67**, 167–72.

Shprintzen, R. J., Schwartz, R. H., Daniller, A. & Hoch, L. (1985) Morphologic significance of bifid uvula. *Pediatrics*, **75**, 553–61.

Valnicek, S. M., Zuker, R. M., Halpern, L. M. & Roy, W. L. (1994) Perioperative complications of superior pharyngeal flap surgery in children. *Plast. Reconstr. Surg.*, **93**, 954–8.

Vantrappen, G., Devriendt, K., Swillen, A. *et al.* (1999) Presenting symptoms and clinical features in 130 patients with the velo-cardio-facial syndrome. The Leuven experience. *Genet. Counsel.*, **10**, 3–9.

Veau, V. & Ruppe, C. (1922) Anatomie chirurgicale de la division palatine. Considérations opératoires. *Rev. Chir.*, **20**, 1–30.

von Langenbeck, B. (1861) Die uranoplastik mittelst ablösung des mucös-periostalen gaumenüberzuges. *Arch. Klin. Chir.*, **2**, 205–87.

Wardill, W. E. M. (1937) The technique of operation for cleft palate. *Br. J. Surg.*, **25**, 117–30.

Williams, M. A., Shprintzen, R. J. & Rakoff, S. J. (1987) Adenoid hypoplasia in the velo-cardio-facial syndrome. *J. Craniofac. Genet. Dev. Biol.*, **7**, 23–6.

Witt, P., Cohen, D., Grames, L. M. & Marsh, J. (1999) Sphincter pharyngoplasty for the surgical management of speech dysfunction associated with velocardiofacial syndrome. *Br. J. Plast. Surg.*, **52**, 613–18.

Zori, R. T., Boyar, F. Z., Williams, W. N. *et al.* (1998) Prevalence of 22q11 region deletions in patients with velopharyngeal insufficiency. *Am. J. Med. Genet.*, **77**, 8–11.

5

Nephro-urologic, gastrointestinal, and ophthalmic findings

Koen Devriendt[1], Nathalie Rommel[2] and Ingele Casteels[3]

[1] Centre for Human Genetics, University Hospital Leuven, Belgium
[2] Centre for Paediatric and Adolescent Gastroenterology, Women's and Children's Hospital, Adelaide, Australia
[3] Department of Ophthalmology, University Hospital Leuven, Belgium

Besides major manifestations such as cardiac defects, ENT-anomalies, and learning difficulties, individuals with a deletion of chromosome 22q11 may present with a large variety of other anomalies. Some of these are probably coincidental, for instance a cleft lip, whereas other malformations are most likely related to the underlying chromosomal aberration, e.g., renal agenesis or anal anomalies. Clinical care for children with multiple congenital anomalies and developmental problems require a personalized approach. Detailed lists of all possible associated anomalies may provoke a blind screening for any potentially hidden disorder. Besides causing an unnecessary financial and physical burden for the child and his family, this often leads to the detection of clinically harmless findings which will cause additional unnecessary anxiety. Examples include the finding of enlarged thrombocytes, or certain structural brain anomalies. As an alternative, it is more appropriate to concentrate on the diagnosis and treatment of clinically important issues, and these will differ from one child to the other, and may vary with age. The best way to provide optimal care is within a multidisciplinary team, where the diagnostic procedures, therapy, and follow-up for each problem are guided by the global needs of the child.

Three systems frequently involved in VCFS are the nephro-urologic and the gastrointestinal systems and the eyes. We will discuss the different manifestations, their pathogenesis and evaluate possible options for diagnosis, treatment and follow-up.

Nephro-urological anomalies in VCFS

Nephro-urological malformations such as vesico-ureteric reflux, renal agenesis, multicystic renal dysplasia (see Table 5.1) are common congenital malformations associated with VCFS. In different studies, their incidence ranged from 10–60%. For instance, Lipson *et al.* (1991) found VUR in 4/38 VCFS patients. Other studies

Velo-Cardial-Facial Syndrome: A Model for Understanding Microdeletion Disorders, ed. Kieran C. Murphy and Peter J. Scambler. Published by Cambridge University Press. © Cambridge University Press, 2005.

Table 5.1. Urinary system manifestations of VCFS

Uropathies
  Vesico-ureteric reflux (VUR)
  Multicystic renal dysplasia
  Renal agenesis
  Renal hypoplasia
  Pelvi-ureteral junction obstruction (PUJ)
  Vesico-ureteric junction obstruction
  Duplex kidney or ureter
  Ectopic kidney
  Horseshoe kidney

Other
  Nephrocalcinosis
  Enuresis nocturna

found an incidence of renal anomalies in 4/39 patients (Devriendt *et al.*, 1996), in 25/67 prospectively studied patients (McDonald-McGinn *et al.*, 1999), in 49/136 patients on whom renal investigations were performed (Ryan *et al.*, 1997), and in 4/13 prospectively studied patients (Stewart *et al.*, 1999). However, these high incidence figures by no means indicate that children with VCFS have a high chance of suffering from clinically significant renal disease. In many instances, these findings are coincidental, and do not cause any symptoms and may even resolve spontaneously. We will discuss the pathogenesis and clinical aspects of these anomalies, and then briefly deal with some other nephro-urological manifestations of VCFS, enuresis, and nephrocalcinosis.

Pathogenesis of congenital nephro-urological malformations

A large spectrum of uropathies are seen in individuals with VCFS, including renal agenesis, multicystic renal dysplasia, vesico-ureteral reflux, megaureter, vesico-ureteric junction obstruction, and pelvi-ureteral junction obstruction (Table 5.1). The same observation of a spectrum of malformations has been made in other syndromic causes of uropathies such as the branchio-oto-renal syndrome (caused by mutations in the EYA1 gene) and the papillo-renal syndrome (caused by mutations in the PAX2 gene). Also, in many patients with VCFS and a bilateral uropathy, contralateral uropathies of a different type are often present, as for instance the observation of unilateral renal agenesis in association with contralateral multicystic renal dysplasia (Devriendt *et al.*, 1997). This indicates that these different urological malformations have a related pathogenesis, i.e., an abnormal development of the ureteric bud (Tanagho, 1976, Moerman *et al.*, 1994). Around four weeks of gestation, the ureteral bud develops as an outgrowth of the meso-nephric duct and cranially invades the metanephric blastema, made of undiffer-entiated mesenchyme. Reciprocal inductive effects between the ureter and metanephric blastema are assumed to lead to the formation of the collecting ducts and ureter from the former and nephrons from the latter. The number of genes shown to be involved in these reciprocal inductive events and subsequent differentiation is rapidly increasing (Patterson & Dressler, 1994). A disruption in the programmed development of the ureteral bud can result in a spectrum of ureteral anomalies, depending on its timing and site (Tanagho, 1976). Some of the genes involved in ureteral bud development, such as the *PAX2* gene, are also expressed in the early stages of metanephric blastema development, and this may explain why renal dysplasia and renal agenesis can belong to the spectrum of uropathies observed in patients with *PAX2* gene mutations (Torres *et al.*, 1995). In the commonly deleted region of 3Mb on chromosome 22q11, 25 genes have been identified to date (Baldini, 2002). Many of these genes are expressed in the developing kidney and are therefore candidate genes for the phenotype. However, large deletions or knock-out studies for genes in the deleted region have not resulted in kidney defects in mice (Baldini, 2002).

An alternative explanation for these nephro-urological malformations is a vascular origin. Robson *et al.* (1994) proposed a vascular disruption as the cause of uropathies, with the variable severity of the disorder related to the timing of the abnormal blood supply to the ureteric bud. This is not unlikely, given the recent finding that the developmental anomalies in VCFS may be related to a vascular defect (Baldini, 2002). A primary vascular malformation is also suggested by the finding that mice lacking a vascular growth factor, the 164-isoform of VEGF, display the major cardiovascular anomalies in VCFS (Stalmans *et al.*, 2002). Conversely, besides those vessels that have a neural crest component, no other vascular anomalies were noted in these mice.

The DiGeorge anomaly can have other causes than VCFS, and interestingly, two of these conditions have a high incidence of renal anomalies. Chromosomal deletions in chromosome 10p feature hypoparathyroidism, immune disturbances, cardiac defects, mental retardation, and frequently also renal anomalies and sensorineural deafness. It is now clear that part of the features are caused by haploinsufficiency of the GATA3 gene, causing the HDR syndrome (hypoparathyroidism-deafness-renal anomalies). Therefore, the DiGeorge phenotype associated with chromosome 10p deletions should be considered a true contiguous gene syndrome (Van Esch *et al.*, 2000).

Teratogenic causes such as maternal diabetes may also cause the DiGeorge anomaly without VCFS, and interestingly, this is frequently associated with renal agenesis (Wilson *et al.*, 1993; Novak & Robinson, 1994; Digilio *et al.* 1995).

Clinical manifestations of congenital uropathies

Congenital uropathies are frequent. For instance, the incidence of vesico-ureteral reflux (VUR) is estimated between 1/100 to 1/1000 (Abbott *et al.*, 1981). Typically, congenital uropathies present during the first years of life with a urinary infection and this may cause significant morbidity. Unless treated, this may result in or add to pre-existing renal damage. As a result, these congenital uropathies are a major cause of childhood hypertension (Wyszynska *et al.*, 1982) and chronic renal failure (Gusmano & Perfuma, 1993). For this reason, several authors have recommended that all individuals with VCFS undergo screening for the presence of a nephro-urological malformation at the time of diagnosis (Devriendt *et al.*, 1996; McDonald-McGinn *et al.*, 1999). In the absence of overt disease, renal ultrasound would be the preferred method. Various anomalies can reliably be detected such as renal agenesis, multicystic renal dysplasia, and hydronephrosis or hydroureter (a general term used to indicate dilated pelvis or ureter, and which can be caused by anomalies such as (severe) vesico-ureteral reflux, megaureter, vesico-ureteric junction obstruction, and pelvi-ureteral junction obstruction). Alternatively, many patients with a 22q11 deletion have a congenital heart defect, and will undergo cardiac catheterization. During this procedure, contrast medium is injected in the circulation, and therefore, renography and pyelography can easily be performed simultaneously.

Mild VUR or PUJ often remains undetected. Even though this can remain asymptomatic and frequently regresses spontaneously, urinary infections often are the first symptom. Therefore, a urinary infection should always be considered in every child with VCFS and a fever of unexplained origin.

Unilateral renal agenesis is a relatively common finding in the normal population. The prognosis is good, but there are reports showing an increased risk of developing proteinuria, hypertension, and renal failure. However, it is not clear whether this represents a true increased risk, or ascertainment bias. Nevertheless, the knowledge that a child has a solitary kidney is a factor to be taken into account in the follow-up (Robson *et al.*, 1995). In a series of 190 patients consecutively diagnosed individuals with VCFS, not a single person suffered from significant renal insufficiency (Devriendt *et al.*, unpublished data). Thus, despite their frequent occurrence in VCFS, it is clear that in most instances, these malformations do not lead to serious clinical complications and with appropriate treatment, major complications seem to be relatively rare.

Prenatal presentation of uropathies

The prenatal presentation of uropathies is a special situation. Most cases with a conotruncal heart defect that have been detected antenatally are isolated, but it may be of interest to detect those cases with VCFS. It has been suggested that besides associated findings such as pulmonary anomalies, polyhydramnios, IUGR and increased nuchal translucency (Boudjemline et al., 2002), a uropathy may be an additional prenatal sign of VCFS (Devriendt et al., 1997; Goodship et al., 1997). However, the prenatal finding of an isolated renal anomaly is not an indication for 22q11 analysis (Goodship et al., 1997).

Bilateral multicystic renal dysplasia or agenesis is not compatible with life. During fetal life, this causes an absent urine production, resulting in oligohydramnios. This will lead to a sequence of events related to a lack of intrauterine space known as the Potter sequence. These fetuses develop lung hypoplasia, the cause of death at delivery, as well as characteristic facial features. No systematic series are reported on the incidence of VCFS in the Potter sequence, except for a small series of 10 patients where no VCFS was detected (Devriendt et al., 1997). However, careful autopsy is necessary in these instances, since the diagnosis can be suspected on additional findings of VCFS such as thymus hypoplasia, cleft palate, or subtle cardiac defects.

Other renal and urological manifestations

Nephrocalcinosis is a pathological deposition of calcium in the kidney. It usually occurs in the context of a primary disorder of calcium metabolism. However, in VCFS it may occur as a complication of treatment of hypoparathyroidism with an inappropriately high dose of calcium supplements and Vitamin D. This is often reversible when diagnosed in time.

In our experience, enuresis nocturna is a frequent complaint in children with VCFS. At present, there are no systematic studies on the incidence of enuresis in children with VCFS. Given their high incidence, nephro-urological anomalies should first be excluded. However, enuresis nocturna is more common in children with developmental delay, and for this reason, it is probably related to the delayed maturation in most individuals with VCFS. Therefore, a conservative approach is indicated.

Gastrointestinal findings

Gastrointestinal manifestations rarely are the presenting sign in VCFS. In a minority of children, congenital malformations of the gastrointestinal tract are present. On the other hand, feeding difficulties are a frequent and important problem. Even though mean birth weight of a child with VCFS is approximately 1 SD below the mean (Devriendt, unpublished observations), failure to thrive is frequently observed during the first year of life (Digilio et al., 2001). Besides the medical problems such as the heart defects, swallowing and feeding difficulties probably are the main cause of this. Thus, even though only a minority of children will present a major gastrointestinal malformation, careful follow-up of feeding is indicated in all infants with the VCFS. Therefore, feeding difficulties will be discussed more extensively.

Congenital malformations of the gastrointestinal system

Congenital malformations of the gastrointestinal system in VCFS are rare, and reported anomalies include congenital anal stenosis of ectopic anus (Worthington et al., 1997), intestinal malrotation (Devriendt, unpublished observation), esophageal atresia (Digilio et al., 1999), Hirschsprung's disease (Kerstjens-Frederikse et al., 1999) and jejunal atresie (Yamanaka et al., 2000).

In our series, anal malformations were observed in 3/190 individuals with VCFS (1.5%) which is much higher than the incidence of 1/5000 in the control population. For the other manifestations, it is not clear whether these anomalies are etiologically related to VCFS or purely coincidental. Hirschsprung's disease is a neurocristopathy, caused by an abnormal migration of vagal neural crest in the hindgut. Since many features in VCFS also are related to abnormalities in the neural crest, it is thought that the reported association of both conditions was not coincidental (Kerstjens-Frederikse et al., 1999). Severe Hirschsprung's disease manifests at birth with failure to pass meconium, but milder cases will only be diagnosed at an older age during an exploration for severe constipation. Constipation is very frequent in VCFS and may last for several years before it resolves (Swillen et al., 1997). The exact cause of the constipation in VCFS is not known, and probably has a multifactorial origin, including factors such as hypotonia. In addition, it is also possible that VCFS individuals have subtle defects in gut innervation and motility and further studies are required to address this.

Feeding and swallowing difficulties

Normal swallowing is usually divided into oral-preparatory, oral, pharyngeal, and esophageal phases (Logemann, 1983). The entire duration of a swallow sequence is about 1.0–1.5 seconds in children (Arvedson & Lefton-Greif, 1998). Children with VCFS are particularly at risk of developing feeding and swallowing problems at a young age (Rommel et al., 1999). This section will describe normal feeding and swallowing development as it relates to the feeding pathology seen in infants and children with VCFS.

Oral preparatory phase

Normal development

The infant's preparatory activities of rooting for a nipple and latching on can be considered as part of the oral preparatory phase. Once infants achieve an effective suck and swallow sequence there is no true oral preparatory phase, since sucking becomes synonymous with the oral phase. As children begin to handle thicker textures, the oral preparatory phase may last several seconds (Arvedson & Lefton-Greif, 1998). The more chewing that is required, the longer it takes for the child to form a bolus. The bolus is modified by chewing and mixing with saliva. During this phase the soft palate is lowered, helping to prevent the bolus from entering the pharynx. This active lowering of the soft palate occurs by contraction of the palatoglossus muscle innervated by the vagus nerve. The larynx and pharynx are at rest. The airway is open and nasal breathing continuous until a swallow is initiated.

VCFS

In case a cleft palate is present, non-nutritive sucking might be compromised in the VCFS infant as positioning of the pacifier in the mouth is difficult due to the structural abnormality and because the baby can create only a limited amount of negative pressure (suction) on the pacifier as no vacuum can be formed in the oral cavity (Rommel *et al.*, 1999).

Oral phase
Normal development

The oral phase is initiated by the tongue with posterior propulsion of the food bolus and ends with deglutition. The onset is voluntary whereas the final stages are involuntary. Infants initiate the oral phase as they begin antero-posterior tongue action with a suckle pattern on the nipple. This is accomplished by a rolling or peristaltic motion of the tongue against the palate. Older children elevate the tongue tip against the maxillary alveolar ridge or the superior incisors. The anterior 1/3 to 2/3 of the tongue forms a depression to contain a semisolid or liquid bolus (Logemann, 1993). As the bolus enters the pharynx, the soft palate contracts, elevates, and comes into contact with the posterior pharyngeal wall. This forms a seal between the chambers of the naso- and oro-pharynx to prevent nasal regurgitation. Palatal motion is accomplished by contraction of the levator veli palatini, tensor veli palatini, and palatopharyngeus muscle. A strong seal at this level helps maintain the propulsive forces necessary to transport the bolus through the hypopharynx, UES (upper esophageal sphincter) and into the esophagus (Tuchman, 1994). In adults, the oral phase lasts about 0.7 s and does not vary with texture (Dodds *et al.*, 1990). In infants, the mean oral transit time is 0.88 s (range 0.26–4.67 s) (Newman *et al.*, 1991).

VCFS

Feeding problems in VCFS are mainly related to this phase of swallowing. The triad 'velo-cardio-facial' expresses the different areas of feeding compromise. Velo: it is well known that oral-facial anomalies such as cleft lip and/or palate interfere with infant feeding. The child with VCFS is specifically at risk as in 10% of these children a cleft is present (Vantrappen *et al.*, 2002). Depending on the type and severity of cleft, including a submucous cleft, breast or bottle feeding needs to be considered. In the case of the absence of a cleft, a velopharyngeal disorder may still be present. Inadequate functioning of the soft palate may be due to insufficient elevation of the velum or the soft palate itself might be too short in order to close off the velopharyngeal cavity during deglutition. This functional or anatomical problem may lead to nasal regurgitation of liquids and insufficient suction during sucking. Poor suction results in limited expression of milk out of the breast or bottle. Cardio: children with congenital heart disease may be easily fatigued and may tire before taking sufficient volume. Depending on the severity of the cardiac lesion and the age of the baby, such an infant may not arouse spontaneously to feed. Since the baseline heart rate may be fast the infant may have limited capacity to increase the heart rate to respond to the energy demands required for feeding. While the baby may be able to respond in the short term, the baby may fatigue quickly and oral intake is insufficient. With decreased energy levels and decreased delivery of oxygen for work, the baby may have inadequate strength to produce an effective suck; the suck may be weak although tongue, lip, and jaw movements are appropriate. Sucking bursts may be short, with longer than average pauses to rest and recover (Wolf & Glass, 1992). The effects of congestive heart failure may play a part in the poor appetite seen in many infants with congenital heart disease. Congestive heart failure can lead to delayed gastric emptying and gastrointestinal hypomotility, which may blunt the baby's appetite (Pittman & Cohen, 1964). Delayed gastric emptying and increases in intra-abdominal pressure from increased work of breathing can result in gastro-esophageal reflux (Wolf & Glass, 1992).

Inadequate intake is not the sole reason for growth failure in infants with congenital heart disease. The undernourished state may partially be due to increased metabolic requirements. Oxygen consumption is higher in patients with congenital heart disease. There are increased metabolic demands from the muscles of respiration and heart muscles. Therefore, decreased endurance, early satiety, and poor growth and nutritional status are causes of feeding problems in children with congenital heart disease, and more specifically those with VCFS. Facial: short upper lip may influence the ability to spoon feed. Taking food from the spoon requires active movement of the upper lip and sufficient range of motion. Children with VCFS present frequently with a short upper lip and therefore might be compromised in their ability to spoon feed.

Pharyngeal phase
Normal development

There are multiple sensory fields within the oropharyngeal region triggering the pharyngeal phase of swallowing. In the infant, swallow initiation occurs when the liquid bolus accumulates in the space between the soft palate and the tongue or when the bolus accumulates in the valleculae, the space between the tongue base and the epiglottis (Arvedson & Lefton-Greif, 1998).

During the pharyngeal phase, the swallow is reflexive and involves a complex sequence of coordinated motions. The pharyngeal swallow response consists of the following four movements: elevation of the soft palate to seal the nasopharynx, laryngeal displacement and laryngeal closure, UES relaxation and opening, and bolus propagation with pharyngeal clearance. Some investigators report that the true vocal folds play only an accessory role in airway protection (Ardran & Kemp, 1967; Eckberg & Hilderfors, 1985), while others indicate that their role is critical (Shin *et al.*, 1988). The function of the false vocal folds in deglutition is not clearly delineated (Arvedson & Lefton-Greif, 1998).

As the glottis and the cricopharyngeus muscle are intimately related with the cricoid cartilage, movement of the larynx in this direction aids opening the UES by traction. In addition, an obliteration of the laryngeal vestibule occurs as the larynx is positioned caudal from the tongue base and a downward tilt of the epiglottis over the laryngeal complex occurs which deflects the bolus laterally and posteriorly towards the UES. The epiglottis is found to be most inverted when the tongue base makes contact with the pharyngeal wall (Logemann *et al.*, 1992). The epiglottis plays an active role although is not essential for glottic closure or for prevention of aspiration in at least some subjects, as demonstrated in a child with congenital absence of the epiglottis (Reyes *et al.*, 1994).

The bolus is propagated by the tongue (Kahrilas *et al.*, 1993) and pharyngeal clearance occurs by contraction of pharyngeal constrictors and elevators (Kahrilas, 1992). Competent pharyngeal phase function results in the simultaneous transport of the bolus into the esophagus and airway protection. Newman *et al.* (1991) studied sucking and oral and pharyngeal transit times in 21 infants referred with feeding problems ranging in age from 3–170 days (mean age = 50 days, SD = 40.3 days). The mean pharyngeal transit time reported is 0.60 ± 0.10 s (range 0.46–0.89 s) and mean sucks per swallow are 1.74 ± 1.45 (range = 1.00 to 7.8).

VCFS

No specific data on the pharyngeal phase of swallowing are available in children with VCFS. From our observations, we believe that silent aspiration as well as the coordination between suck-swallow and breath are two major problems in VCFS. Silent aspiration is defined as aspiration of the bolus below the true vocal folds without triggering a protective cough reflex. In infant feeding, sucking, swallowing and breathing needs to be well coordinated as it is essential for oral intake as well as for prevention of aspiration. Deglutition of a wet bolus always has an interruption of the airflow of 1 s (Wilson *et al.*, 1980) as well as a dry swallow following after sucking (Weber *et al.*, 1986). These findings have led to the view that sucking, swallowing, and breathing must be coordinated in infant feeding (Wolf & Glass, 1992). In preterm infants sucking and respiratory patterns are still maturing. There is evidence that coordination between respiration and swallowing improves with maturation which then may be reflected in better coordination between sucking and swallowing (Shivpuri et al., 1983). These factors may contribute to the development of feeding skills of the child with VCFS.

Esophageal phase
Normal development

Normal swallowing requires the precise coordination of lingual propulsion and pharyngeal contraction with relaxation and opening of the UES (Jacob et al., 1989), described as the initiation of the esophageal phase. This final phase involves the coordinated relaxation of two sphincters, one at each end of the esophagus, and peristaltic action to propel the bolus towards the stomach (Code & Schlegel, 1986). The UES and lower esophageal sphincter are tonically closed at rest. The resting cricopharyngeal pressure protects the pharynx from reflux and the esophagus from air insufflation (Donner et al., 1985). Schechter (1990) describes the beginning of UES relaxation when the larynx is pulled forward and upward. The bolus is then carried into the esophagus by a series of contraction waves sweeping down from the pharynx. The esophageal phase promptly follows each pharyngeal phase given there is a definite time delay between each swallow. However, an immediate and complete inhibition of the esophageal phase is noted when a second pharyngeal swallow occurs while the bolus remains in the striated muscle segment of the esophagus (Vanek & Diamant, 1987). If a bolus is in the esophageal smooth muscle segment when the next swallow occurs, it will progress for several seconds before disappearing in the stomach. Depending on bolus size, the amplitude and velocity of subsequent swallows will be altered for as long as 10 seconds. A series of rapid swallows results in an inactive esophageal body and lower esophageal sphincter relaxation (Vanek & Diamant, 1987). During normal suckle feeding, when infants perform rapid consecutive swallows, peristaltic waves in the esophagus tend to summate. The esophagus remains filled and is slightly distended throughout with the undersurface of the UES well outlined. The final swallow will be followed by a solitary normal peristaltic wave that clears the esophagus (Clark, 1993).

VCFS

Achalasia of the upper esophageal sphincter (UES) in children is extremely rare, with only 12 cases reported in the literature since 1919. Patients usually present with dysphagia. We have observed a 10-month-old boy with VCFS, who was referred to our clinic because of severe feeding problems. The boy was born at term with weight 3810 g, length 52 cm, head circumference 36 cm and APGAR scores 2, 7, 10. A right pes equinovarius and art. lusoria were present which in combination with mild facial dysmorphism led to the diagnosis of VCFS. Other abnormalities included axial hypotonia, hypertelorism, retrognathia, frequent upper airway infections and recurrent pneumonias, obstructive apnea, inhalation stridor, nasal obstruction, tracheomalacia, diastasis of mm. rectus, hernia umbilicalis, and delayed motor development. Feeding observation showed minor nasal regurgitation with liquids. However, feedings of a thicker consistency were regurgitated for the most part through the nose. Despite normal oral motor and oral sensory functions, severe dysphagia was present. A 24 h pH study was normal. ENT assessment showed no submucous cleft. An upper barium failed to disclose anatomical abnormalities because of the dysphagia but videotaped modified barium swallow clearly demonstrated inefficient relaxation of the m. cricopharyngeus. Stationary pull-through manometry of the UES showed no relaxation. Because of the risk for aspiration, liquid bolus feedings were recommended in anticipation of further treatment. Based on the clinical and radiological findings, a myotomy of the upper esophageal sphincter was performed. This is the first report of UES achalasia in VCFS. Since this syndrome has only recently been delineated, reassessment of previous patients with achalasia is warranted. Severe feeding problems in combination with nasal regurgitation of semi-solids may suggest achalasia of the UES. More accurate evaluation techniques of swallowing in infants and young children with feeding problems are needed to ensure earlier diagnosis of underlying structural and functional disorders.

Developmental influence

In approximately 20–50% of infants with congenital heart disease, the heart defect occurs along with other major extracardiac malformations, a syndrome or chromosomal defect such as VCFS (Kramer *et al.*, 1987). Infants with these types of defects frequently have difficulties in multiple sensory and motor systems and may demonstrate developmental delay (Davenport, 1988). Developmental delay, if present, will impact the rate of acquisition of normal feeding skills or may influence the baby's persistence at feeding (Wolf & Glass, 1992).

Breastfeeding in VCFS

Breastfeeding is a natural biological process but is known not to be instinctive or simple in the compromised child (Naylor & Wester, 1987). Several factors can interfere with the success of breastfeeding in the child with VCFS: limited energy and endurance due to heart disease and insufficient compression (positive pressure) on the nipple influences milk expression from the breast as well as the continuation of milk supply. The possibility to create negative pressure and to maintain suction is the major underlying mechanism in the positioning of the nipple in the mouth and in latching. Specifically in those children with VCFS and a cleft, this skill might be compromised and breastfeeding insufficient.

Conclusions

To our knowledge, feeding problems in the child with VCFS are mainly temporary and seen in young infants up to one year of age. Nevertheless, some of these children may require extra nutritional support by tubefeeding in order to provide the optimal nutrients for their development. In case long-term tubefeeding is expected, transition from nasogastric to gastrostomy feeding may be indicated as this type of alternative feeding is less traumatizing for the child and its oropharyngeal cavity. At the same time an oral stimulation program needs to be started to maintain oral skills and responsivity. We believe that early diagnosis by an accurate clinical oral assessment and videofluoroscopic swallow study in case of aspiration risk will lead to more effective treatment and less secondary behavioral feeding problems in the long term.

Ophthalmic findings

Reports in literature on the incidence and type of ophthalmological findings in VCFS patients are rare. In the first report on VCFS, Shprintzen describes narrow palpebral fissures in 68% and blue suborbital coloring in 42% of his 39 patients (Shprintzen *et al.*, 1978). However, even though the narrow palpebral fissures may help in establishing a clinical diagnosis, this is of no functional significance. The suborbital coloring in some of the VCFS patients, also described in other reports, is an atypical finding thought to accompany mouth-breathing in those children.

In a retrospective study by Motzin *et al.* (1993), ophthalmological findings were diagnosed in 70% of patients with VCFS and monosomy for the chromosome region 22q11. In a review of ocular findings in 22 patients with VCFS by Mansour *et al.* (1987), frequent ocular findings include moderate to severe retinal vascular tortuosity (36%), posterior embryotoxon, narrow palpebral fissures, and small optic discs. Refractive errors were present in 59% of the patients, particularly hypermetropia and astigmatism. In isolated cases iris nodules, prominent corneal nerves, cataract and strabismus were diagnosed. Visual acuity in this patient group was good, usually between 20/20 and 20/30.

Tortuosity of the retinal vessels affecting the large and medium sized arterial and venous circulation is a common finding and is present in about 30% of patients with VCFS (Fitch, 1983, Beemer *et al.*, 1986) (Figure 5.1). However, tortuosity of retinal vessels has been described in many other genetic and acquired disorders. To establish the association of a given syndrome or disorder with retinal vascular tortuosity, several acquired etiologies need to be excluded: anemia, premature birth, hypoxia from cyanotic heart disease, hypermetropia, and hyperviscosity states. In VCFS, tortuosity does not correlate with those known etiologies, suggesting a primary association. Therefore, this reflects a primary developmental defect of these vessels. There is evidence that neural crest cells contribute to the

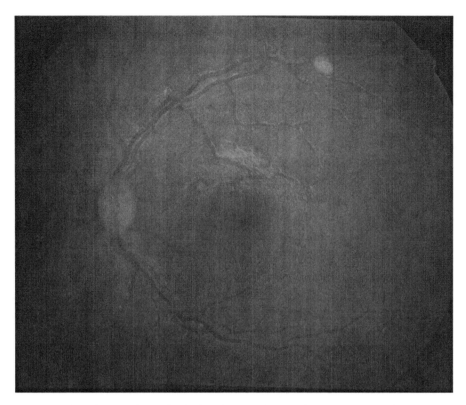

Figure 5.1   Fundus of the right eye of an individual with VCFS, showing the tortuous retinal vessels. See color plate.

phenotype, and for this reason, it is of interest that the periendothelial cells of the retinal vessels are also derived from the cranial neural crest cells (Etchevers *et al.*, 2001). A primary vascular malformation is also suggested by the finding that these vascular anomalies are also seen in a recently described animal model of the DiGeorge syndrome; i.e. mice lacking the VEGF-164 isoform (Stalmans *et al.*, 2002).

Iris and chorioretinal coloboma are not a typical finding in VCFS but were described in two patients. The child reported by Devriendt and colleagues had an iris coloboma but had characteristics of both the VCFS and the CHARGE association (Devriendt *et al.*, 1998). Another neonate with VCFS reported by Digilio *et al.* (1997) had bilateral chorioretinal coloboma.

In VCFS learning disability is reported in virtually 100% of cases, although IQ is often normal (Shprintzen *et al.*, 1978). Typically, verbal skills are better preserved than nonverbal skills; in particular spatial abilities are weaker compared with verbal capacities (see Chapter 8). In a prospective study it was shown that children with the 22q11.2 deletion syndrome displayed a selective deficit in visual-spatial memory which is mirrored by deficits in arithmetic and general visuo-spatial cognition. Further, a dissociation between visuo-spatial and object memory was observed. The authors suggest that this region of chromosome 22q11 may harbor a gene or genes relevant to the etiology of nonverbal learning deficits (Bearden *et al.*, 1999; Swillen *et al.*, 1999). An abnormal visual function may contribute to the poor visuo-spatial performance in VCFS patients. It is surprising that to date, there are only a few studies on the systematic assessment of the visual function in this patient population. Visual function in VCFS was evaluated by Kok *et al.* (1996) using conventional clinical binocular tests and analysis of the visually evoked potential, to understand possible influences on learning and reading difficulties within this patient population. VCFS subjects seemed to have deficiencies in the ocular and central nervous system components of their visual function. The authors describe hyperoptic refractive errors in the great majority of the patients studied; astigmatism was seen in the older patient group. They suggest that the weakness in accommodation and convergence may be a further expression of the hypotonia of much of the body musculature which characterizes this syndrome (Kok *et al.*, 1996). Poor accommodation and convergence in comparison with control data and mild to moderate hypermetropia was also described by Abel & O'Leary (1997) in their study of 10 children with VCFS. Correction of refractive errors can help the child's reading performance, whatever other problem they have (Abel & O'Leary 1997; Crewther *et al.*, 1998).

Brain abnormalities in VCFS were diagnosed with magnetic resonance imaging of the brain in nine of eleven consecutively referred patients with the VCFS, cerebellar lesions being the most frequently diagnosed. Unfortunately, in this study no mention was made of the ocular findings, including visual acuity, fundus appearance, ocular motility, and refractive errors (Mitnick *et al.*, 1994).

In conclusion, despite the frequent finding of various ophthalmological manifestations in velo-cardio-facial syndrome, serious ocular involvement is uncommon. It is clear that further research is needed to evaluate the frequency of visual impairment in patients with the VCFS. Every patient with the VCFS should be examined ophthalmologically at an early age to detect refractive errors, amblyopia, and eye motility abnormalities. Treatment and follow-up at regular intervals is necessary. A prospective study of the ophthalmological together with the brain MRI findings will give us a better insight in the underlying causes of the visual-spatial problems these individuals frequently experience.

Acknowledgements

We thank the other members of the multidisciplinary VCFS team at the University Hospital Leuven for helpful discussions (Benedicte Eyskens, Marc Gewillig, Mia

Laeremans, Marleen Peeters, Ann Swillen, Vincent Vanderpoorten, and Annick Vogels).

REFERENCES

Abbott, G. D., Taylor, B. & Maling, T. M. J. (1981) Incidence of vesicoureteral reflux in infants with sterile urine. *Br. J. Urol.*, **53**, 73.

Abel, H. P. & O'Leary, D. J. (1997) Optometric findings in velocardiofacial syndrome. *Optom. Vis. Sci.*, **74**, 1007–10.

Ardran, G. & Kemp, F. (1967) The mechanism of the larynx. II. The epiglottis and closure of the larynx. *Br. J. Radiol.*, **40**, 372–89.

Arvedson, J. & Lefton-Greif, M. (1998) Anatomy, physiology and development of deglutition. In Arvedson, J. & Lefton-Greif, M., eds., *Pediatric Videofluoroscopic Swallow Studies* TX: Communication Skill Builders, San Antonio, pp. 13–37.

Baldini, A. (2002) DiGeorge syndrome: the use of model organisms to dissect complex genetics. *Hum. Mol. Genet.*, **11**, 2363–9.

Bearden, C. E., Woodin, M. F., Wang, P. P. *et al.* (1999) The neurocognitive phenotype of the 22q11.2 deletion syndrome: selective deficit in visual-spatial memory. *Neuropsychol. Dev. Cogn. Sect. C. Child. Neuropsychol.*, **5**, 230–41.

Beemer, F. A., de Nef, J. J. E. M., Delleman, J. W., Bleeker-Wagemakers, M. D. & Shprintzen, R. J. (1986) Letter to the Editor: Additional eye findings in a case of velo-cardio-facial syndrome. *Am. J. Med. Genet.*, **24**, 541–2.

Boudjemline, Y., Fermont, L., Le Bidois, J., Villain, E., Sidi, D. & Bonnet, D. (2002) Can we predict 22q11 status of fetuses with tetralogy of Fallot? *Prenat. Diagn.*, **22**, 231–4.

Clark, J. (1993) Anatomy and physiology of the esophagus. In Wyllie, R. & Hyams, J., eds., *Pediatric Gastrointestinal Disease: Pathophysiology, Diagnosis, Management* Philadelphia, WB Saunders. pp. 311–17.

Code, J. & Schlegel, J. (1986) Motor action of the esophagus and its sphincters. In Code, C., ed., *Handbook of Physiology: Alimentary Canal* Washington, DC: American Physiology Society, 1821–39.

Crewther, S. G., Kiely, P. M., Kok, L. L. & Crewter, D. P. (1998) Anomalies of genetic development as predictors of oculo-cardio-facial syndrome. *Optom. Vis. Sci.*, **75**, 749–57.

Davenport, S. (1988) Multiple congenital anomalies: an approach to management. *Pediatrician*, **15**, 37–44.

Devriendt, K., Swillen, A., Proesmans, W., Gewillig, M. & Fryns, J. P. (1996) Renal and urological tract malformations caused by a 22q11 deletion. *J. Med. Genet.*, **33**, 349.

Devriendt, K., Moerman, Ph., Van Schoubroeck, D., Vandenberghe, K. & Fryns, J. P. (1997) Chromosome 22q11 deletion presenting as the Potter sequence. *J. Med. Genet.*, **34**, 423–5.

Devriendt, K., Swillen, A. & Fryns, J. P. (1998) Deletion in chromosome 22q11 in a child with CHARGE association. *Clin. Genet.*, **53**, 408–10.

Digilio, M. C., Marino, B., Formigari, R. & Giannotti, A. (1995) Maternal diabetes causing DiGeorge anomaly and renal agenesis. *Am. J. Med. Genet.*, **55**, 513–14.

Digilio, M. C., Giannotti, A., Marino, B., Guadagni, A. M., Orzalesi, M. & Dallapiccola, B. (1997) Radial aplasia and chromosome 22q11 deletion. *J. Med. Genet.*, **34**, 942–4.

Digilio, M. C., Marino, B., Bagolan, P., Giannotti, A. & Dallapiccola, B. (1999) Microdeletion 22q11 and oesophageal atresia. *J. Med. Genet.*, **36**, 137–9.

Digilio, M. C., Marino, B., Cappa, M., Cambiaso, P., Giannotti, A. & Dallapiccola, B. (2001) Auxological evaluation in patients with DiGeorge/velocardiofacial syndrome (deletion 22q11.2 syndrome). *Genet. Med.*, **3**, 30–3.

Dodds, W., Stewart, E. & Logemann, J. (1990) Physiology and radiology of the normal oral and pharyngeal phases of swallowing. *Am. J. Roentgenol.*, **154**, 953–63.

Donner, M., Bosma, J. & Robertson, D. (1985) Anatomy and physiology of the pharynx. *Gastroint. Radiol.*, **10**, 196–212.

Eckberg, O. & Hilderfors, H. (1985) Defective closure of the laryngeal vestibule. *Am. J. Radiol.*, **145**, 1159–64.

Etchevers, H. C., Vincent, C., Le Douarin, N. M. & Couly, G. F. (2001) The cephalic neural crest provides pericytes and smooth muscle cells to all blood vessels of the face and forebrain. *Development*, **128**, 1059–68.

Fitch, N. (1983) Letter to the Editor: Velo-cardio-facial syndrome and eye abnormality. *Am. J. Med. Genet.*, **15**, 669.

Jacob, P., Kahrilas, P., Logemann, J., Shah, V. & Ha, T. (1989) Upper esophageal sphincter opening and modulation during swallowing. *Gastroenterology*, **97**, 1469–78.

Kahrilas, P. (1992) Pharyngeal clearance during swallowing: a combined manometric and videofluoroscopic study. *Gastroenterology*, **103**, 128–36.

Kahrilas, P., Lin, S., Logemann, J., Ergun, G. & Facchini, F. (1993) Deglutitive tongue action: volume accommodation and bolus propulsion. *Gastroenterology*, **104**, 152–63.

Goodship, J., Robson, S. C., Sturgiss, S., Cross, I. E. & Wright, C. (1997) Renal abnormalities on obstetric ultrasound as a presentation of DiGeorge syndrome. *Prenat. Diagn.*, **17**, 867–70.

Gusmano, R. & Perfuma, F. (1993) Worldwide demographic aspects of chronic renal failure in children. *Kidney Int.* **43** (**Suppl. 41**), S31–5.

Kerstjens-Frederikse, W. S., Hofstra, R. M., van Essen, A. J., Meijers, J. H. & Buys, C. H. (1999) A Hirschsprung disease locus at 22q11? *J. Med. Genet.*, **36**, 221–4.

Kok, L. L., Crewther, S. G., Crewther, D. P. & Klistorner, A. (1996) Visual function in velocardiofacial syndrome. *Aust. N.Z. J. Ophthalmol.*, **24**, 53–5.

Kramer, H., Majewski, F., Trampisch, H., Rammos, S. & Bourgeois, M. (1987) Malformation patterns in children with congenital heart disease. *Am. J. Dis. Child.*, **141**, 789–95.

Lipson, A. H., Yuille, D., Angel, M., Thompson, P. G., Vandervoord, J. G. & Beckenham, E. J. (1991) Velocardiofacial (Shprintzen) syndrome: an important syndrome for the dysmorphologist to recognize. *J. Med. Genet.*, **28**, 596–604.

Logemann, J. (1983) *Manual for the Videofluorographic Study of Swallowing*. Austin, TX: Pro Ed.

Logemann, J., Kahrilas, P., Cheng, J. *et al.* (1992) Closure mechanisms of laryngeal vestibule during swallow. *Am. J. Physiol.*, **262**, G338–44.

Mansour, A. M., Goldberg, R. B., Wang, F. M. & Shprintzen, R. J. (1987) Ocular findings in the velo-cardio-facial syndrome. *J. Pediatr. Ophthalmol. Strabismus.*, **24**, 263–6.

McDonald-McGinn, D. M., Kirschner, R., Goldmuntz, E., *et al.* (1999) The Philadelphia story: the 22q11.2 deletion: report on 250 patients. *Genet. Couns.*, **10**, 11–24.

Mitnick, R. J., Bello, J. A. & Shprintzen, J. (1994). Brain anomalies in velo-cardio-facial syndrome. *Am. J. Med. Genet.*, **54**, 100–6.

Moerman, Ph., Fryns, J. P., Sastrowijoto, Sh., Vandenberghe, K. & Lauweryns, J. M. (1994) Hereditary renal adysplasia: new observations and hypotheses. *Ped. Pathol.*, **14**, 405–10.

Motzin, B., Marion, R., Goldberg, R., Shprintzen, R. & Saenger, P. (1993) Variable phenotypes in velocardiofacial syndrome with chromosomal deletion. *J. Pediatr.*, **123**, 406–10.

Naylor, A. & Wester, R. (1987) Providing professional lactation management consultation. *Clin. Perinatol.*, **14**, 33–8

Newman, L., Cleveland, R., Blickman, J., Hellman, R. & Jaramillo, D. (1991). Videofluoroscopic analysis of the infant swallow, *Invest. Radiol.*, **26**, 870–3.

Novak, R. W. & Robinson, H. B. (1994) Coincident DiGeorge anomaly and renal agenesis and its relation to maternal diabetes. *Am. J. Med. Genet.*, **50** (4), 311–12.

Patterson, L. T. & Dressler, G. R. (1994) The regulation of kidney development: new insights from an old model. *Curr. Opin. Genet. Develop.*, **4**, 696–702.

Pittman, J. & Cohen, P. (1964) The pathogenesis of cardiac cachexia. *N. Engl. J. Med.*, **271**, 403–8.

Reyes, B., Arnold, J. & Brooks, L. (1994) Congenital absence of the epiglottis and its potential role in obstructive apnea. *Int. J. Pediatr. Otorhinolaryngol.*, **30**, 223–6.

Robson, W. L., Rogers, R. C. & Leung, A. K. C (1994) Renal agenesis, multicystic renal dysplasia, and uretero-pelvic junction obstruction – a common pathogenesis? Letter to the editor. *Am. J. Med. Genet.*, **53**, 302.

Robson, W. L., Leung, A. K. & Rogers, R. C. (1995) Unilateral renal agenesis. *Adv. Pediatr.*, **42**, 575–92.

Rommel, N., Vantrappen G., Swillen A., Devriendt K., Feenstra L. & Fryns, J. P. (1999) Retrospective analysis of feeding and speech disorders in 50 patients with VCFS. *Genet. Couns.*, **10**, 71–8.

Ryan, A. K., Goodship, J. A., Wilson, D. I. *et al.* (1997). Spectrum of clinical features associated with interstitial chromosome 22q11 deletions: a European collaborative study. *J. Med. Genet.*, **34**, 798–804.

Schechter, G. (1990) Physiology of the mouth, pharynx and esophagus. In Bluestone, C., Stool, S. & Scheetz, M., eds., *Pediatric Otolaryngology*, Vol. 2 Philadelphia, PA: WB Saunders, pp. 816–22.

Shin, T., Maeyama, T. & Morikawa, I. (1988) Laryngeal reflex mechanisms during deglutition: observation of subglottal pressure and afferent discharge. *Otolaryng. Head Neck*, **99**, 465–71.

Shivpuri, C., Martin, R., Carlo, W. & Fanaroff, A. (1983) Decreased ventilation in preterm infants during oral feeding. *J. Pediatr.*, **103**, 285–9.

Shprintzen, R. J., Goldberg, R. B., Lewin, M. L. *et al.* (1978) A new syndrome involving cleft palate, cardiac anomalies, typical facies, and learning disabilities: velo-cardio-facial syndrome. *Cleft Palate J.*, **15**, 56–62.

Stalmans, I., Ng, Y. S., Rohan, R. *et al.* (2002) Arteriolar and venular patterning in retinas of mice selectively expressing VEGF isoforms. *J. Clin. Invest.*, **109**, 327–36.

Stewart, T. L., Irons, M. B., Cowan, J. M. & Bianchi, D. W. (1999) Increased incidence of renal anomalies in patients with chromosome 22q11 microdeletion. *Teratology*, **59**, 20–2.

Swillen, A., Devriendt, K., Legius, E. *et al.* (1997) Intelligence and psychosocial adjustment in velocardiofacial syndrome: a study of 37 children and adolescents with VCFS. *J. Med. Genet.*, **34**, 453–8.

Swillen, A., Vandeputte, L., Cracco, J. *et al.* (1999) Neuropsychological, learning and psychosocial profile of primary school aged children with the velo-cardio-facial syndrome (22q11 deletion): evidence for a nonverbal learning disability? *Neuropsychol. Dev. Cogn. Sect. C. Child. Neuropsychol.*, **5**, 230–41.

Tanagho, E. A. (1976) Embryologic basis for lower ureteral anomalies: a hypothesis. *Urology*, **7**, 451–64.

Torres, M., Gomez-Pardo, E., Dressler, G. R. & Gruss, P. (1995) Pax2 controls multiple steps of urogenital development. *Development*, **121**, 4057–65.

Tuchman, D. (1994) Physiology of the swallowing apparatus. In Tuchman, D. & Walter, R., eds., *Disorders of Feeding and Swallowing in Infants and Children: Pathophysiology, Diagnosis and Treatment* San Diego: Singular Publishing Group.

Vanek, A. & Diamant, N. (1987) Responses of the human esophagus to paired swallows. *Gastroenterology*, **92**, 643–50.

Van Esch, P., Groenen, M. A., Nesbit S. *et al.* (2000) GATA3 haplo-insufficiency causes human HDR syndrome. *Nature*, **406**, 419–22.

Weber, F., Woolridge, M. & Baum, J. (1986) An ultrasonographic study of the organization of sucking and swallowing by newborn infants. *Dev. Med. Child Neurol.*, **28**, 19–24.

Wilson, S., Thach, B., Brouillette, R. & Abu-Osba, Y. (1980) Upper airway patency in the human infant: influence of airway pressure and posture. *J. Appl. Physiol.*, **48**, 500–4.

Wilson, T. A., Blethen, S. L., Vallone, A. *et al.* (1993) DiGeorge anomaly with renal agenesis in infants of mothers with diabetes. *Am. J. Med. Genet.*, **47**, 1078–82.

Wolf, L. & Glass, R. (1992) Special diagnostic categories. In Wolf, L. & Glass, R., eds., *Feeding and Swallowing in Infants and Children: Pathophysiology, Diagnosis and Treatment* San Diego, CH: Singular Publishing Group, pp. 297–386.

Worthington, S., Colley, A., Fagan, K., Dai, K. & Lipson, A. H. (1997) Anal anomalies: an uncommon feature of velocardiofacial (Shprintzen) syndrome? *J. Med. Genet.*, **34**, 79–82.

Wyszynska, T., Chichocka, T., Wieteska-Kimczak, A., Jobs, K. & Januszewicz, P. (1982) A single pediatric center experience with 1025 children with hypertension. *Acta Paediatr.*, **81**, 244–6.

Yamanaka, S., Tanaka, Y., Kawataki, M., Ijiri, R., Imaizumi, K. & Kurahashi, H. (2000). Chromosome 22q11 deletion complicated by dissecting pulmonary arterial aneurysm and jejunal atresia in an infant. *Arch. Pathol. Lab. Med.*, **124**, 880–2.

6

Immunodeficiency in velo-cardio-facial syndrome

Kathleen E. Sullivan

The Children's Hospital of Philadelphia, PA, USA

Overview

Velo-cardio-facial syndrome (VCFS) is one of a number of syndromes which are associated with monosomic deletions of chromosome 22q11.2 (Kelley *et al.*, 1982, Kelley *et al.*, 1993, Driscoll *et al.*, 1992). It is estimated that 80–100% of patients with the clinical features of VCFS have a chromosome 22q11.2 deletion and 90% of those with the deletion carry an identical 2.5–3 megabase deletion (Motzkin *et al.*, 1993). DiGeorge syndrome, conotruncal anomaly face syndrome, and occasional patients with Opitz GBBB, CHARGE association, and Noonan's syndrome are also associated with chromosome 22q11.2 deletions. Although the immunodeficiency was generally believed to be associated with DiGeorge syndrome, most patients with the deletion will have compromise of T-cell production regardless of their other phenotypic features. The clinical findings are generally not related to the specific genes encompassed by the breakpoints and family studies confirm that twins and siblings with the same deletion may have very discordant clinical features (Kasprzak *et al.*, 1998; Yamagishi *et al.*, 1998; Vincent *et al.*, 1999). The deletion is mediated by homologous recombination between low copy number repeats (Edelmann *et al.*, 1999) and includes several genes implicated in development. Some patients with VCFS have been identified as having monosomic deletions of chromosome 10p (Schuffenhauer *et al.*, 1998; Daw *et al.*, 1996). The more proximal region appears to mediate immunodeficiency while the distal region mediates hypocalcemia. A related disorder called hypoparathyroidism, sensorineural hearing deafness, renal anomaly syndrome (HDR) maps to this distal region and is due to heterozygous mutations/deletions of GATA3 (Van Esch *et al.*, 2000). Finally, a VCFS locus has been identified at 4q31-ter (Lin *et al.*, 1988). Patients with defects at this locus, do not appear to have significant immunodeficiency. Therefore, there is significant heterogeneity amongst patients with the classic deletion and there can be multiple etiologies for the clinical phenotype known as VCFS. The immunodeficiency is known to be associated

Velo-Cardial-Facial Syndrome: A Model for Understanding Microdeletion Disorders, ed. Kieran C. Murphy and Peter J. Scambler. Published by Cambridge University Press. © Cambridge University Press, 2005.

with the chromosome 22q11.2 deletion and the 10p deletion. Various terms have been applied to patients who carry the monosomic deletion of chromosome 22q11.2 and VCFS has been applied primarily to patients with cardiac lesions and palatal defects. The terminology which seems to be most straightforward is to use "chromosome 22q11.2 deletion syndrome" for those patients with the named deletion and to use VCFS when the etiology is not known. This review will focus on VCFS patients with the chromosome 22q11.2 deletion.

A multidisciplinary approach

Patients with VCFS are often diagnosed shortly after birth at the time the cardiac lesion is identified. Three-quarters of patients with the deletion will have a cardiac defect (Ryan et al., 1997; Goldmuntz et al., 1998; McDonald-McGinn et al., 1999). Most patients will require a multidisciplinary evaluation to define their medical, social, economic, and educational needs (Hopkin et al., 2000). The cardiac lesion is usually their most serious medical issue in the first week or two of life. Hypocalcemia is present in 17–60% patients with the deletion and is typically most serious in the immediate newborn period. These significant clinical issues, transfusions, stress, impaired nutrition, and vascular access issues often impede the assessment of the immunologic status of the patient in the first few days of life. For this reason, it is typical to recommend conservative measures for patients with VCFS. The use of CMV negative, irradiated blood products, protective isolation from potential pathogens, and protection from live viral vaccine exposure (either primary exposure or secondary) should be instituted. It is helpful to have the coordinated involvement of cardiologists, cardiothoracic surgeons, geneticists, endocrinologists, and immunologists in the immediate newborn period.

Older infants and toddlers are susceptible to recurrent infection even when their host defense is normal. Thus, it is no surprise that this age group of VCFS patients experiences the most frequent infections. The phenotypic diversity in VCFS is extraordinary and this extends to the infection pattern. Seizures, aspiration, palatal dysfunction, reflux, and immunodeficiency can all contribute to recurrent infections and cardiac disease can contribute to severity. Any one child may have multiple risk factors. Constipation and feeding problems are not often described but are extremely common and can lead to poor nutrition which further impairs cellular immunity (Eicher et al., 2000). Significant developmental delay can be independently associated with infections and may contribute to the infectious morbidity in VCFS.

In the older child, school issues are common and the physician can often provide insight into the optimal learning environment for the child; however, this seldom is affected by the presence of immunodeficiency. Very few school-age children require active management of their immunodeficiency and most have no contact or activity restrictions. Therefore, the immunodeficiency is one of the more common phenotypic features in VCFS/chromosome 22q11.2 deletion syndrome and the presence of significant immunodeficiency frequently impacts on the management of other medical issues.

Overview of the immunodeficiency

Most VCFS patients with the 22q11.2 deletion have a mild to moderate immunodeficiency. The population as a whole has relatively preserved T-cell function, as measured by in vitro proliferative assays, and normal production and function of immunoglobulins (Junker & Driscoll, 1995). Responses to immunizations are usually normal. In individual patients, both T-cell and B-cell deficits can be significant, however (Schubert & Moss, 1992; Gennery et al., 2002). The T-cell repertoire is largely intact in spite of substantial reductions in T-cell numbers, however, increasing effects on the repertoire are seen with increasing decrements in T-cell numbers (Pierdominici et al., 2000). The most commonly defined abnormality is a diminution in T-cell numbers. This is most marked in infancy and ameliorates with time. Across the entire population of patients with the deletion, the spectrum of immunodeficiency is enormous. Approximately 0.5–1.0% have a profound immunodeficiency with absent or nearly absent T-cells. Another 20–30% have normal T-cell numbers with the majority of the others having a mild to moderate defect in T-cell numbers (Figure 6.1).

Initially, the immunodeficiency was described in patients with DiGeorge syndrome and was considered to be very severe. Fungal infections were common and survival rates were low (Lischner & Huff, 1975; Conley et al., 1979). Infection caused the majority of deaths. Graft versus host disease was also described in patients with severe immunodeficiency. Subsequently, it became apparent that the majority of patients with chromosome 22q11.2 deletion have a mild to moderate immunodeficiency regardless of whether they have the clinical phenotype of DiGeorge syndrome or VCFS (Junker & Driscoll, 1995; Ryan et al., 1997; Sullivan et al., 1998). Patients often have prolonged respiratory viral infections and frequent secondary bacterial infections. Autoimmune disease is increased (see below) and there may be an increased incidence of lymphomas suggesting the immunodeficiency is medically significant. There are surprisingly few data on infections and immunodeficiency. Early case reports of patients with DiGeorge syndrome emphasized the immunodeficiency and the infectious morbidity. Case reports and small series of patients with VCFS did not note an increase in infections. When the entire population with the deletion was considered, one large European study suggested that serious infections were infrequent in this

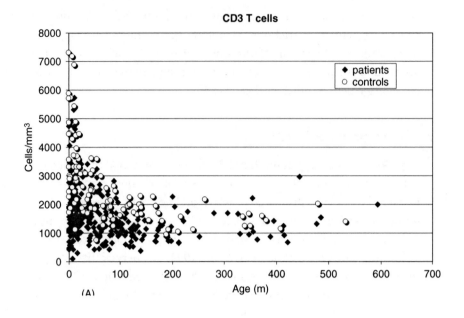

(A)

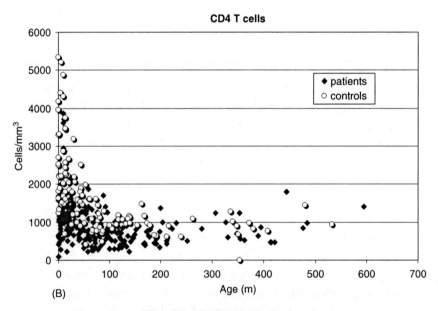

(B)

Figure 6.1   T-cell counts in patients with chromosome 22q11.2 deletion syndrome and controls. Absolute T-cell counts are displayed on the vertical axis and the age in months is displayed on the horizontal axis. (A) CD3 (total) T cells; (B) CD4 T-cell counts; (C) CD8 T-cell counts.

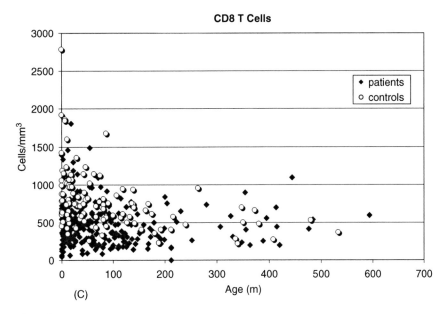

Figure 6.1 (*cont.*)

population (Ryan *et al.*, 1997). An American cohort examined 55 patients over the age of 9 years. Only 40% were considered to be as healthy as their peers with respect to infections. Seven patients had autoimmune disease, 27% had recurrent sinusitis (more than twice a year), 25% had recurrent otitis media, and 7% had recurrent bronchitis (Jawad *et al.*, 2001). Therefore, older patients continue to develop infections but they are infrequently serious.

The immunodeficiency is independent of other phenotypic features

The immunodeficiency does not correlate with any other clinical feature. This makes it difficult to determine which infants should be screened for immunodeficiency. Thymus transplantation and bone marrow transplantation are used only for the most severely affected infants, but for that minority of patients, timely diagnosis and treatment are essential.

The immunologic features in patients defined as having classic DiGeorge syndrome and patients considered to have VCFS are no different. Immunocompromise was found in 77% of patients with chromosome 22q11.2 deletions regardless of their other clinical features. There was no correlation between frequency or severity of immunocompromise and any specific clinical feature or combination of clinical features (Sullivan *et al.*, 1998). Similarly, when T-cell repertoires were examined, there were no differences in patients considered to have DiGeorge syndrome versus those with VCFS (Pierdominici *et al.*, 2000). These studies demonstrate that there is no substitution for performing the appropriate immunologic evaluations in patients with the deletion. The decision to perform an immunologic evaluation in patients with VCFS but who do not have either the 10p or 22q11.2 deletion is difficult to address. Some of these patients may have a small deletion or mutation of a single gene within the commonly deleted region. Others may have a phenocopy disorder with a completely different genetic basis. For this reason, it is difficult to assess the likelihood of immunodeficiency in these cases. The most conservative approach would be to perform simple screening studies for T-cell defects .

Natural history of the immunodeficiency

The immunodeficiency occurs as a consequence of thymic hypoplasia. The role of the thymus is to support the maturation of functional T cells. Thus, the typical defect is an impaired production of T cells. T-cell functional defects and antibody defects are seen less commonly and are usually a consequence of the T-cell production abnormality. T-cell numbers are normally highest at birth and decline rapidly in the first year and more slowly thereafter. Thus the T-cell production defect in patients is most notable in infancy when the normal production is highest. Patients with VCFS/chromosome 22q11.2 deletion exhibit some catch-up T-cell production in the first year of life and subsequently their T-cell numbers decline at a rate slightly slower than that of non-deleted children. The conse-quences of the decline over many years are not understood but could compromise host defense as patients age. Thus, there can be marked change in the first year of life and less extreme changes after the first year or two of life. Patients with the worst T-cell production improved the most in the first year of life, however, patients with absent T cells typically do not improve (Markert *et al.*, 1998; Sullivan *et al.*, 1999; Jawad *et al.*, 2001).

In contrast to T-cell defects, lymphocyte lineages which have thymic independent maturation such as B cells and natural killer cells are quantitatively preserved in VCFS/chromosome 22q11.2 deletion syndrome. In fact, B-cell numbers can often be elevated in the first 2 years of life (Jawad *et al.*, 2001). This presumably reflects impaired T-cell regulation of B cells and has been seen in murine thymectomy models. The relationship of this B-cell expansion to autoimmune disease is not known.

Parents of patients often ask about the long-term outlook, but there are few data on this topic. The continued decline of T-cell numbers could compromise responses to infection and surveillance for malignancy. With so few adults known in the literature, it is difficult to make recommendations regarding their care. It is reassuring, however, that the infections seen in patients over 9 years of age are seldom life-threatening.

Specifics of the immunodeficiency

The T-cell defect is typically characterized by quantitating the T-cell numbers in a patient. The most common problem is a diminution in T-cell numbers with preserved T-cell function, as measured by proliferative assays, and preserved antibody production and function. Mean CD3 counts from patients are 1977 ± 1106 cells/mm^3 at 0–6 months of age, 1913 ± 914 cells/mm^3 at 6 m–3 y of age, 1537 ± 650 cells/mm^3 at 3–9 years of age and 1188 ± 482 cells/mm^3 at > 9 years of age. Mean CD4 counts from patients are 1383 ± 839 cells/mm^3 at 0–6 months of age, 1333 ± 672 cells/mm^3 at 6 m–3 y of age, 953 ± 432 cells/mm^3 at 3–9 years of age and 687 ± 302 cells/mm^3 at > 9 years of age (Jawad et al., 2001). These are approximately 50% of normal in infancy and approximately 30% less than normal in the older ages. Patients with the most severe production defect may have accompanying defects in function, largely attributable to very few responding cells in the assay. Patients with significant T-cell deficiency have abnormalities in their repertoire (Collard et al., 1999; Pierdominici et al., 2000); however the relationship of repertoire defects with infection is still theoretical.

In contrast to the diminished T-cell numbers in patients with the deletion, B-cell numbers and natural killer cell numbers are often increased. Both the fraction and the absolute number are often increased (Muller et al., 1988, 1989). Antibody production and avidity is usually normal (Junker & Driscoll, 1995). Older patients often have elevated levels of immunoglobulins. A minority of patients have humoral deficits and these may be secondary to the T-cell defects. IgA deficiency may be seen in 2–10% of patients with the deletion (Smith et al., 1998) and it may be more common in patients with autoimmune disease (Davies et al., 2001).

Consequences of the immunodeficiency

Autoimmune thyroiditis, juvenile rheumatoid arthritis, idiopathic thrombocytopenia purpura, aplastic anemia, and hemolytic anemia have been described in the literature (Ham Pong et al., 1985; Tuvia et al., 1988; Pinchas-Hamiel et al., 1994; DiPiero et al., 1997; Sullivan et al., 1997). One series found 10% of patients with the deletion had autoimmune cytopenias and these occurred in patients with the most disordered T-cell function (Duke et al., 2000). Another study found that 9% of all patients had autoimmune disease and 13% of the patients over the age of nine had autoimmune disease. This suggested that the frequency of autoimmune disease may rise with age (Jawad et al., 2001). Juvenile rheumatoid arthritis is seen 20 times more frequently than in the general population and idiopathic thrombocytopenia purpura is seen 200 times more frequently than in the general population. Thus, autoimmune disease is significantly associated with chromosome 22q11.2 deletion syndrome. Another predicted consequence of T-cell compromise is an increased frequency of malignancy. This has not been observed in large cohorts although the populations under study were relatively young. It is possible that as the population ages, malignancies will become more apparent. The two most important clinical consequences of the immunodeficiency are autoimmune disease and infections. While the infections and autoimmune disease are seldom life-threatening, they contribute significantly to the morbidity in VCFS/chromosome 22q11.2 deletion syndrome. Fortunately, recent mortality rates are only approximately 5–8% and deaths are infrequently due to infection (Ryan et al., 1997; McDonald-McGinn et al., 1999).

Management

Infants suspected of having VCFS/chromosome 22q11.2 deletion syndrome should have FISH analyses performed. The 22q11.2 deletion and the 10p deletion should be sought and can be tested simultaneously (Berend et al., 2000). When the diagnosis is uncertain, most centers would treat conservatively with isolation, withholding vaccines, and the use of CMV negative, irradiated blood products. If the patient has a normal lymphocyte count, it may be possible to liberalize these precautions. The lymphocyte count is a useful indicator of T-cell numbers because the majority of lymphocytes are T cells. In infancy, a lymphocyte count should be at least 2800 cells/mm^3. Computerized tomography scans or echocardiography can be used to determine whether a normal anatomical thymus is present, although absence of a thymus does not predict immunodeficiency (Moran et al., 1999). Once the diagnosis is established either on clinical grounds or on the basis of genetic studies, immunologic evaluations should be obtained. Typically, CD3$^+$, CD4$^+$, CD8$^+$, CD19$^+$, and CD3$^-$/16$^+$/56$^+$ subset analyses are obtained and lymphocyte proliferation responses to phytohemagglutinin, pokeweed mitogen, and concanavalin A are measured. If proliferative responses are less than 10% of the control or the T-cell subsets are markedly diminished (i.e., CD3 < 200 cells/mm^3), patients should be immediately started on Pneumocystis carinii prophylaxis and evaluated for a transplant. Intravenous immunoglobulin (IVIG) may also be necessary. A few patients will have a significant immunodeficiency but are not so severely affected as to require a transplant. They require careful individualized management and aggressive treatment of infections. Patients with a mild to moderate immunodeficiency may be observed with some restrictions. Parents are advised on how to minimize infectious exposures and are advised to withhold live viral vaccines initially. Respiratory Syncytial Virus (RSV) prophylaxis and influenza vaccination may be helpful, particularly in patients with cardiac disease.

If there is no evidence of immunodeficiency, parents are advised that the child should not receive live viral vaccines in the first year of life. This conservative measure is predicated on the belief that the immunologic testing performed shortly after birth is limited and may not reflect subsequent function. Thus, patients should be reevaluated at 1 year of age because there can be substantial changes in the first year of life. If a complete humoral and T-cell evaluation at 1 year of age is completely normal, then no further restrictions are imposed. It is important to optimize nutrition during the first year of life and to try to perform laboratory evaluations when the child has no acute illness and is in a positive nitrogen balance.

The patients with severe immunodeficiency have a high mortality unless treated with thymic transplantation or a fully matched bone marrow transplant. Serial evaluations of T-cell numbers should establish with certainty that the immuno-deficiency is not spontaneously improving and that intervention is required. Thymic transplants are performed at very few centers and require experience with organ culture. They are usually partially matched to the host. Host T cells appear in the peripheral blood as early as 30 days post-transplant and T cell function typically appears at approximately 90 days post transplant (Markert *et al.*, 1997, 1999). This treatment modality can be lifesaving. When fully matched bone marrow transplants are performed, T cells appear immediately and function normalizes rapidly. Due to the absence of thymic tissue, it is not completely certain how durable these special bone marrow transplants are. Stem cell transplants are ineffective in the absence of thymic tissue.

Management of the immunodeficiency often impacts on the other clinical issues. The use of CMV negative, irradiated blood is recommended for patients undergoing surgery with known or suspected significant immunodeficiency. This is not always possible, but it is the only strategy to prevent the rare but potentially fatal complications of graft versus host disease or bloodborne CMV infection.

It is becoming increasingly common for patients to be recognized with delayed or atypical presentations. When patients are seen after the first year of life, the laboratory studies need to be individualized. For example, a healthy 15-year-old probably needs only education about the syndrome. A young school-age child with recurrent infections, should have lymphocyte subset analyses, proliferative studies (which may include recall antigen responses after the first year of life), and measures of antibody production.

Humoral immunity should be assessed in patients with recurrent infections. Although chromosome 22q11.2 deletion syndrome is classically considered a T-cell defect, there may be secondary antibody deficits (Smith *et al.*, 1998; Duke *et al.*, 2000; Davies *et al.*, 2001; Gennery *et al.*, 2002). IgA deficiency (2–10%) and delayed production of IgG (5%) seem to be most common. Few patients require IVIG to replace immunoglobulin and IVIG is contraindicated for patients with isolated IgA deficiency. Interventions for patients with a mild to moderate T-cell immunodeficiency include vaccination, prophylactic antibiotics and other measures that one would typically use for other moderately immunocompromised patients. Live viral vaccines may be withheld for safety and nonimmune patients exposed to varicella treated with either VZIg or acyclovir.

Summary

Immunodeficiency is one of the more common manifestations of VCFS, although it infrequently causes death. Prolonged viral infections are common, and older patients may have recurrent sinusitis and recurrent bronchitis. Autoimmune disease occurs in a significant subset. For patients with serious immunodeficiency, thymic transplantation or fully matched bone marrow transplantation are required.

REFERENCES

Berend, S. A., Spikes, A. S., Kashak, C. D. *et al.* (2000) Dual-probe fluorescence in situ hybridization assay for detecting deletions associated with VCFS/DiGeorge syndrome I and DiGeorge syndrome II loci. *Am. J. Med. Genet.*, **91**, 313–17.

Collard, H. R., Boeck, A., McLaughlin, T. M. *et al.* (1999) Possible extrathymic development of nonfunctional T cells in a patient with complete DiGeorge syndrome. *Clin. Immunol.*, **91**, 156–62.

Conley, M. E., Beckwith, J. B., Mancer, J. F. & Tenckhoff (1979) The spectrum of the DiGeorge syndrome. *J. Pediatr.*, **94**, 883–90.

Davies, K., Stiehm, E. R., Woo, P. & Murray, K. J. (2001) Juvenile idiopathic polyarticular arthritis and IgA deficiency in the 22q11 deletion syndrome. *J. Rheumatol.*, **28**, 2326–34.

Daw, S. C. M., Taylor, C., Kraman, M. *et al.* (1996) A common region of 10p deleted in DiGeorge and velocardiofacial syndromes. *Nat. Genet.*, **13**, 458–60.

DiPiero, A. D., Lourie, E. M., Berman, B. W., Robin, N. H., Zinn, A. B. & Hostoffer, R. W. (1997) Recurrent immune cytopenias in two patients with DiGeorge/velocardiofacial syndrome. *J. Pediatr.*, **131**, 484–6.

Driscoll, D. A., Budarf, M. L. & Emanuel, B. S. (1992) A genetic etiology for DiGeorge syndrome: consistent deletions and microdeletions of 22q11. *Am. J. Hum Genet.*, **50**, 924–33.

Duke, S. G., McGuirt, W. F., Jr. Jewett, T. & Fasano, M. B. (2000) Velocardiofacial syndrome: incidence of immune cytopenias. *Arch. Otolaryn. Head Neck Surg.*, **126**, 1141–5.

Edelmann, L., Pandita, R. K. & Morrow, B. E. (1999) Low-copy repeats mediate the common 3-Mb deletion in patients with velo-cardio-facial syndrome. *Am. J. Hum. Genet.*, **64**, 1076–86.

Eicher, P. S., McDonald-McGinn, D. M., Fox, C. A., Driscoll, D. A., Emanuel, B. S. & Zackai, E. H. *et al.* (2000) Dysphagia in children with a 22q11.2 deletion: unusual pattern found on modified barium swallow. *J. Pediatr.*, **137**, 158–64.

Gennery, A. R., Barge, D., O'Sullivan, J. J., Flood, T. J., Abinun, M. & Cant, A. J. *et al.* (2002) Antibody deficiency and autoimmunity in 22q11.2 deletion syndrome. *Arch. Dis. Child.*, **86**, 422–5.

Goldmuntz, E., Clark, B. J., Mitchell, L. E. *et al.* (1998) Frequency of 22q11 deletions in patients with conotruncal defects. *J. Am. Coll. Cardiol.*, **32**, 492–8.

Ham Pong, A. J., Cavallo, A., Holman, G. H., & Goldman, A. S. (1985) DiGeorge syndrome: long term survival complicated by Graves disease. *J. Pediatr.*, **106**, 619–20.

Hopkin, R. J., Schorry, E. K., Bofinger, M. & Saal, H. M. (2000) Increased need for medical interventions in infants with velocardiofacial (deletion 22q11) syndrome. *J. Pediatr.*, **137**, 247–9.

Jawad, A. F., McDonald-McGinn, D. M., Zackai, E. & Sullivan, K. E. (2001) Immunologic features of chromosome 22q11.2 deletion syndrome (DiGeorge syndrome/velocardiofacial syndrome). *J. Pediatr.*, **139**, 715–23.

Junker, A. K. & Driscoll, D. A. (1995) Humoral immunity in DiGeorge syndrome. *J. Pediatr.*, **127**, 231–7.

Kasprzak, L., Der Kabustian, V. M., Elliott, A. M., Shevell, M., Lejtenyi, C. & Eydoux, P., (1998) Deletion of 22q11 in two brothers with different phenotype. *Am. J. Med. Genet.*, **75**, 288–91.

Kelley, D., Goldberg, R., Wilson, D. *et al.* (1993) Confirmation that the velo-cardiofacial syndrome is associated with haplo-insufficiency of genes at chromosome 22. *Am. J. Med. Genet.*, **45**, 308–12.

Kelley, R. I., Zackai, E. H., Emanuel, B. S., Kistenmacher, M., Greenberg, F. & Punnett, H. H. (1982) The association of the DiGeorge anomalad with partial monosomy of chromosome 22. *J. Pediatr.*, **101**, 197–200.

Lin, A. E., Gavver, K. L., Diggans, G. *et al.* (1988) Interstitial and terminal deletions of the long arm of chromosome 4: further delineation of phenotypes. *Am. J. Med. Genet.*, **31**, 533–48.

Lischner, H. W. & Huff, D. S. (1975) T-cell deficiency in DiGeorge syndrome. *Birth Defects: Orig. Art. Ser.*, **11**, 16–21.

Markert, M. L., Kostyu, D. D., Ward, F. E. *et al.* (1997) Successful formation of a chimeric human thymus allograft following transplantation of cultured postnatal human thymus. *J. Immunol.*, **158**, 998–1005.

Markert, M. L., Hummell, D. S., Rosenblatt, H. M. *et al.* (1998) Complete DiGeorge syndrome: persistence of profound immunodeficiency. *J. Pediatr.*, **132**, 15–21.

Markert, M. L., Boeck, A., Hale, L. P. *et al.* (1999) Transplantation of thymus tissue in complete DiGeorge syndrome. *N. Engl. J. Med.*, **341**, 1180–9.

McDonald-McGinn, D. M., Kirschner, R., Goldmuntz, E. *et al.* (1999) The Philadelphia story: the 22q11.2 deletion: report on 250 patients. *Genet. Counsel.*, **10**, 11–24.

Moran, A. M., Colan, S. D., Mayer, J. E., Jr. & Van der Velde, M. E. (1999) Echocardiographic identification of thymic hypoplasia in tetralogy of fallot/tetralogy pulmonary atresia. *Am. J. Card.*, **84**, 1268–71.

Motzkin, B., Marion, R., Goldberg, R., Shprintzen, R. & Saenger, P. (1993) Variable phenotypes in velocardiofacial syndrome with chromosomal deletion. *J. Pediatr.*, **123**, 406–10.

Muller, W., Peter, H. H., Wilken, M. *et al.* (1988) The DiGeorge syndrome. I. Clinical evaluation and course of partial and complete forms of the syndrome. *Eur. J. Pediatr.*, **147**, 496–502.

Muller, W., Peter, H. H., Kallfelz, H. C., Franz, A. & Rieger, C. H. (1989) The DiGeorge sequence. II. Immunologic findings in partial and complete forms of the disorder. *Eur. J. Pediatr.*, **149**, 96–103.

Pierdominici, M., Marziali, M., Giovannetti, A. *et al.* (2000) T cell receptor repertoire and function in patients with DiGeorge syndrome and velocardiofacial syndrome. *Clin. Exp. Immunol.*, **121**, 127–32.

Pinchas-Hamiel, O., Engelberg, S., Mandel, M. & Passwell, J. H. (1994) Immune hemolytic anemia, thrombocytopenia and liver disease in a patient with DiGeorge syndrome. *Israel J. Med. Sci.*, **30**, 530–2.

Ryan, A. K., Goodship, J. A., Wilson, D. I., *et al.* (1997) Spectrum of clinical features associated with interstitial chromosome 22q11 deletions: a European collaborative study. *J. Med. Genet.*, **34**, 798–804.

Schubert, M. S. & Moss, R. B. (1992) Selective polysaccharide antibody deficiency in familial DiGeorge syndrome. *Ann. All.*, **69**, 231–8.

Schuffenhauer, S., Lichtner, P., Peykar-Derakhshandeh, P. *et al.* (1998) Deletion mapping on chromosome 10p and definition of a critical region for the second DiGeorge syndrome locus (DGS2). *Eur. J. Hum. Gen.*, **6**, 213–25.

Smith, C. A., Driscoll, D. A., Emanuel, B. S., McDonald-McGinn, D. M., Zackai, E. H. & Sullivan, K. E. (1998) Increased prevalence of immunoglobulin A deficiency in patients with the chromosome 22q11.2 deletion syndrome (DiGeorge syndrome/velocardiofacial syndrome). *Clin. Labor Diag. Immunol.*, **5**, 415–17.

Sullivan, K., McDonald-McGinn, D., Driscoll, D. *et al.* (1997) Juvenile rheumatoid arthritis-like polyarthritis in chromosome 22q11.2 deletion syndrome (DiGeorge anomalad/velocardio-facial syndrome/conotruncal anomaly face syndrome). *Arthritis Rheum*, **40**, 430–6.

Sullivan, K. E., Jawad, A. F., Randall, P. *et al.* (1998) Lack of correlation between impaired T-cell production, immunodeficiency and other phenotypic features in chromosome 22q11.2 deletion syndrome (DiGeorge syndrome/velocardiofacial syndrome). *Clin. Immunol. Immunopathol.*, **84**, 141–6.

Sullivan, K. E., McDonald-McGinn,D., Driscoll, D., Emanuel, B. S., Zackai, E. H. & Jawad, A. F. (1999) Longitudinal analysis of lymphocyte function and numbers in the first year of life in chromosome 22q11.2 deletion syndrome (DiGeorge syndrome/velocardiofacial syndrome). *Clin. Labor Diag. Immunol.*, **6**, 906–11.

Tuvia, J., Weisselberg, B., Shif, I. & Keren, G. (1988) Aplastic anaemia complicating adenovirus infection in DiGeorge syndrome. *Eur. J. Pediatr.*, **147**, 643–4.

Van Esch, H., Groenen, P., Nesbitt, M. A. *et al.* (2000) GATA3 haplo-insufficiency causes human HDR syndrome. *Nature*, **406**, 419–22.

Vincent, M. C., Heitz, F., Tricoire, J., *et al.* (1999) 22q11 deletion in DGS/VCFS monozygotic twins with discordant phenotypes. *Genet. Counsel.*, **10**, 43–9.

Yamagishi, H., Ishii, C., Maeda, J. *et al.* (1998) Phenotypic discordance in monozygotic twins with 22q11.2 deletion. *Am. J. Med. Genet.*, **78**, 319–21.

7

Behavioral and psychiatric disorder in velo-cardio-facial syndrome

Angela F. Stevens[1] and Kieran C. Murphy[2]

[1] Institute of Psychiatry, King's College London, UK
[2] Department of Psychiatry, Royal College of Surgeons in Ireland, Dublin, Ireland

In their earliest description of velo-cardio-facial syndrome, Shprintzen *et al.* (1978) reported "A new syndrome involving cleft palate, cardiac anomalies, typical facies and learning disabilities." Therefore, in addition to the physical abnormalities described in previous chapters, the brain is also very commonly involved in VCFS and this involvement was recognized in some of the earliest descriptions of this syndrome. In Chapter 8, Campbell and Swillen discuss how such involvement leads to characteristic cognitive profiles in VCFS while in Chapter 9, Eliez and van Amelsvoort discuss the brain structural abnormalities observed using magnetic resonance imaging in children and adults with VCFS. In this chapter, we will discuss another component of the behavioral phenotype in VCFS, namely, the high rates of behavioral and psychiatric disorder seen in VCFS children and adults.

Behavioral and psychiatric disorder in children with VCFS

There have been relatively few studies of behavioral and psychiatric disorder in children or adults with VCFS. Moreover, many are confounded by methodological constraints including lack of operational criteria for psychiatric diagnosis, sample heterogeneity (with children and adults included in the same sample), small sample size, and lack of control groups. Nevertheless, several common behavioral and temperamental features have been reported in studies of children and adolescents with VCFS. These include a stereotypic personality with poor social interaction (quantitatively and qualitatively), a bland affect with minimal facial expression and extremes of behavior, notably uninhibited and impulsive or serious and shy (Golding-Kushner *et al.*, 1985; Swillen *et al.*, 1997).

In a study of 15 children and adolescents, Papolos *et al.* (1996) reported high rates of bipolar II disorder (47%), attention deficit with hyperactivity disorder (ADHD) (27%), and attention deficit disorder without hyperactivity (13%). In addition, other studies have reported high rates of autistic spectrum disorders,

Velo-Cardial-Facial Syndrome: A Model for Understanding Microdeletion Disorders, ed. Kieran C. Murphy and Peter J. Scambler. Published by Cambridge University Press. © Cambridge University Press, 2005.

anxiety disorders, and emotional instability in VCFS children (Goldberg *et al.*, 1993; Swillen *et al.*, 1997; Niklasson *et al.*, 2001; Stevens *et al.*, 2003).

In a cross-sectional study of a cohort of 60 Flemish children and adolescents with VCFS, Swillen (1999a) found that, up to the age of 3 years, parents of such children most often reported somatic complaints (eating problems and constipation) and withdrawn behavior. From early school age to adolescence, parents and teachers most frequently reported social difficulties (problematic peer relationships), social withdrawal and attention problems with no significant gender differences. Swillen (1999b) postulated that the poor social skills and social withdrawal might at least in part be a function of the adolescents' impaired communication abilities. Allied with this is the impairment in visuo-perceptual skills, problems with new situations and their non-verbal learning disabilities (discussed in Chapter 8), all of which could contribute to this pattern of poor social interaction.

From the age of 11 years, parents also reported increased levels of anxiety and depressed mood in adolescents with VCFS. Swillen *et al.* (1999b; Swillen, 2001) have proposed that hormonal changes during puberty and increased social demands, allied with a genetic predisposition may play a role in the development of these anxieties and depressive traits in affected individuals. In order to exclude the potential confounding effects of learning disability, Swillen (2001) compared primary school children with VCFS with a group of children matched for learning disorder and speech and language impairment (children with IQ < 70 were excluded from both groups). They found that, while both groups behaved similarly with respect to problematic social interaction, poor attention and anxieties, the 22q11.2 children were more withdrawn whilst the control group were more aggressive. This suggests that VCFS children may be more likely to choose internalizing behaviors compared with children with similar developmental levels.

Conversely, a study by Feinstein *et al.* (2002) evaluated the rates and types of psychiatric disorder in children with VCFS and compared them to those found in children matched for age and cognitive ability. They reported that there were no differences in either the rate or the type of disorder found in the two groups, although both groups had greatly increased levels of psychopathology when compared with the normal population. They suggested that the explanation for this finding may be that subtle phenotypic differences in behavior found in VCFS may not be observed using standard symptom inventories.

Psychiatric disorder in adults with VCFS

Table 7.1 summarizes the principal studies of the psychiatric phenotype in VCFS individuals. As the first recognized cohort of children and adolescents with VCFS was followed up into adulthood, high rates of major psychiatric disorder were

Table 7.1. Rates of psychiatric disorder in studies of VCFS individuals

Reference	No of VCFS individuals	Age of sample (years)	Psychiatric disorder
Shprintzen *et al.* (1992)	> 90 children/ adults	Unspecified	"Chronic paranoid schizophrenia" (∼10%) (not operationally defined)
Pulver *et al.* (1994)	14 adults	17–41	Schizophrenia or schizoaffective disorder (29%)
Papolos *et al.* (1996)	15 children/ adolescents	5–16	Bipolar II disorder (47%) Attention deficit hyperactivity disorder (27%) Attention deficit disorder without hyperactivity (13%)
	10 adults	17–34	Psychosis (40%), Schizoaffective disorder (20%) Bipolar I disorder (30%), Bipolar II disorder (30%)
Murphy *et al.* (1999)	50 adults	17–52	Psychosis (30%): Schizophrenia or schizoaffective disorder (26%), Bipolar disorder (2%), Psychosis not otherwise specified (2%), Major depressive disorder (12%)

Source: From Murphy & Owen (2001).

observed. Shprintzen *et al.* (1992) suggested that more than 10% had developed psychiatric disorders that mostly resembled chronic schizophrenia with paranoid delusions, although operational criteria were not used. Subsequently, in a small study of VCFS adults (n = 14), 11 (79%) were found to have a psychiatric diagnosis of which 4 (29%) had DSM–III–R schizophrenia or schizoaffective disorder (Pulver *et al.*, 1994). In a further study, of 10 VCFS adults, Papolos *et al.* (1996) reported that 4 (40%) of their sample had psychotic symptoms, 2 (20%) had schizoaffective disorder, 3 (30%) had bipolar I disorder while 3 (30%) had bipolar II disorder.

In a large study, Murphy *et al.* (1999) found that 18 (36%) of a sample of 50 VCFS adults had a major psychiatric disorder; 15 (30%) had a psychotic disorder with 12 (24%) fulfilling DSM–IV criteria for schizophrenia while a further 6 (12%) had major depression without psychotic features. The individuals with schizophrenia had fewer negative symptoms (symptoms such as apathy, loss of initiative, and social withdrawal) and a relatively later age of onset (mean age = 26 years) compared with nondeleted controls. Using different ascertainment strategies, however, Bassett *et al.* (1998) reported a relatively early age of onset (mean age = 19 years) in their sample of 10 individuals with VCFS and schizophrenia. More recently, Bassett *et al.* (2003) reported no significant differences in age at onset, positive or negative symptoms, or global functioning in a sample of 16 individuals with VCFS and schizophrenia compared with 46 adults with schizophrenia without VCFS. However, in an accompanying editorial, Kendler (2003) suggested that this sample of VCFS individuals with schizophrenia were probably not a representative sample since most were selected because they were first diagnosed with schizophrenia and only later shown to have the deletion. In addition, as the two groups were not well matched for IQ, this lack of matching may also have confounded their results. Clearly, larger and more representative samples using properly IQ matched controls are required to resolve the differing results between these studies.

VCFS and schizophrenia – a valid association?

The most reliable criteria to determine whether the association between VCFS and schizophrenia is valid should involve at least two, or preferably all, of the following: (1) increased frequency of schizophrenia in VCFS individuals, (2) increased frequency of VCFS in people with schizophrenia and (3) susceptibility locus for schizophrenia should map to 22q11.2.

Is the frequency of schizophrenia increased in VCFS individuals?

The studies outlined above certainly suggest that people with VCFS have extremely high rates of schizophrenia. Such high rates of schizophrenia are not explained by the potential confounding effects of ascertainment bias or learning disability and suggest that apart from being a monozygotic co-twin of an individual with schizophrenia or a child of two affected parents, deletion of chromsome 22q11.2 represents the highest known risk factor for the development of schizophrenia yet identified. What is the true prevalence of schizophrenia in VCFS? Although Murphy *et al.* (1999) reported that 12 (24%) of 50 VCFS adults fulfilled DSM–IV criteria for schizophrenia, 80% were younger than 40 years and were therefore still within the age of risk. In addition, there is an ascertainment bias implicit in any study of VCFS adults as they will have been selected for a less severe phenotype to have survived into adulthood. If this is the case, the true lifetime prevalence of schizophrenia in VCFS may be considerably higher than the 24% reported in this study. Consequently, longitudinal studies of VCFS children are required to determine the true lifetime prevalence of schizophrenia in VCFS individuals and these are currently being undertaken.

It is unsurprising that studies of children with VCFS do not report high rates of schizophrenia as the mean age of onset for the development of schizophrenia in the general population is in the late teenage years. Furthermore, as social withdrawal and affective disorder are features that often precede the onset of psychosis in schizophrenia, Murphy et al. (1999) have suggested that the apparently conflicting findings of high rates of affective disorder in VCFS children might reflect the pathoplastic effects of age, with the psychiatric disorder in VCFS tending to evolve into schizophrenia or schizoaffective disorder (in a proportion of individuals) as the subjects get older.

Is there increased frequency of VCFS in people with schizophrenia?

Several studies have reported an increased prevalence of chromosome 22q11.2 deletions in populations of people with schizophrenia. Karayiorgou et al. (1995) reported that 2 of 100 randomly ascertained individuals with schizophrenia were found to have a 22q11.2 deletion. No deletions were found in a sample of 200 healthy controls. More recently, in a study of 47 individuals with childhood-onset schizophrenia, Usiskin et al. (1999) reported that 6% (n = 3) were found to have a 22q11.2 deletion.

A more targeted approach to detecting 22q11.2 deletions involves screening individuals with schizophrenia for the presence of clinical features consistent with VCFS. Gothelf (1997) screened the records of two major general hospitals for patients with abnormalities characteristic of VCFS, such as cardiac anomalies and cleft palate, and cross-referenced these data with the register of psychiatric hospitalizations in four psychiatric hospitals. Of the seven individuals with schizophrenia meeting selection criteria, one (14%) was found to have a 22q11.2 deletion. Using a similar approach, Bassett et al. (1998) examined a sample of 15 individuals with schizophrenia who had been selected for 22q11.2 deletion studies using fluorescent in situ hybridization (FISH) as they exhibited two or more of the following features: palatal abnormalities (hypernasal speech or history of cleft palate), congenital heart disease, dysmorphic features, learning disability or other physical congenital abnormalities (e.g., talipes or slender hand with tapered fingers). Eight individuals (53%) were found to have a previously undetected chromosome 22q11.2 deletion.

In summary, there appears to be robust evidence for an increased prevalence of chromosome 22q11.2 deletions in populations of people with schizophrenia. Although it is difficult to estimate the true prevalence of VCFS in schizophrenia, the available evidence suggests that the minimum prevalence rate is at least 2%. The differences in prevalence rates between studies (2–53%) are likely to be a reflection of the differing ascertainment strategies adopted, with increased rates of 22q11.2 deletions reported where studies have selectively targeted subpopulations of people with schizophrenia.

Is there a susceptibility locus for schizophrenia mapping to 22q11?

Although replication has been inconsistent, linkage studies do provide evidence for a susceptibility locus for non-VCFS related schizophrenia on 22q11. Markers telomeric to the VCFS region have been implicated in some of the earlier studies (Schizophrenia Collaborative Linkage Group, 1996) and linkage to chromosome 22q11 has also been reported for an inhibitory phenotype associated with schizophrenia (Myles Worsley et al., 1999). In addition, a recent meta-analysis of 20 schizophrenia genome scans revealed significant evidence for linkage to chromosome 22q11 (Lewis et al., 2003).

As the gene coding for catechol-O-methyltransferase (COMT), an enzyme catalyzing the O-methylation of catecholamine neurotransmitters (dopamine, adrenaline, and noradrenaline), maps to the VCFS region of chromosome 22q11, this is an outstanding candidate gene for schizophrenia in VCFS. An amino acid polymorphism (Val-108-met) determines high and low activity of this enzyme. Dunham et al. (1992) postulated that VCFS individuals with a single copy of the low activity allele might be predisposed to the development of schizophrenia as a result of increased brain dopamine levels. However, Murphy et al. (1999) were unable to demonstrate an association between the low-activity COMT allele and schizophrenia in a sample of 50 VCFS adults.

In a series of 175 individuals with (non-VCFS) schizophrenia, Egan et al. (2001) reported that COMT genotype was related in an allele dosage fashion to performance on the Wisconsin Card Sorting Test of executive cognition. In addition, in a family-based association analysis of 104 trios, they found a significant increase in transmission of the Val allele to the schizophrenic offspring. They postulated that the COMT Val allele, by increasing prefrontal dopamine catabolism, impairs prefrontal cognition and physiology and consequently slightly increases the risk for schizophrenia. More recently, Shifman et al. (2002) found a significant association between schizophrenia and a COMT haplotype in a large case-control sample. In a further development, Bray et al. (2003) have reported that this haplotype is associated with lower expression of COMT mRNA in human brain.

Liu et al. (2002) recently reported a complex pattern of associations between several SNPs in the proline dehydrogenase (PRODH) gene, which also maps to chromosome 22q11, and schizophrenia. This finding was of particular interest as mice with inactivated PRODH have abnormalities of sensorimotor gating similar to those found in people with schizophrenia (Gogos et al., 1999). Although these results are tantalizing, the PRODH finding has not yet been replicated by other groups (Williams et al., 2003).

In another exciting new development, three groups have recently reported that the T-box transcription factor Tbx1 is responsible for the cardiovascular defects found in VCFS using a mouse model (see Chapter 2). Studies are currently underway to examine the role of Tbx1 in the etiology of schizophrenia in VCFS and in the wider population.

VCFS and schizophrenia – what is the mechanism?

There is compelling evidence that a defect in early embryonic development is the cause of many of the abnormalities present in VCFS individuals. The importance of cephalic neural crest-derived cells in the development of the conotruncal region of the heart, thymus, parathyroid glands, and the palate, all structures that are affected in VCFS, has been demonstrated by microablation and transplantation studies in avian embryos.

Evidence from neuroimaging and neuropathological studies suggest that schizophrenia is a neurodevelopmental disorder associated with aberrant neuronal migration and abnormal synaptic connectivity. In addition, structural neuroimaging studies of individuals with schizophrenia report enlarged ventricles, reduced total brain volume, and midline brain abnormalities, features that have also been described in VCFS (see Chapter 9). Based on these observations, it is therefore reasonable to hypothesize that a gene or genes located within the 22q11.2 deleted region is involved in the process of neural cell migration or differentiation in the pharyngeal arches and that haploinsufficiency of such a gene(s) disrupts proper development of these systems leading to multiple organ and tissue abnormalities.

In addition to the COMT and PRODH genes mapping to chromosome 22q11 described above, recent papers have also reported five additional susceptibility genes mapping to other chromosomal loci (Chowdhari *et al.*, 2002; Chumakov *et al.*, 2002; Straub *et al.*, 2002; Stefansson *et al.*, 2003). All these genes are associated with glutamatergic transmission with particular involvement of N-methyl-D-aspartate (NMDA) receptors (Harrison & Owen, 2003). Specifically, PRODH potentially affects glutamatergic synapses via several mechanisms (Gogos *et al.*, 1999; Liu *et al.*, 2002). COMT acts directly on monoaminergic neurotransmission and will likely affect other synaptic populations, including glutamatergic ones, via the many links between dopamine and aminoacid transmitter systems.

Assessment and treatment of psychiatric disorders in individuals with VCFS

It is now well recognized that the early treatment of mental illness, and psychosis in particular, is essential to minimize future psychiatric morbidity and social isolation or exclusion. Indeed, this fact was recognized as early as 1912 by Bleuler who wrote "The sooner the patients can be restored to an earlier life and the less they are allowed to withdraw into the world of their own ideas, the sooner do they become socially functional" (Bleuler, 1912).

A major goal of psychiatric and especially schizophrenia research over the past three decades has been the identification of precursor symptoms and areas of dysfunction in children and adolescents which precede the later development of major psychiatric disorder in adults. Longitudinal studies of children with VCFS are currently being undertaken to identify precursor symptoms and areas of dysfunction which precede the later development of major psychiatric disorder. Identification of such prodromal features in VCFS may have enormous implications for the clinical management of major psychiatric disorder in children and adults with VCFS.

Adults

A comprehensive assessment is essential before a reliable diagnosis of mental illness in individuals with VCFS can be established. In particular, the potentially confounding effects of learning disability or mental retardation must be noted, as this may significantly impair effective communication of underlying symptoms. For those patients with an IQ < 50, the Psychiatric Assessment Schedule for Adults with Developmental Disability (Moss et al., 1993) is a particularly useful diagnostic tool. For those found to be learning disabled, their assessment and subsequent treatment should be carried out by a psychiatric team experienced in the care of people with learning disability.

To date, there have been few clinical trials examining the efficacy of treatment of psychiatric disorders in children or adults with VCFS. Although Gothelf et al. (1999) reported that VCFS individuals respond poorly to conventional antipsychotics, Murphy et al. (1999) reported no differences in treatment response between individuals with schizophrenia with or without VCFS. Gothelf et al. (1999) favor the early introduction of clozapine and our clinical experience suggests that schizophrenia associated with VCFS also responds well to clozapine. In contrast to Gothelf et al. (1999) however, our experience suggests that the newer atypical neuroleptics such as olanzepine and risperidone are also effective. In addition to the use of pharmacological treatment, psychological interventions e.g., cognitive-behavioral therapy (CBT) may also be useful.

Modern antidepressants such as the selective serotonin reuptake inhibitors (SSRIs) are probably the drugs of choice for those VCFS individuals with depressive illnesses. In addition, the use of psychological interventions such as CBT should also be considered as a useful adjunct in treatment of severe depression and as an alternative in milder cases.

Children and adolescents

The psychiatric assessment of young people with VCFS merits a different approach to that of adults as, by necessity, there must be an appraisal of their educational needs, in addition to the psychiatric assessment. Thus a comprehensive neuro-psychological assessment is essential in order to delineate any specific areas of disability. Treatment programs should include, where appropriate, pharmacological therapy and psychotherapy, and should address specific social and educational needs. Compared with the adult patients there is usually far greater involvement of the young person's family, with whom the clinician must work closely to achieve the maximum response to treatment.

The treatment of psychosis in adolescence is similar to that for adult patients although special efforts should be made to ensure minimum disruption to the individual's education. Likewise, the treatment of depression in adolescents with VCFS is also similar to that for adults, with fluoxetine being the preferred pharmacological option. Cognitive-behavioral therapy should also be considered as a useful adjunct/alternative to medication.

Approaches that have proven to be of value in the treatment of ADHD in children include educational measures, CBT, pharmacological therapy, dietary advice/management and the use of supplementary treatments for associated problems, if present (e.g. social skills training, family therapy/support). Drug treatments should be considered only when other avenues have been adequately explored and found (or considered) to be unsuccessful. This is particularly true for children with VCFS as many of the drugs used to treat ADHD may have an adverse effect in individuals with pre-existing cardiac conditions (although this relates more to arrhythmias than to structural abnormalities). In addition, the use of the psychostimulant methylphenidate, which is frequently used in the treatment of ADHD, is problematic in patients with schizophrenia and other psychoses as it may exacerbate thought disorder and behavioral disturbances in these individuals. However, in an open-label study of methylphenidate, Gothelf and colleagues (2003) reported that no psychotic symptoms were induced in a series of 12 VCFS children and adolescents with ADHD.

Other pharmacological approaches that are used to treat ADHD include tricyclic antidepressants (e.g. imipramine), bupropion (a non-tricyclic antidepressant), and atomoxetine (a noradrenergic specific reuptake inhibitor that has recently been licenced for the treatment of ADHD and appears to be well tolerated). Of these drugs, imipramine should be used with caution in VCFS patients because of its cardiac effects. Bupropion on the other hand appears to be well tolerated and does not have the cardiac conduction problems observed with imipramine. In summary, the pharmacological treatment of ADHD in children with VCFS should be undertaken by clinicians who are experienced child psychiatrists with expertise in the treatment of ADHD in the general population.

Difficult behaviors seen in children with VCFS (e.g., temper outbursts, aggression, poor sleep patterns, dietary idiosyncrasies) can be approached using behavioral modification techniques including the use of token economies and reward schemes. Anger management programs and social skills training may be as effective in this group as in other non-learning disabled groups providing that their disabilities are taken into account when devising the schemes. Appropriate educational provision is essential for children with VCFS and mental health professionals working with such children should liaise closely with those responsible for providing such education. The majority of children with VCFS are able to attend mainstream school, with varying degrees of additional help in the classroom. However, it should be recognized that, depending on their level of intellectual ability, a minority of children with VCFS will benefit more from a placement at a school specializing in providing education for children with special needs, both in terms of their academic requirements and in terms of their behavioral difficulties.

Conclusions

People with VCFS have high rates of psychiatric and behavioral disorders. While VCFS children have high rates of ADHD, anxiety and affective disorders, adults have high rates of psychotic disorders, particularly schizophrenia. Early detection and treatment of mental illness in these individuals is of paramount importance as this will have a major effect in determining the outcome and hence the prognosis. The identification of genes associated with schizophrenia and other major psychiatric disorders may have a profound effect on our understanding of the underlying pathophysiology of these disorders and will pave the way for a new generation of novel and even more effective treatments in the future.

REFERENCES

Bassett, A. S., Hodgkinson, K., Chow, E. W. C. et al. (1998) 22q11 deletion syndrome in adults with schizophrenia. *Am. J. Med. Genet.*, **81**, 328–37.

Bassett, A. S., Chow, E. W. C., AbdelMalik, P. et al. (2003) The schizophrenia phenotype in 22q11 deletion syndrome. *Am. J. Psychiatry*, **160**, 1580–6.

Bleuler, E. (1912) *The Theory of Schizophrenic Negativism, Nervous and Mental Disease. Monograph Series No. 11*, New York.

Bray, N. J., Buckland, P. R., Williams, N. M. *et al.* (2003) A haplotype implicated in schizophrenia susceptibility is associated with reduced COMT expression in human brain. *Am. J. Hum. Genet.*, **73**, 152–61.

Chowdhari, K. V., Mirnics, K., Semwal, P. *et al.* (2002) Association and linkage analyses of RGS4 polymorphisms in schizophrenia. *Hum. Mol. Genet.*, **11**, 1373–80.

Chumakov, I., Blumenfeld, M., Guerassimenko, O. *et al.* (2002) Genetic and physiological data implicating the new human gene G72 and the gene for D-amino acid oxidase in schizophrenia. *PNAS*, **99**, 13675–80.

Dunham, I., Collins, J., Wadey, R. & Scambler, P. (1992) Possible role for COMT in psychosis associated with velo-cardio-facial syndrome. *Lancet*, **340**, 1361–2.

Egan, M. F., Goldberg, T. E., Kolachana, B. S. *et al.* (2001) Effect of COMT Val 108/158 Met genotype on frontal lobe function and risk for scizophrenia. *PNAS*, **98**, 6917–22.

Feinstein, C., Eliez, S., Balsey, C. & Reiss, A. L. (2002) Psychiatric disorders and behavioral problems in children with velo-cardio-facial syndrome: usefulness as phenotypic indicators of schizophrenia risk. *Biol. Psychiatry*, **51**, 312–18.

Gogos, J. A., Santha, M., Takacs, Z. *et al.* (1999) The gene encoding proline dehydrogenase modulates sensorimotor gating in mice. *Nat. Genet.*, **21**, 434–9.

Goldberg, R., Motzkin, B., Marion, R. *et al.* (1993) Velo-cardio-facial syndrome: a review of 120 patients. *Am. J. Med. Genet.*, **45**, 313–19.

Golding-Kushner, K. J., Weller, G. & Shprintzen, R. J. (1985) Velo-cardio-facial syndrome: language and psychological profiles. *J. Craniofac. Genet. Devel. Biol.*, **5**, 259–66.

Gothelf, D., Frisch, A., Munitz, H. *et al.* (1997) Velocardiofacial manifestations and microdeletions in schizophrenic inpatients. *Am. J. Med. Genet.*, **72**, 455–61.

(1999) Clinical characteristics of schizophrenia associated with velo-cardio-facial syndrome. *Schiz. Res.*, **35**, 105–12.

Gothelf, D., Gruber, R., Presburger, G. *et al.* (2003). Methylphenidate treatment for attention-deficit/hyperactivity disorder in children and adolescents with velocardiofacial syndrome: an open-label study. *J. Clin. Psych.*, **60** (**10**), 1163–9.

Harrison, P. J. & Owen, M. J. (2003) Genes for schizophrenia? Recent findings and their pathophysiological implications. *Lancet*, **361**, 417–19.

Karayiorgou, M., Morris, M. A., Morrow, B. *et al.* (1995) Schizophrenia susceptibility associated with interstitial deletions of chromosome 22q11. *PNAS*, **92**, 7612–16.

Kendler, K. S. (2003) The genetics of schizophrenia: chromosomal deletions, attentional disturbances and spectrum boundaries. *Am. J. Psychiatry*, **160**, 1549–53.

Lewis, C. M., Levinson, D. F., Wise, L. H. *et al.* (2003) Genome scan meta-analysis of schizophrenia and bipolar disorder. Part 11: Schizophrenia. *Am. J. Hum. Genet.*, **73**, 34–48.

Liu, H., Heath, S. C., Sobin, C. *et al.* (2002) Genetic variation at the 22q11 PRODH2/DGCR6 locus presents an unusual pattern and increases susceptibility to schizophrenia. *PNAS*, **99**, 3717–22.

Moss, S. C., Patel, P., Prosser, H. *et al.* (1993) Psychiatric morbidity in older people with moderate and severe learning disability (mental retardation), part 1: development and reliability of the patient interview (the PAS-ADD). *Br. J. Psychiatry*, **163**, 471–80.

Murphy, K. C. & Owen, M. J. (2001) Velo-cardio-facial-syndrome (VCFS): a model for understanding the genetics and pathogenesis of schizophrenia. *Br. J. Psychiatry*, **178**, 397–402.

Murphy, K. C., Jones, L. A. & Owen, M. J. (1999) High rates of schizophrenia in adults with velo-cardio-facial syndrome. *Arch. Gen. Psychiatry*, **56**, 940–5.

Myles Worsley, M., Coon, H., McDowell, J. *et al.* (1999) Linkage of a composite inhibitory phenotype to a chromosome 22q locus in eight Utah families. *Am. J. Med. Genet.*, **88**, 544–50.

Niklasson, L., Rasmussen, P., Oskarsdottir, S. & Gillberg, C. (2001) Neuropsychiatric disorders in the 22q11 deletion syndrome. *Genet. Med.*, **3**, 79–84.

Papolos, D. F., Faedda, G. L., Veit, S. *et al.* (1996) Bipolar spectrum disorders in patients diagnosed with velo-cardio-facial syndrome: does a hemizygous deletion of chromosome 22q11 result in bipolar affective disorder? *Am. J. Psychiatry*, **153**, 1541–7.

Pulver, A. E., Nestadt, G., Goldberg, R. *et al.* (1994) Psychotic illness in patients diagnosed with velo-cardio-facial syndrome and their relatives. *J. Nerv. Ment. Dis.*, **182**, 476–8.

Schizophrenia Collaborative Linkage Group (1996) A combined analysis of D22S278 marker alleles in affected sib-pairs: support for a susceptibility locus for schizophrenia at chromosome 22q12. *Am. J. Med. Genet.*, **67**, 40–5.

Shifman, S., Bronstein, M., Sternfeld, M. *et al.* (2002) A highly significant association between a COMH haplotype and schizophrenia. *Am. J. Hum. Genet.*, **71**, 1296–302.

Shprintzen, R. J., Goldberg, R. B., Lewin, M. L. *et al.* (1978) A new syndrome involving cleft palate, cardiac anomalies, typical facies and learning disabilities: velo-cardio-facial syndrome. *Cleft Palate J.*, **15**, 56–62.

Shprintzen, R. J., Goldberg, R., Golding-Kushner, K. J. & Marion, R. (1992) Late-onset psychosis in the velo-cardio-facial syndrome. *Am. J. Med. Genet.*, **42**, 141–2.

Stefansson, H., Sarginson, J., Kong, A. *et al.* (2003) Association of Neuroregulin 1 with schizophrenia confirmed in a Scottish population. *Am. J. Hum. Genet.*, **72**, 83–7.

Stevens, A. F., Campbell, L. E., Morris, R. *et al.* (2003) Psychiatric profile of children with velo-cardio-facial syndrome (VCFS). *Am. J. Med. Genet.*, **122B**, P84.

Straub, R. E., Jiang, Y., Maclean, C. J., *et al.* (2002) Genetic variation in the 6p22.3 gene DTNBPI, the human ortholog of the mouse Dysbindin gene, is associated with schizophrenia. *Am. J. Hum. Genet.*, **71**, 337–48.

Swillen, A. (2001). *The Behavioural Phenotype in Velo-cardio-facial Syndrome: from Infancy to Adolescence*. Department of Psychology and Educational Sciences. Leuven: Acco Leuven, University of Leuven.

Swillen, A., Devriendt, K., Legius, E. *et al.* (1997) Intelligence and psychological adjustment in velocardiofacial syndrome: a study of 37 children and adolescents with VCFS. *J. Med. Genet.*, **34**, 453–8.

Swillen, A., Devriendt, K., Legius, E. *et al.* (1999a) The behavioural phenotype in velocardiofacial syndrome (VCFS): from infancy to adolescence. *Genet. Couns.*, **10**, 79–88.

Swillen, A., Vandeputte, L., Cracco, J. *et al.* (1999b) Neuropsychological, learning and psychosocial profile of primary school aged children with the velo-cardio-facial syndrome (22q11 deletion): evidence for a non-verbal learning disability? *Child Neuropsychol.*, **5**, 230–41.

Usiskin, S. I., Nicolson, R., Krasnewich, D. M. *et al.* (1999) Velocardiofacial syndrome in childhood-onset schizophrenia. *J. Am. Acad. Child Adolesc. Psychiatry*, **38**, 1536–43.

Williams, H. J., Williams, N., Spurlick, G. *et al.* (2003) Association between PRODH and schizophrenia is not confirmed. *Mol. Psychiatry*, **8**, 644–5.

8

The cognitive spectrum in velo-cardio-facial syndrome

Linda Campbell[1] and Ann Swillen[2]

[1] Institute of Psychiatry, King's College London, UK
[2] Centre for Human Genetics, University Hospital Gasthuisberg, Leuven, Belgium

Introduction

A major challenge in both clinical practice and research in the field of intellectual disabilities and of learning disorders is to identify the underlying causes: the genetic, chromosomal, and environmental factors that have important influences on a person's development and behavior. Advances in clinical genetics have led to an increased recognition of specific syndromes. In recent years, cytogenetic and molecular genetic tools have resulted in the identification of the underlying genetic defects in a large number of disorders e.g., the 22q11.2 microdeletion in velo-cardio-facial syndrome (VCFS).

For many years, interest was focused on the delineation of the somatic aspects of the phenotypes and their underlying pathogenetic mechanisms. However, in the last decade, researchers have paid more attention to the cognitive and behavioral features of various genetic conditions, the so-called "behavioral phenotype." A behavioral phenotype is broadly defined as "a behavioural pattern, including cognitive processes and social interaction style, consistently associated with, and specific to, a syndrome with a chromosomal or a genetic aetiology" (Flint, 1996). This definition does not propose a simple, one-to-one or universal relationship link between the behavioral phenotype and the associated biological/genetic disorder. On the contrary, the relationships are complex and varied.

It was not until 1992 that submicroscopic deletions on chromosome 22q11 were identified, confirming that VCFS is indeed a specific syndrome (Scambler *et al.*, 1991; Driscoll *et al.*, 1992). This discovery made it possible to use cytogenetic testing to confirm the clinical diagnosis of VCFS. Hence, studies investigating the cognitive profile of VCFS predating this discovery may have included individuals without the 22q11.2 deletion, making it difficult to interpret data and to draw reliable conclusions from these studies. However, the early literature (Golding-Kushner *et al.*, 1985) did point out the wide range of developmental and behavioral expressions

Velo-Cardial-Facial Syndrome: A Model for Understanding Microdeletion Disorders, ed. Kieran C. Murphy and Peter J. Scambler. Published by Cambridge University Press. © Cambridge University Press, 2005.

displayed by individuals with VCFS, and later research has continued to investigate and expand these early findings. Despite the wide range of expressions of the phenotype, there are indications that there is a cognitive profile characteristic of individuals with VCFS and independent of associated medical conditions, e.g., cardiac and palatal problems (Swillen et al., 1997; Gerdes et al., 1999; Solot et al., 2001; De Smedt et al., 2003). In this chapter we review the different studies of cognition in VCFS, in order to delineate the cognitive phenotype of individuals with VCFS.

Cognition

Intelligence

Throughout the course of neuropsychological research into VCFS, one of the most well established features of the syndrome is a general intellectual impairment. In fact, the prevalence of learning disabilities has been reported to be as high as 82% (Lipson et al., 1991) to 100% (Shprintzen et al., 1981). Full-scale IQ (FSIQ) scores tend to range from normal to moderately learning disabled with a mean FSIQ of about 70 (Swillen et al., 1997; Moss et al., 1999) while severe learning disabilities in this condition appear rare. Gerdes et al., (2001) reported that 41% of their sample of 40 young children (aged 13–63 months) with VCFS was significantly delayed and 32% mildly delayed on major developmental milestones, including speech and language, cognition, and motor skills. Those individuals who were most delayed in infancy were also those more likely to go on to receive a later diagnosis of mild (IQ: 50–70) or moderate learning disability (IQ: 35–49).

So far, no direct link between cardiac status and intellectual outcome has been established in the del22q11.2 population. Gerdes et al. (2001) found no association between cardiac diagnosis and developmental scores in their study of preschool children, and Swillen et al. (1997) reported no statistically different FSIQ scores in their child and adolescent subjects with and without a congenital heart defect. It should be noted however that, until now, no study had specifically focused on the precise role of cardiac defects on neurocognitive processes. The only contributing factor identified to date to the variability in intelligence in VCFS is the presence of a de novo versus familial occurrence of the deletion. In a study of 37 consecutively diagnosed children and adolescents with VCFS (age range: 8 months to 20 years), Swillen et al. (1997) found that the mean FSIQ of individuals with a deletion inherited from their parent was significantly lower than the mean FSIQ of the individuals with a de novo deletion. This finding is not unexpected, in that the more severe learning disabilities in familial cases can partly be explained by lower educational level and FSIQ of the affected parent. In addition, the unaffected parent has been found to achieve a lower educational level than the unaffected parents in nonfamilial cases of VCFS (Swillen et al., 1997), suggesting assortative mating.

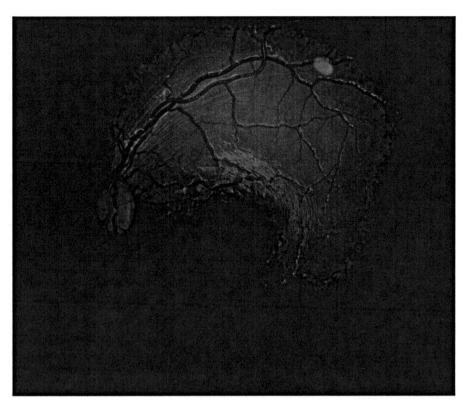

Plate 1   Relative deficits (yellow) and excesses (blue) in white matter volume in velo-cardio-facial syndrome compared with controls. The maps are oriented with the right side of the brain shown on the left side of each panel. The z-coordinate for each row of axial slices in the standard space of Talairach & Tournoux (1988) is given in millimetres.

Plates 1 and 2 in this section are available for download in colour from www.cambridge.org/9780521184328

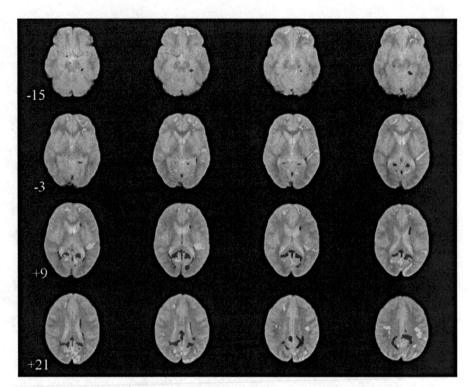

Plate 2   Relative deficits (yellow) and excesses (blue) in white matter volume in velo-cardio-facial syndrome compared with controls. The maps are oriented with the right side of the brain shown on the left side of each panel. The z-coordinate for each row of axial slices in the standard space of Talairach & Tournoux (1988) is given in millimetres.

Intellectual profile

In a study of 33 children and adults with VCFS (6–27 years old) using the WISC-III, Moss *et al.* (1999) found that while individuals with VCFS were relatively good at the "information" and "comprehension" subtests involving general knowledge and understanding of everyday problems and social rules, they were most impaired on the subtests involving visual-perceptual abilities and planning, such as "picture completion," "object assembly" and "picture arrangement." This profile can be interpreted according to the model of intelligence postulated by Horn & Cattell (1966) which would indicate a relatively preserved crystallized intelligence in the VCFS group as reflected by the comparatively higher score on the Verbal Comprehension (VC) factor with deficits within fluid intelligence manifested by impairments on the Perceptual Organisation (PO) factor. Crystallized intelligence is viewed as a set of acquired skills and knowledge strongly influenced by education, while fluid intelligence is conceptualized as a general relation-perceiving capacity strongly loading abstract, nonverbal, and culture-fair tests (e.g., analogies, matrices, numbers, and letters series) which is considered as largely innately and physiologically determined (Horn, 1985). This profile, however, of relatively preserved crystallized intelligence versus deficits within fluid intelligence is also seen in persons with general intellectual impairment, and in other genetic syndromes such as Turner syndrome and Williams–Bueren syndrome (Udwin & Yule, 1991; Swillen *et al.*, 1993; Rovet *et al.*, 1994). This profile does not, therefore, seem to be unique to VCFS. Several studies report that children and adolescents with VCFS have a discrepancy between verbal IQ (VIQ;) i.e. verbal conceptualization, knowledge and expression, and number ability and performance IQ (PIQ;) i.e. non-verbal thinking, visual-motor coordination and response speed, and sequential processing (where VIQ is greater than PIQ), which can be indicative of a nonverbal learning disability (NVLD) (Swillen *et al.*, 1997; Gerdes *et al.*, 1999; Moss *et al.*, 1999; Woodin *et al.*, 2001). The group differences between VIQ and PIQ reported in these studies are between 8–10 points, and although this reaches statistical significance it does not reach clinical significance (11.3 points for $\alpha = 0.05$). When investigating individual discrepancies in the samples, it has been found that, although some individuals do show a clinically significant VIQ > PIQ discrepancy, an even smaller minority also show a clinically significant PIQ > VIQ discrepancy. Since standard US population norms for the WISC-III/WPPSI-R reveal that 44.5% of children demonstrate a VIQ/PIQ difference of 10 points or more, albeit in the normal range, the discrepancies in these samples could simply be due to normal variance (Wechsler, 1989, 1991). In one of the few studies of adults with VCFS (n = 19) Henry *et al.* (2002) failed to find a consistent VIQ > PIQ discrepancy in their sample. In fact, 6 (31.5%) of the sample showed a significant discrepancy between VIQ and PIQ (11 points or more) in favor of PIQ while only 3 (16%) had a significant discrepancy in favor of VIQ.

Another method of distinguishing between verbal and nonverbal abilities is to compare Verbal Comprehension (VC) and Perceptual Organization (PO) where the subtests of arithmetic and coding have been excluded. This may give a more accurate picture of the true abilities of individuals with VCFS, due to their problems with mathematics. Some researchers have done this in their VCFS samples and have found that the VC > PO difference is indeed larger than the VIQ > PIQ discrepancy (Moss et al., 1999; Swillen et al., 1999b). This indicates that a closer inspection of the index scores and perhaps even subtest scores may shed more light on the verbal and nonverbal abilities in VCFS than global scores (Moss et al., 1999).

To conclude, although discrepancies between verbal and performance abilities are common in the general population, there appear to be some instances where a clinically significant VIQ/PIQ discrepancy may be indicative of a specific learning disability in individuals with VCFS. Hence, clinicians ought to take this into consideration when evaluating an individual's educational needs. Interestingly, the VIQ/PIQ discrepancies have been more observed among children and adolescents with VCFS than in adults with the syndrome. These findings could indicate an atypical development in childhood of the skills involved in these particular measures, where the visuo-spatial abilities develop at a slower rate than their peers while their verbal abilities remain stable. This latter hypothesis is supported by a preliminary study by Campbell et al. (2002) in a study of 26 children and adolescents (6–16 years old) with VCFS, where it was found that FSIQ decreased with age and that this decline could be attributed to decreases in PIQ while no changes in VIQ were found over time. No such differences occurred among the control group of "typically" developing siblings. However, further longitudinal studies will enable a closer inspection of the developmental trajectory of VIQ and PIQ skills in VCFS.

Academic achievement

Over the years it has been well established that children with VCFS perform better at reading and spelling than arithmetic (Swillen et al., 1999a; Wang et al., 2000). When investigating mathematical skills in their sample, Moss et al. (1999) report that both orally presented mathematical reasoning and 'rote' calculation (paper and pencil equations, e.g., $3 + 3$) skills appeared equally impaired in comparison with reading comprehension and single-word reading. In addition, reading comprehension and single-word reading yielded similar results. However, other studies of verbal academic skills report better performance on single-word reading than reading comprehension (Woodin et al., 2001). In order to explore whether the psychoeducational profile reported in VCFS is simply due to differences in FSIQ, Moss et al. (1999) excluded individuals with a FSIQ lower than 70 from the analysis. The same psychoeducational patterns, e.g., VIQ > PIQ, VC > PO, reading and spelling > maths, appeared in this more homogenous group as for the whole group, indicating that this profile is indeed characteristic of a 22q11.2 deletion rather than a consequence of general learning disability. However, it would be interesting to know whether the same profile is similarly found in the group of individuals with a FSIQ below 70. One could hypothesize that the differences between verbal and nonverbal skills become less pronounced as the level of intellectual ability decreases.

In conclusion, the reviewed literature suggests that many children with VCFS display a characteristic intellectual and achievement profile with particular verbal, visuo-spatial and mathematical impairments, which must be taken into consideration when evaluating educational remediation strategies. However, there are a wide variety of skills and impairments exhibited by individuals with VCFS, highlighting the importance of individual assessments. Studies with larger sample sizes, more homogenous groups, and appropriate IQ-matched controls are necessary to characterize the whole spectrum of the syndrome. In addition, larger studies and/ or longitudinal studies can elucidate the developmental trajectory of global intellectual, VIQ/PIQ profiles as well as educational abilities in VCFS.

Cognitive functions

In order to investigate the underlying basis of the observed impairments as well as areas of relative proficiency in intellectual and academic ability, it is important to use tasks specifically designed to tap into these neuropsychological functions. In VCFS these investigations are still in their infancy but there already exist some interesting findings that further strengthen our understanding of the behavioral phenotype in this complex syndrome.

Mathematics and numerical skills

Academic achievement tests have established that mathematics pose a problem for individuals with VCFS. In the only published functional magnetic resonance imaging (fMRI) study of eight children with VCFS, it was found that the VCFS children showed a significantly different pattern of neural activation than age and gender-matched controls during an 'easy' and a 'difficult' mathematical task (Eliez et al., 2001). In particular, it was found that the VCFS children showed an increase in activation of the left supramarginal gyrus (SMG) during the "difficult" task while the controls showed comparable levels of activation during both tasks. It is, however, only during the "difficult" task that the VCFS group show a significantly higher activation of the left SMG than controls. The conclusions from this first fMRI study of VCFS are interesting although the paradigm could be improved using a more similar "on" and "off" stimulus. In addition, the lack of a large sample size but primarily the lack of an IQ-matched control group makes it complicated to discern whether the differences in activations of the left SMG during the "difficult" task were not simply an effect due to the lower intellectual ability in the VCFS group. Indeed, the VCFS group showed a lower performance on both tasks but especially on the "difficult" task. It could be the case that the control population would have shown a similar activation pattern if sufficient pressure had been put on their mathematical ability.

Although the conclusions from this study are limited, the findings are of special interest in the search to delineate the basis and structure of the mathematical impairments observed in this group. It has been suggested, based on neuropsychological and functional neuroimaging studies in adults, that mathematical skills are dependent on two functionally and anatomically separate processing systems: language-specific (symbolic) used for exact arithmetic (i.e., storage and retrieval of rote arithmetic facts) and a language independent (analog) format (quantity manipulation and approximation) (Dehaene, 1997; Dehaene & Cohen, 1997). The verbal system involves, for instance, the left temporal lobe while the system said to be underlying at least the nonverbal component of numerical skill has been suggested to be dependent on visuo-spatial networks located in the parietal lobe (Dehaene & Cohen, 1997; Butterworth, 1999). Interestingly, the SMG implicated in the abnormal activation pattern in the study by Eliez and colleagues (2001) is located in the (inferior) parietal lobe. A very recent study by Simon and colleagues (Simon et al., in press), gives further evidence of visuo-spatial and numerical cognitive deficits in children with the 22q11.2 deletion syndrome. Relative to a group of typically developing controls (siblings of the del22q11.2 children and typically developing controls) children with del22q11.2 performed more poorly on tests of visual attentional reasoning, visual enumeration, and relative magnitude judgment. The results of the study indicate that the visuo-spatial and numerical deficits in children with del22q11.2 may be due, at least in part, to inferior parietal dysfunction.

Although it is appealing to apply theories about number modules to VCFS, one has to bear in mind that, as VCFS is a neurodevelopmental disorder, one cannot easily generalize from findings of dissociations in the mature normal brain. Instead, Karmiloff-Smith et al. (unpublished) suggest that it is vital to take into account the developmental emergence of function. The impairment of mathematics in VCFS is also of interest from a cross-syndrome approach since similar profiles with better language skills than arithmetic have been well documented in other developmental disorders e.g., Williams syndrome (Bellugi et al., 1988; Udwin et al., 1996). It has been hypothesized that perhaps number skills are more vulnerable to early neural disruptions than language skills (Karmiloff-Smith et al., unpublished). However, to increase the understanding of numeracy problems in VCFS, further in-depth studies of visuo-spatial and language functions are important in order to specify the exact developmental nature of these problems in the VCFS population.

In addition, it has been hypothesized that (mathematical) problem solving is linked to executive functions, especially with the ability of reducing the accessibility of irrelevant information in memory (Bull & Scerif, 2001; Passolunghi & Siegel, 2001). These future studies should focus not only on the end-state of functions but also investigate the early emergence and development of cognition in order to properly assess if there are any particular aspects of mathematics that pose more specific problems to people with VCFS than other groups.

Visual object and spatial cognition

From the previous reported deficits of nonverbal and mathematical abilities from psychoeducational measures, it is clear that further analysis of spatial cognition in this population is required. However, to date only one study has attempted to study this in VCFS. Henry *et al.* (2002) utilized the visual object and space perception battery (VOSP) (Rapport *et al.*, 1998) in a group of 19 adults with VCFS. They reported object-perceptual impairments, specifically on the subtests of silhouettes (recognition of objects from unusual views) and object decision (object recognition) in the VCFS group. Unfortunately, as no object-naming task was used in this study, no conclusions regarding the origin of the VCFS group's worse performance on the object perceptual subtests can be drawn. Interestingly, no group differences between the VCFS group and IQ-matched controls were found on the visual spatial domains.

Memory

Several studies have suggested that "rote" (repetitive) verbal learning and memory are an area of strength for individuals with VCFS while visuo-spatial memory and complex verbal memory such as story recall are impaired. Swillen *et al.* (1999b) tested auditory memory in 9 children with VCFS and found normal group performance on the "15 words of Rey" (Rey, 1958), which measures rote verbal learning (Swillen *et al.*, 1999b). Recently, Bearden and colleagues (2001) published a study investigating more specific memory abilities in 29 children with VCFS. The VCFS group demonstrated selective deficits in visuo-spatial immediate and delayed memory when compared with 'rote' verbal memory. In addition, the VCFS group performed significantly better on an object memory test compared with a pure visual spatial memory task indicating a dissociation between these two domains. Wang *et al.* (2000) also reported that, in their sample of 36 VCFS children, the majority (67%) of children appeared to be better at number recall than spatial memory, although 20% did show an opposite pattern of performance with higher scores on spatial memory than number recall. Both scores correlated significantly with the children's performance on mathematics subtests. However, Henry *et al.* (2002), using the 'Executive Golf' task (Owen *et al.*, 1996; Morris *et al.*, 1988), investigated spatial working memory (WM) and strategy formation in adult VCFS individuals and found no significant difference between the VCFS group and IQ matched controls.

Although studies of memory function in children and adults with VCFS are relatively few, they seem to indicate that there are specific deficits within visual spatial memory (at least in children) and the complex verbal memory domain, while individuals with VCFS perform well in "rote" verbal memory. Whether this is specific to VCFS or due to the lower intellectual abilities in the VCFS will need further investigation using intellectually comparable control groups especially when considering the findings from Henry *et al.* (2002) who did not find any differences when using intellectually matched controls. The findings from these studies are important in order to delineate the mathematical impairments observed in this syndrome since there appears to be a relationship between memory skills and arithmetic in VCFS (Wang *et al.*, 2000). In addition, a number of non-VCFS studies have suggested a link between mathematical difficulties and working- or short-term memory difficulties (Siegel & Ryan, 1989; Geary *et al.*, 1991; Ashcraft, 1995).

Executive functions (EF)

The term "executive functions" (EF) has been widely used in cognitive neuropsychology to describe the coordination of the cognitive processes involved in the execution of complex tasks. Intact EF is necessary for planning, generation of strategies for action, and the monitoring of behavior in response to environmental feedback. It has been proposed that EF dysfunction leads to failure to inhibit inappropriate responding, and an inability to generate novel responses or to devise strategies for problem solving.

There have been a small number of studies specifically investigating EF in VCFS. Swillen *et al.* (1999b) used the Wisconsin Card Sorting Test (WCST) (Heaton, 1981), devised to study "abstract behavior" and "shift of set" in a study of nine VCFS children (6–12 years old) and found no significant impairments on Perseverative Errors, although six out of nine children had weak performance on Categories Achieved i.e., difficulties in finding correct solution strategies. Similarly, there were no significant differences in performance between adults with VCFS and a group of IQ-matched controls on the WEIGL's test (Weigl, 1941), designed to measure sorting and shifting i.e., cognitive flexibility (Henry *et al.*, 2002). However, Henry *et al.* (2002) did find that the VCFS adults used more moves to solve problems in a computerized 3-D Tower of London (TOL) task (Shallice, 1982; Morris *et al.*,

1988, 1990;) and less planning time, which may indicate increased impulsivity and less thought-through strategies to solve problems. Further studies are required using specific tasks to dissect further the EF abilities in VCFS, although at the very least there appear to be problems in the domain of planning in adults with VCFS.

Attention

Attention, concentration, and tracking are mechanisms that are difficult to differentiate from each other in neuropsychological investigations. Intact attention is an essential precondition of both concentration and mental tracking tasks and pure attentional deficits appear to manifest themselves as distractibility or in an impaired ability for focused behavior (Lezak, 1995). Concentration deficits can be caused by attentional impairments or by an inability to maintain "purposeful" attentional focus, while conceptual tracking can be interrupted by attention or concentration difficulties, focused attention on problem-solving or following a sequence of ideas (Lezak, 1995).

Attention problems have been implicated in the behavioral profile of individuals with VCFS in a wide range of questionnaire studies (Swillen *et al.*, 1997; Gerdes *et al.*, 1999; Eliez *et al.*, 2000; Woodin *et al.*, 2001). Additionally, thought problems such as muddled thinking, being easily confused, ruminations and repetitive thoughts have also been reported in children with VCFS (Swillen *et al.*, 1999a; Woodin *et al.*, 2001). Thought problems may be indicators of problems with divided and/or shifting attention (Lezak, 1995). So, do neuropsychological findings support the behavioral attentional problems found in VCFS? Although research has only just begun to answer this question, Woodin *et al.* (2001) have reported that, in a group of 50 children with VCFS (6–12 years old), the VCFS group scored significantly higher on Trails A (Trail-Making Test) compared with Trails B (Lezak, 1995; Woodin *et al.*, 2001). Although Trails A is a more straightforward spatial arrangement task than Trails B, it has been suggested that individuals who display significantly worse performance on Trails B compared with Trails A are likely to have problems with complex (double or multiple) conceptual tracking involving divided and/or shifting attention (Lezak, 1995). Problems with sustained visual attention have also been found when using the Bourdon-Vos dot test (Vos, 1988) in a group of nine children with VCFS (Swillen *et al.*, 1999b). However, in a further study, Henry *et al.* (2002) used the Continuous Performance Task (CPT) (Rapport *et al.*, 1998) in their adult sample of individuals with VCFS (n = 19) and found no significant differences in attention and impulsivity in the VCFS group compared with IQ-matched controls. Therefore, while the behavioral pattern of children and adolescents with VCFS is suggestive of attentional problems, cognitive studies of attention in VCFS have been few and no IQ-matched controls have been used in the studies of children.

Consequently, it is difficult to know whether these difficulties are simply attributed to learning difficulties, as suggested by the findings from Henry *et al.* (2002).

Communication skills and language

Delayed speech and language development is one of the most consistent features in VCFS and a major concern to parents of children with VCFS (Golding-Kushner *et al.*, 1985; Gerdes *et al.*, 1999). First words generally do not emerge until 2 years or later (Wang *et al.*, 2000). In addition, most young children with VCFS have speech abnormalities including high-pitched voice, hoarseness, and compensatory articulation errors (see Chapter 10). This delayed speech and language development has multifactorial origins such as velopharyngeal insufficiency and developmental delay. In a small study, Scherer and colleagues (2001) tested four VCFS children on five occasions over 24 months using several different measures. They reported deficits in vocabulary and speech acquisition, receptive and expressive language in VCFS children when compared with children with Down syndrome. Similar findings have also been reported when comparing VCFS children with normally developing children and to children with cleft lip and palate (Scherer *et al.*, 1999) suggesting a specific language impairment in some children with VCFS. It was also noted by the authors that the VCFS children followed a different developmental trajectory of communication skills from the other groups, where the severity of impairments increased from birth to 3 years of age and by the age of 12–18 months their language abilities were distinctly different from children with clefts (Scherer *et al.*, 1999). In further studies, Gerdes *et al.* (1999) reported that 40% of a sample of 40 VCFS children (age range: 13–63 months) were significantly delayed, 44% mildly delayed and 16% average, on total language development. Although both expressive and receptive language showed a high degree of delay, expressive language was more impaired than receptive language among these young children. In addition, such delays of expressive language remained significant even after controlling for their cognitive levels (measured by the onset of speech). Indeed, Moss *et al.* (1999) found that specific language impairments (including both receptive and expressive language deficit) could be diagnosed in approximately 50% (n = 10) in their sample of 20 VCFS school-aged subjects. Conversely however, Glaser *et al.* (2002) recently reported that VCFS children in their sample (n = 27; 6–19 years old) had significantly lower receptive than expressive language skills compared with IQ-matched controls with idiopathic learning disability while no differences in word association were found. The authors argued that the conflicting findings of receptive/expressive language abilities might be due to differences in the administration of specific language tests over age groups since the mean ages in the studies are dissimilar. However, they also suggested a developmental explanation whereby, as the children with VCFS mature, they continue to improve on expressive language skills while their receptive language skills are more stable. This is possibly due to speech/language therapy or that a relative immaturity in abstract reasoning could effect the level of receptive language, becoming more noticeable among older children (Glaser *et al.*, 2002). Interestingly, Glaser and colleagues further reported that the origin of deletion might influence the language development of children with VCFS. They found that individuals with a deletion of paternal origin (n = 9, de novo) had higher scores on receptive language than children with a maternally (n = 12, de novo) derived deletion (Glaser *et al.*, 2002). This finding may have implications for all future studies of cognition in VCFS, particularly as brain anatomy also may be influenced by imprinting (Eliez *et al.*, 2001).

VCFS and non-verbal learning disability (NVLD)

Several studies have suggested that the pattern of cognitive impairment seen in VCFS is consistent with a nonverbal learning disability (NVLD) (Fuerst *et al.*, 1995; Swillen *et al.*, 2000; Woodin *et al.*, 2001). Rourke (1995) has suggested that NVLD is a white matter syndrome, i.e., that NVLD develops as a result of a primary processing dysfunction associated with early white matter abnormalities primarily in the right hemisphere. The characteristic features of NVLD are (1) impairments of bilateral tactile perception, (2) discrimination and recognition of visual detail and visual relationships, (3) bilateral psychomotor coordination and (4) problem solving with novel stimuli (Rourke, 1987, 1988, 1989, 1995; Rourke *et al.*, 1989). Consequently, children with NVLD develop difficulties with visual attention, social competence, emotional distress, concept formation, and problem solving. In addition, NVLD children often exhibit initial developmental delays in language development, followed by rapid acquisition of verbal skills. Affected children develop good cognitive and functional abilities in auditory perception and memory, simple motor tasks, and learning of rote material. Problems with social perception, judgment and interactive skills are also reported in children with NVLD.

In a small study of the neuropsychological, learning, and psychosocial profile of nine Flemish primary school aged children with VCFS and FSIQ higher than 70, Swillen *et al.* (1999b) found that 56% (n = 5) had a NVLD-profile characterized by a VIQ–PIQ discrepancy (in favor of the VIQ), significantly better scores on reading (decoding) and spelling compared with arithmetic, deficient tactile-perceptual skills (more problems on the left side of the body), weak but not deficient visuo-perceptual abilities, deficient visuo-spatial skills, extremely poor psychomotor skills (gross motor skills more deficient than fine motor skills), problems with processing of new and complex material, poor visual attention, good auditory memory, and relatively good language skills. These findings correspond to the pattern of neuropsychological assets and deficits that has been described for the syndrome of NVLD

(Rourke, 1995). In addition, the psychosocial profiles of all the nine children with VCFS correspond to those of children with NVLD with more internalizing than externalizing problem behavior, in particular social problems (especially in relationships with peers), withdrawn behavior, and attention problems.

It is, however, important to emphasize that the term "nonverbal learning disability" (NVLD) does not mean that the learning problems of these children with VCFS only involve "non-verbal" functions. A substantial number of these children also have language difficulties, for example, difficulties in comprehending instructions, assessing and retrieving language (i.e., word finding), receptive language, and oral expression (Woodin *et al.*, 2001). In clinical practice, it is worthwhile exploring in greater depth the neuropsychological functions of children with VCFS to rule out NVLD, since they may benefit from specific remediation following the learning principles of the NVLD-treatment as described by Rourke (1995).

Summary

The majority of studies of cognition in VCFS have focused on psychoeducational profiles and communicative skills in children with VCFS in order to identify appropriate remedial approaches to the needs of this group. The studies suggest a complex pattern of areas of strengths and weaknesses in VCFS. The psychoeducational profile suggests that children with VCFS have problems mainly with nonverbal tasks, but specific language impairments are also commonly observed. Mathematical skills, associated with both language and visuo-spatial abilities, have been found to be impaired in individuals with VCFS. A subgroup of children with VCFS appears to exhibit a NVLD profile with specific language problems. Investigations of underlying cognitive problems have recently begun and specific deficits have been identified e.g., visuo-spatial memory and planning. In addition, recent findings point to a link between visuo-spatial and numerical cognitive deficits and inferior parietal dysfunction.

Discussion and future directions

Our review of the literature of the cognitive phenotype in VCFS suggests that the characterization of this very complex disorder is gradually improving with an increasing number of research studies being published each year. At this point it is important to seriously consider the direction in which the research is proceeding and to remember that it is extremely important to use a dynamic approach to this type of research on neurodevelopmental disorders. Children with and without disorders are all developing individuals and as such one cannot directly employ static adult neuropsychological models and solely focus on the end-state in school-age children and adults (Karmiloff-Smith, 1998). VCFS is associated with a deletion of chromosome 22q11.2 and haploinsufficiency (reduced gene dosage) of one or several genes in the deleted region is thought to lead to a disturbance in brain development. This disturbance may then result in several behavioral outcomes, which may explain the varied pattern of impairments found in this group. In addition, the origin and size of the deletion, and the occurrence of metabolic modifiers such as VEGF (Stalmans *et al.*, 2003), may be important to further delineate the spectrum of the syndrome. Hence, studies of the whole developmental trajectory of infants, children, and adults with VCFS are necessary.

With the increased characterization of the behavioral phenotype in VCFS, it seems likely that VCFS individuals do indeed have a specific cognitive profile. However, as with other developmental disorders, there is invariably considerable phenotypic variability within the group, as a consequence of both genetic and environmental factors. Hence studies of more homogenous groups of individuals with VCFS would be informative. This has been done in studies by Swillen *et al.* who have concentrated on children with an IQ higher than 70. However, future research should also try to gain insight into the cognitive processes of children with VCFS with a mild to moderate learning disability. Appropriate instruments must be developed in order to meet this goal, since many instruments and questionnaires are aimed at children with an FSIQ > 70.

Another important issue is the specificity and the developmental course of the cognitive phenotype i.e., is this cognitive phenotype specific for VCFS itself or due to confounding variables, and what is the natural course of the phenotype? These questions can be answered by longitudinal, multi-center studies with multiple appropriate (IQ-matched, chronological age-matched, siblings, controls matched for cardiac status) control groups. "It is crucial for developmental cognitive neuroscientists to launch an array of studies at first understanding and then possibly remediating some of these problems" (Simon *et al.*, in press).

Furthermore, the focus of future studies in VCFS should not only be on cognition and behavior, but also on other aspects of development such as social skills, self-image, and self-perception. An important challenge for the future is to enable monitoring of the psychological health of children and adolescents with VCFS.

From a more fundamental point of view, this type of research would enable investigations of the relative influences of genetic and environmental factors on the behavioral phenotype. Until now most research on behavioral phenotypes in genetic syndromes has focused on the child with the genetic disorder. However, the observed behaviors are also influenced by other factors such as development and environment, e.g., "parenting" and "interaction styles within families." In this view, a more interactive and dynamic approach would be valuable in the study of the behavioral phenotype.

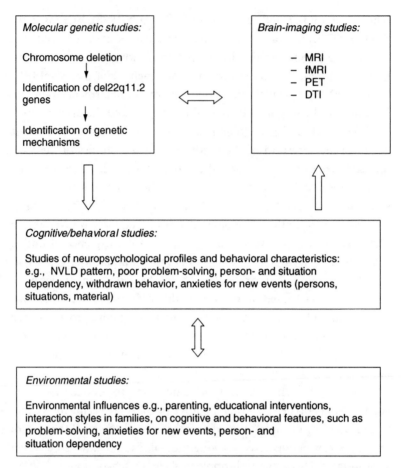

Figure 8.1   Schematic representation of different research strategies to investigate the VCFS (del 22q11.2) behavioral phenotype during childhood and adolescence (Swillen, 2001). MRI, magnetic resonance imaging; FMRI, functional MRI; PET, position emission tomography; DTI, diffusion tensor imaging.

Researchers should also try embracing a more collaborative strategy in order to focus on the establishment of links between gene(s) and brain development, and brain functioning and behavioral phenotype (neuro-cognition and behavior) (see Figure 8.1). This collaborative research would involve different disciplines (e.g., molecular geneticists, radiologists, and psychiatrists, developmental-, educational- and behavioral psychologists). The aims of these studies would be to understand brain-behavior relationships, contribute to developmental theory, and finally to understand the genetic basis of behavior in VCFS.

REFERENCES

Ashcraft, M. (1995) Cognitive psychology and simple arithmetic: a review and summary of new directions. *Math. Cogn.*, **1**, 3–34.

Bellugi, U., Marks, S., Bihrle, A. *et al.* (1988) Dissociations between language and cognitive functions in Williams syndrome. In Bishop, D. & Mogford, K., eds., *Language Development in Exceptional Circumstances*. London: Churchill Livingstone.

Bull, J. & Scerif, G. (2001) Executive functioning as a predictor of children's mathematics ability: inhibition, switching and working memory. *Dev. Neuropsychol.*, **19**, 273–93.

Butterworth, B. (1999) *The Mathematical Brain.* London: Macmillan.

Campbell, L., Stevens, A., Morris, R. *et al.* (2002) Cognitive phenotype of children with velo-cardio-facial syndrome (VCFS). In 8th Annual Meeting of the Velo-Cardio-Facial Syndrome Educational Foundation, 26–28 July, Northampton, UK.

De Smedt, B., Swillen, A., Ghesquiere, P. *et al.* (2003) Pre-academic and early academic achievement in children with velocardiofacial syndrome (del22q11.2) of borderline or normal intelligence. *Genet. Counsel.*, **14**, 15–29.

Dehaene, S. (1997) *The Number Sense.* Oxford: Oxford University Press.

Dehaene, S. & Cohen, L. (1997) Cerebral pathways for calculation: double dissociation between rote verbal and quantitative knowledge of arithmetic. *Cortex*, **33**, 219–50.

Driscoll, D. A., Spinner, N. B., Budarf, M. L. *et al.* (1992) Deletions and microdeletions of 22q11 in velo-cardio-facial syndrome. *Am. J. Med. Genet.*, **44**, 261–8.

Eliez, S., Palacieo-Espasa, F., Spira, A. *et al.* (2000) Young children with velo-cardio-facial syndrome (CATCH-22) psychological and language phenotypes. *Eur. Child. Adolesc. Psychiatry*, **9**, 109–14.

Eliez, S., Antonarakis, S. E., Morris, M. A. *et al.* (2001) Parental origin of the deletion 22q11.2 and brain development in velocardiofacial syndrome (VCFS): a preliminary study. *Arch. Gen. Psychiatry*, **58**, 64–8.

Flint, J. (1996) Annotation: behavioural phenotypes: a window onto the biology of behaviour. *J. Child Psychol. Psychiatry Allied Disc.*, **37**, 355–67.

Fuerst, K. B., Dool, C. B. & Rourke, B. P. (1995) Velocardiofacial syndrome. In Rourke, B., ed., *Syndrome of Nonverbal Learning Disabilities; Neurodevelopmental Manifestations*. New York: Guilford Press.

Geary, D., Brown, S. & Va, S. (1991) Cognitive addition: a short longitudinal study of strategy choice and speed-of-processing differences in normal and mathematically disabled children. *Dev. Psychol.*, **27**, 787–97.

Gerdes, M., Solot, C., Wang, P. P. *et al.* (1999) Cognitive and behaviour profile of pre-school children with chromosome 22q11.2 deletion. *Am. J. Med. Genet.*, **85**, 127–33.

(2001) Taking advantage of early diagnosis: preschool children with the 22q11.2 deletion. *Genet. Med.*, **3**, 40–4.

Glaser, B., Mumme, D. L., Blasey, C. *et al.* (2002) Language skills in children with velocardio-facial syndrome (deletion 22q11.2). *J. Pediatr.*, **140**, 753–8.

Golding-Kushner, K., Weller, G. & Shprintzen, R. (1985) Velo-cardio-facial syndrome: language and psychological profiles. *J. Craniofac. Genet. Dev. Biol.*, **5**, 259–66.

Heaton, R. (1981) *Wisconsin Card Sorting Test Manual*. Odessa, FL: Psychological Assessment Resources.

Henry, J. C., van Amelsvoort, T., Morris, R. G. *et al.* (2002) An investigation of the neuropsychological profile in adults with velo-cardio-facial syndrome (VCFS). *Neuropsychologia*, **40**, 471–8.

Horn, J. (1985) Remodeling old models of intelligence. In Wolman, B. B., ed., *Handbook of Intelligence, Theories, Measurements and Applications*. Chichester: John Wiley & Sons.

Horn, J. & Cattell, R. (1966) Refinement and test of the theory of fluid and crystallized intelligence. *Acta Psychol (Amst)*, **26**, 107–29.

Karmiloff-Smith, A. (1998) Development itself is the key to understanding developmental disorders. *Trends Cogn. Sci.*, **2**, 389–98.

Lezak, D. (1995) *Neuropsychological Assessment*, Third Ed. Oxford: Oxford University Press.

Lipson, A. H., Yuille, D., Angel, M. *et al.* (1991) Velo-cardio-facial (Shprintzen) syndrome: an important syndrome for the dysmorphologist to recognise. *J. Med. Genet.*, **28**, 596–604.

Morris, R., Downes, J., Sahakian, J. *et al.* (1988) Planning and spatial working memory in Parkinson's disease. *J. Neurol. Neurosurg. Psychiatry*, **51**, 757–66.

Morris, R., Downes, J. & Robbins, T. (1990) The nature of the dysexecutive syndrome in Parkinson's disease. In Gilhhly, K., Keane, M., Logie, R. & Erdos, G., eds., *Lines of thinking*. New York, NY: John Wiley & Sons Ltd.

Moss, E. M., Batshaw, M. L., Solot, C. B. *et al.* (1999) Psychoeducational profile of the 22q11.2 microdeletion: a complex pattern. *J. Pediatr.*, **134**, 193–8.

Owen, A., Morris, R., Sahakian, J. *et al.* (1996) Double dissociation of memory and executive functions in working memory tasks following frontal lobe excisions, temporal lobe excisions or amygdalo-hippocampectomy in man. *Brain*, **119**, 1597–615.

Passolunghi, M. & Siegel, L. (2001) Short-term memory, working memory and inhibitory control in children with difficulties in arithmetic problem solving. *J. Exp. Child Psychol.*, **80**, 44–57.

Rapport, L. J., Millis, S. R. & Bonello, P. J. (1998) Validation of the Warrington theory of visual processing and the visual object and space perception battery. *J. Clin. Exp. Neuropsychol.*, **20**, 211–20.

Rey, A. (1958) *L'Examen Clinique en Psychologie*. Paris: Presses Universitaires de Frances.

Rourke, B. (1987) Syndrome of nonverbal learning disabilities. The final common pathway of white-matter disease/dysfunction? *Clin. Neuropsychol.*, **1**, 209–34.

(1988) Syndrome of nonverbal learning disabilities. Developmental manifestations in neurological disease, disorder, and dysfunction. *Clin. Neuropsychol.*, **2**, 293–330.

(1989) *Nonverbal Learning Disabilities: the Syndrome and the Model*. New York, NY: Guilford Press.

(1995) *Syndrome of Nonverbal Learning Disabilities: Neurodevelopmental Manifestations*. New York, NY: Guilford Press.

Rourke, B., Young, G. & Leenaars, A. (1989) A childhood learning disability that predisposes those afflicted to adolescent and adult depression. *J. Learn. Disabil.*, **22**.

Rovet, J., Szekely, C. & MN, H. (1994) Specific arithmetic calculation deficits in children with Turner syndrome. *J. Clin. Exp. Neuropsychol.*, **16**, 820–39.

Scambler, P., Carey, A., Wuse, R. *et al.* (1991) Microdeletions within 22q11 associated with sporadic and familial DiGeorge syndrome. *Genomics*, **10**, 201–6.

Scherer, N. J., D'Antonio, L. L. & Kalbfleisch, J. H. (1999) Early speech and language development in children with velo-cardio-facial syndrome. *Am. J. Med. Genet.*, **88**, 714–23.

Shallice, T. (1982) Specific impairments of planning. *Philos. Trans. R. Soc. Lond. Biol Sci*, 199–209.

Shprintzen, R. J., Goldberg, R. B., Young, D. *et al.* (1981) The velo-cardio-facial syndrome: a clinical and genetic analysis. *Pediatrics*, **67**, 167–72.

Siegel, S. & Ryan, E. (1989) The development of working memory in normally achieving and subtypes of learning disabled children. *Child Dev.*, **60**, 973–80.

Simon, T., Bearden, C. E., McGinn, D. *et al.* (2005) Visuospatial and numerical cognitive deficits in children with chromosome 22q11.2 deletion syndrome. *Cortex.*, **41**, 145–55.

Solot, C. B., Gerdes, M., Kirschner, R. E. *et al.* (2001) Communication issues in 22q11.2 deletion syndrome: children at risk. *Genet. Med.*, **3**, 67–71.

Stalmans, I., Lambrechts, D., De Smet, F. *et al.* (2003) VEGF: a modifier of the del22q11 (DiGeorge) syndrome? *Nat. Med.*, **9**, 173–82.

Swillen, A. (2001) The behavioural phenotype in velo-cardio-facial syndrome: from infancy to adolescence [Doctoral thesis]. Leuven: Acco Leuven, University of Leuven.

Swillen, A., Fryns, J., A, K. *et al.* (1993) Intelligence, behaviour and psychosocial development in Turner syndrome. A cross-sectional study of 50 pre-adolescent and adolescent girls (4–20 years). *Genet. Couns.*, **4**, 7–18.

Swillen, A., Devriendt, K., Legius, E. *et al.* (1997) Intelligence and psychosocial adjustment in velo-cardio-facial syndrome: a study of 37 children and adolescents with VCFS. *J. Med. Genet.*, **34**, 453–8.

Swillen, A., Devriendt, K., Legius, E. *et al.* (1999a) The behavioral phenotype in velo-cardio-facial syndrome (VCFS): from infancy to adolescence. *Genet. Couns.*, **10**, 79–88.

Swillen, A., Vandeputte, L., Cracco, J. *et al.* (1999b) Neuropsychological, learning and psychosocial profile of primary school aged children with the velo-cardio-facial syndrome (22q11 deletion): evidence for a nonverbal learning disability? *Child Neuropsychol.*, **5**, 230–41.

Swillen, A., Vogels, A., Devriendt, K. *et al.* (2000) Chromosome 22q11 deletion syndrome: update and review of the clinical features, cognitive-behavioral spectrum, and psychiatric complications. *Am. J. Med. Genet.*, **97**, 128–35.

Udwin, O. & Yule, W. (1991) A cognitive and behavioral phenotype in Williams syndrome. *J. Clin. Exp. Neuropsychol.*, **13**, 232–44.

Udwin, O., Davies, M. & Howlin, P. (1996) A longitudinal study of cognitive and education attainment in Williams syndrome. *Dev. Med. Child Neurol.*, **38**, 1020–9.

Vos, P. (1988) *Bourdon Vos test: Handleiding*. Lisse: Swets & Zeitlinger.

Wang, P. P., Woodin, M. F., Kreps-Falk, R. *et al.* (2000) Research on behavioral phenotypes: velocardiofacial syndrome (deletion 22q11). *Dev. Med. Child Neurol.*, **42**, 422–7.

Wechsler, D. (1989) *Wechsler Preschool and Primary Scales of Intelligence-Revised*. San Antonio, TX: Psychological Corporation.

(1991) *Wechsler Intelligence Scales for Children – Third Edition*. San Antonio, TX: The Psychological Corporation.

Weigl, E. (1941) On the psychology of so-called processes of abstraction. *J. Abnorm. Social Psychol.*, **36**, 3–33.

Woodin, M., Wang, P., Aleman, D. *et al.* (2001) Neuropsychological profile of children and adolescents with the 22q11.2 microdeletion. *Genet. Med.*, **3**, 34–9.

9

Neuroimaging in velo-cardio-facial syndrome

Stephan Eliez[1] and Therese van Amelsvoort[2]

[1] Division of Child and Adolescent Psychiatry, Geneva University School of Medicine, Switzerland
[2] Department of Psychiatry, Academic Medical Centre, Amsterdam, Holland

Introduction

An increase in the number of publications reporting on the neuropsychiatric aspects of VCFS has been observed over the past 5 years and this is likely attributable to data suggesting that VCFS may represent a homogenous genetic subtype of schizophrenia (Bassett & Chow, 1999). The understanding of brain function and development, similar to investigating other neurogenetic or psychiatric conditions, is a necessary step for our comprehension of the cognitive, behavioral, and psychiatric phenotypes associated with VCFS (see Chapters 7 and 8). In this chapter we will discuss the currently available neuroimaging literature in people with VCFS, and how this contributes to our understanding of the neurobiology of schizophrenia in the general population.

Qualitative MRI studies in VCFS

Early neuroimaging reports emphasized qualitative differences in brain structures associated with VCFS (Mitnick *et al.*, 1994). In addition to overall brain and cortical atrophy, a high prevalence of midline defects like small corpus callosum, cavum septum pellucidum or cavum vergae, enlarged ventricles, cysts adjacent to the frontal horns of the ventricles, small posterior fossa and vermal atrophy, and white matter hyperintensities (WMHIs) have been described (Mitnick *et al.*, 1994; Lynch *et al.*, 1995; Vataja & Elomaa, 1998; Chow *et al.*, 1999; van Amelsvoort *et al.* 2001). However, these brain abnormalities are also observed in non-VCFS schizophrenia or other people with a learning disability, and their clinical significance is not known (Schaefer & Bodensteiner, 1999; Rivkin *et al.*, 2000; van Amelsvoort *et al.*, 2001; Rajarethinam *et al.*, 2001). Interestingly, recent results of a diffusion tensor imaging (DTI) study have demonstrated that WMHIs may be of vascular origin and associated with white matter tract disruption (Taylor *et al.*, 2001). Studies using these newer techniques are needed

Velo-Cardial-Facial Syndrome: A Model for Understanding Microdeletion Disorders, ed. Kieran C. Murphy and Peter J. Scambler. Published by Cambridge University Press. © Cambridge University Press, 2005.

in VCFS individuals to investigate the underlying pathogenetic mechanism of WMHIs in VCFS.

More recently, several cases of cortical dysgenesis including uni/bilateral fronto-parietal polymicrogyria have been reported in children with VCFS (Bingham *et al.*, 1998; Bird & Scambler, 2000; Kawame *et al.*, 2000; Worthington *et al.*, 2000; Ghariani *et al.*, 2002), possibly resulting in hemiplegia and seizures in the most severely affected patient. It is still unclear what the underlying pathogenetic mechanism for VCFS associated cortical dysgenesis is. Abnormal neuronal migration is one proposed explanation, but vascular disruption has also been suggested as a potential mechanism (Shprintzen *et al.*, 1997; Bird & Scambler, 2000). Classification of polymicrogyria depends on histological characterization (unlayered vs. four-layered) reflecting early (10–18th week of gestation) or later (13–24th week of gestation) developmental disorder (Guerrini *et al.*, 2000). To date no neuro-histological studies characterizing the histological type of poly-microgyria have been published on VCFS individuals. The frequency of vascular problems in VCFS, recently related to haploinsufficiency of the gene TBX1(see Chapter 2) (Merscher *et al.*, 2001), could be related to polymicrogyria resulting from perfusion failure, usually limited to the territory of a main artery or the watershed between major arterial territories (e.g., parietal lobe). Magnetic resonance angiography (MRA) of cerebral arteries revealed minor posterior arterial anomalies commonly confined to the circle of Willis, posterior cerebral artery, and the vertebral artery (Chow *et al.*, 1999).

Thus, one could hypothesize that in people with VCFS, WMHIs and cortical dysgenesis share a common pathogenetic mechanism (vascular compromise) which future studies will need to address further.

Quantitative MRI studies of children and adolescents with VCFS

Several publications have investigated quantitative volumetric changes in VCFS children and adolescents. The first study published by Eliez *et al.* (2000) reported regional brain volumes and tissue compositions for a sample of 5 females and 10 males (n = 15) with VCFS (mean age = 10.5, SD 3.1) and 15 typically developing comparison subjects (mean age = 10.8, SD 2.7). All affected subjects had been recruited through parent associations and web-based advertisement. In an attempt to limit recruitment bias toward more severely affected subjects, none of the subjects had been medically referred to the research team. Images used for analyses were high-resolution (0.94 × 0.94 × 1.5mm voxel resolution) 3D coronal SPGR type images acquired on a 1.5 Tesla GE scanner. Findings indicated that people with VCFS experience: (1) a decrease in overall brain volume due to diminution in volumes of both cerebral gray and white matter; (2) a relative enlargement of the frontal lobe after adjusting for total brain volume; (3) a decrease in tissue volume in the left parietal lobe primarily attributable to disproportionate reduction of gray matter in this region; (4) a decrease in right cerebellar tissue volume due to a disproportionate reduction in white matter for this area.

Authors underlined that, consistent with the finding of overall brain volume differences, previous clinical studies have reported a higher rate of microcephaly (40%) in individuals with VCFS (Goldberg et al., 1993). Relative frontal lobe brain volume preservation/enlargement in affected individuals might explain why, despite significant overall brain volume reduction, the majority of children and adolescents with VCFS have borderline intellectual quotients (IQ) rather than the more severe mental retardation (Swillen et al., 1997) observed in other disorders associated with microcephaly, e.g., Rett (Reiss et al., 1993) or Williams (Lenhoff et al., 1997; Reiss et al., 2000) syndrome.

This publication was also the first report implicating parietal lobe abnormalities in sensorimotor or cognitive deficits, such as learning and language difficulties, and lower performance in abstract reasoning tasks such as arithmetic (Golding-Kushner et al., 1985; Goldberg et al., 1993; Kok & Solman, 1995; Swillen et al., 1997; Eliez et al., 2001b), observed in VCFS individuals. Thus, at least part of the cognitive phenotype associated with VCFS could be explained by parietal lobe dysfunction. In addition, the crucial role of the parietal lobe in memory has been demonstrated in functional imaging studies (Ungerleider, 1995). Increased activity has been observed in the parietal lobe region during episodic memory retrieval (Shallice et al., 1994), working memory tasks, implicit or explicit recognition memory (Rugg et al., 1998), and long-term memory consolidation (Shadmehr & Holcomb, 1997). Consequently, parietal lobe aberration may damage information storage and retrieval and may contribute to learning difficulties in VCFS. Specific deficits in language or in phonological processing could also be partially explained by an alteration in parietal lobe function.

Another study by Kates et al. (2001) compared ten subjects with VCFS (mean age $= 10.1 \pm 1.8$) with ten typically developing age- and gender-matched controls. The authors found white matter reduction in the posterior brain regions (parietal and occipital lobes). An association between full-scale IQ and total cerebral tissue was demonstrated in both groups.

Using functional MRI (fMRI) methods, the same group of researchers, using a subsample of individuals previously published (Eliez et al., 2001b), explored differences in brain activation patterns between eight persons with VCFS (three females and five males; mean age 15.5 ± 3.6 years) and eight matched typically developing controls (three females and five males; mean age 15.8 ± 4.1 years) during a mathematical reasoning task hypothesized to activate the parietal lobe. Experimental epochs consisted of five, two (easy) or three (hard) operand addition/subtraction problems with either a correct or an incorrect resultant (e.g., $6 - 3 + 5 = 8$ or $6 + 2 = 5$). Half of the results were correct and required a button press, and the other half were incorrect. When comparing left supramarginal gyrus (SMG) activation by task condition, results indicated a significant group difference in the patterns of activation during the "easy" and "difficult" conditions of the math task. People with VCFS showed a distinct increase in activation during the "difficult" condition, whereas controls showed equivalent levels of activation during both conditions. Results comparing the mean percent activation in the left SMG indicated significant group differences only during the "difficult" math task and not during the "easy" math task. Voxel-based analyses contrasting the "difficult" three operand computation with the control task pointed to two large clusters or regions that showed significantly more activation in subjects with VCFS than controls. The maximum difference was observed in the posterior left precentral gyrus. Extending from this region, activation was observed at the juncture between the left lateral fissure (Brodman's Area (BA) 4/6) and the left SMG (BA 40). The second area of activation centered in the right insular gyri and parietal operculum and extended into the right intraparietal sulcus and the right SMG.

In summary, a significant increase in neuronal activity in the left supramarginal gyrus was observed during the more difficult arithmetic problems in subjects with VCFS. This finding supports our a priori hypothesis that parietal lobe function is altered in VCFS individuals and is consistent with the previous report of structural abnormalities in this region (Eliez et al., 2000). Accordingly, alteration in parietal lobe morphology may contribute to decreased math performance commonly reported among children with VCFS.

Structural alteration of the cerebellum in children and adolescents with VCFS was congruent with several qualitative studies reporting reduction in posterior fossa, cerebellum, or vermis (Mitnick et al., 1994; Lynch et al., 1995; Devriendt et al., 1996; Chow et al., 1999). Eliez et al. (2001d) have reported that the reduction of cerebellar volume was associated with a decrease of the vermis (segment VI–VII) and the pons.

Developmentally, the pons and the cerebellum share a common cellular ancestry. During embryogenesis, the pons and the cerebellum arise primarily from the metencephalon, the most anterior region of the hindbrain (rombencephalon), developmentally distinct from both the midbrain and the medulla (Moore & Persaud, 1993; Rowitch et al., 1999). Interestingly, the cerebellar hemispheres and posterior vermis are predominantly derived from metencephalic tissue, while the tissue of the anterior vermis, like the midbrain, is of mesencephalic origin (Martinez & Alvarado-Mallart, 1989; Hallonet et al., 1990; Millet et al., 1996; Rowitch et al., 1999). This may explain why no significant differences were found in volumes of the anterior vermis of VCFS individuals.

In addition, the pons and the cerebellum are cytoarchitecturally linked. The basal pontine nuclei project major afferent pathways to the cerebellar cortex (Yachnis & Rorke, 1999). These projections are in the form of mossy fibers from the basis pontis which synapse on Purkinje cells early in development (Grishkat & Eisenman, 1995; Yachnis & Rorke, 1999). In addition, all of the neurons in the basis pontis project exclusively to the cerebellum while the corticopontocerebellar pathway is the primary method of communication between cerebrum and cerebellum (Schmahmann & Pandya, 1991). Since a lack of adequate stimulation can cause neuron death during development (LeVay et al., 1978; Cabelli et al., 1995), it is possible that damage to the pons may in turn result in a degeneration of cerebellar tissue.

VCFS is not the first neurogenetic condition to reportedly have an aberrant posterior fossa and cerebellar vermal size. Specifically, Joubert syndrome and Fragile X both have been shown to have decreased vermal areas (Holroyd et al., 1991; Guerreiro et al., 1998; Mostofsky et al., 1998). Subjects with both Joubert syndrome and Fragile X also typically present with social and communication problems resembling autistic behavior (Cohen et al., 1988, 1991; Holroyd et al., 1991). Conversely, subjects with Williams syndrome, who are unusually socially outgoing and overly friendly, show a significant increase in the posterior vermis and the neocerebellar hemispheres relative to normal controls (Reiss et al., 2000; Schmitt et al., 2001). Thus, there appears to be a possible relationship between posterior vermis size and level of social drive as evidenced by comparing neurogenetic disorders with prominent affective components.

These observations are concordant with the description of specific social difficulties in VCFS (see Chapter 7). All the studies reporting observations of social behavior point to poor social interaction, shyness, behavioral inhibition, and withdrawal (Golding-Kushner et al., 1985; Swillen et al., 1997, 1999; Gerdes et al., 1999). Social, communication, and depression problems described in the samples of children with VCFS could be a prelude to the later development of psychiatric disorders like schizophrenia (Nicolson & Rapoport, 2000; Ichimiya et al., 2001). Additionally, an alteration of the cortico-cerebellar-thalamic-circuit (CCTCC) potentially leading to "cognitive dysmetria" (Andreasen et al., 1998; Nopoulos et al., 1999) could be responsible for the disruption of the fluid, coordinate sequences of normal thought processes observed in subjects with VCFS.

Given the overlap in psychiatric features between the VCFS and schizophrenia, Eliez et al. analyzed the similarities between the present imaging findings in VCFS and earlier reports concerning structural changes in the brains of individuals with schizophrenia (Shenton et al., 2001). Previous studies on schizophrenia have reported a decrease in overall brain size especially in early-onset schizophrenia (Jacobsen et al., 1996, 1998). Frontal and temporal lobe abnormalities have been observed as slight reductions in persons with schizophrenia. Subjects with VCFS also showed an alteration in the frontal lobe although the changes were counter-intuitive as authors found that this region was actually enlarged. Contrary to what was hypothesized by the authors, no reduction of temporal lobe was demonstrated in this sample. This rather unexpected finding triggered further studies (Eliez *et al.*, 2001c) on a larger sample (23 subjects, 8 females and 15 males age- and gender-matched with 23 typically developing controls; ages ranged from 5.8–21.0 years: VCFS =12.7 ± 3.9; control =12.9 ± 4.1). Using cross-sectional data analysis, changes of temporal and mesio-temporal lobe structures in individuals with VCFS compared with typically developing subjects were investigated. According to the authors, VCFS children and adolescents experience marked neuroanatomical alterations in the temporal lobe region, and that these aberrations occur within the context of a reduction of total brain volume. Specifically, temporal gray matter volume and left hippocampal gray were reduced with age. Superior temporal gyrus or amygdala did not change significantly with age between groups.

Quantitative MRI studies of VCFS adults

Compared with the literature in children and adolescents with VCFS, there are relatively few quantitative MRI studies of VCFS adults. In the first quantitative MRI study of VCFS adults, van Amelsvoort *et al.* (2001) reported that, when compared with IQ-matched controls, VCFS adults have a smaller cerebellar volume. This finding is in agreement with findings from earlier mentioned qualitative MRI studies (Mitnick *et al.*, 1994; Lynch *et al.*, 1995), and from a quantitative study of VCFS children and adolescents (Eliez *et al.*, 2001). In contrast to Eliez *et al.* (2001), while they did not quantify cerebellar hemispheres and vermis separately, they found a significantly reduced gray matter volume in left cerebellar hemisphere suggesting that not only vermis but also cerebellar hemispheres are affected in VCFS. Furthermore, cerebellar dysfunction could also partially explain VCFS associated deficits in cognitive domains such as planning, problem solving, and visuo-spatial functioning (Henry *et al.*, 2002), via cortico-cerebellar circuits.

Although the authors did not find a significant reduction in total volume of gray, and white matter and CSF, they found widespread deficits in white matter, extending bilaterally in frontal, temporal, and occipito-parietal regions (Figure 9.1).

This finding supports findings observed in a study by Kates *et al.* (2001) who found white matter reduction in posterior brain regions in VCFS children. These findings, taken together in addition to the high prevalence of WMHIs in VCFS individuals, suggest that white matter may be particularly compromised in people with VCFS. Localized gray matter differences were also reported by van Amelsvoort *et al.* (2001); deficits in right temporal and left cerebellar regions,

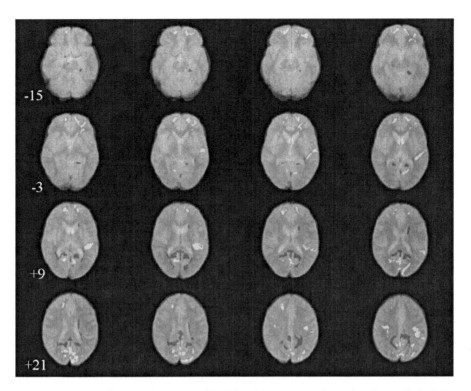

Figure 9.1   Relative deficits (yellow) and excesses (blue) in white matter volume in velo-cardio-facial syndrome compared with controls. The maps are oriented with the right side of the brain shown on the left side of each panel. The z-coordinate for each row of axial slices in the standard space of Talairach & Tournoux (1988) is given in millimetres. See color plate.

and excesses in left insula and frontal region. The authors point out that their results are unlikely confounded by the impaired level of intellectual functioning of people with VCFS because they used IQ-matched controls in contrast to other MRI studies in people with VCFS. However, they point out that their results could have been confounded by the presence of psychosis because their VCFS population included both people with and without schizophrenia.

More recently, Chow *et al.* (2002) reported that adults with VCFS and schizophrenia, compared with healthy non-VCFS controls, had a smaller volume of total gray matter, regional differences in gray and white matter in frontal, temporal, parietal, and occipital lobes, and an increased volume of ventricular and sulcal CSF bilaterally. Although this study is an important first step, their control group was not matched for IQ and so the differences they report may be confounded by differences in subject intelligence e.g., IQ is positively correlated with cortical gray matter (Reiss *et al.*, 1996). In addition, they studied subjects with VCFS and schizophrenia only, and not those with VCFS who did not develop schizophrenia.

In order to control for these confounding factors, studies examining brain anatomy within VCFS and comparing those with and without schizophrenia are necessary.

Preliminary results of an extended study by van Amelsvoort *et al.* (2004) suggest that within VCFS, adults with schizophrenia have a reduced total brain volume and increased CSF volume compared with those without schizophrenia, and regional differences particularly in frontal regions. Furthermore white matter seems to be more affected than gray matter. Even though they are only preliminary results, they are the first to make comparisons within the VCFS population. The results are in agreement with the large body of neuroimaging literature in the general population with schizophrenia. The most consistently reported structural brain abnormalities in people with schizophrenia are an increased volume of cerebral ventricles and a reduced volume of total brain (and gray matter) volume (Shenton *et al.*, 2001). In addition, localized volume reductions have been frequently reported in temporo-limbic and frontal neocortical regions. There are fewer studies reporting on white matter in schizophrenia but using newer techniques such as DTI, decreased white matter integrity has also been reported in people with schizophrenia (Lim *et al.*, 1999).

An interesting observation is that MRI studies in children report relatively larger frontal lobe volumes (Eliez *et al.*, 2000; Kates *et al.*, 2001), whereas those in adults find no difference in volume albeit with differences in tissue composition (van Amelsvoort *et al.*, 2001), or reduced volume of frontal lobes (Chow *et al.*, 2002; van Amelsvoort *et al.*, 2002). Since the process of brain maturation (i.e., reduction of gray matter volume as a result of increased synaptic pruning, and increase in white matter volume as a result of increased myelination), takes last place in the frontal regions, dysmaturation in people with VCFS could underlie increased liability for psychosis (Giedd *et al.*, 1999; Sowell *et al.*, 1999; van Amelsvoort *et al.*, 2002).

A recent study investigating white matter in VCFS using DTI neuroimaging methods (Barnea-Goraly *et al.*, 2003) compared 19 children and young adults with age- and gender-matched controls. Compared with the control group, the VCFS group had reduced white matter anisotropy in the frontal, parietal, and temporal regions, as well as in tracts connecting the frontal and temporal lobes (Filley, 2001) (left external/extreme capsule including the superior and inferior longitudinal fasiculus). This finding suggests disrupted fronto-temporal connectivity in VCFS, which is of interest considering recent findings reported in samples of patients with schizophrenia. Preliminary studies using structural and functional imaging modalities reported that fronto-temporal connectivity could be disrupted in schizophrenia (Friston & Frith, 1995; Ford *et al.*, 2002). Investigating white matter tract integrity, a recent DTI study demonstrated aberrant connectivity in the uncinate fasciculus, one of the fronto-temporal pathways, in individuals with schizophrenia (Kubicki *et al.*, 2002). It has been hypothesized that disruption in fronto-temporal connectivity may underlie failure to recognize inner speech as self-generated (Feinberg & Guazzelli, 1999; Ford et al., 2002). Multimodal neuro-imaging studies (DTI and fMRI) will have to investigate the impact of fronto-temporal white matter tract disruption on auditory hallucination symptoms in schizophrenia and VCFS.

In summary, even though the available literature is still limited, and methodo-logical differences between the existing studies make it difficult to draw conclu-sions, the current literature suggests that the adult VCFS population has brain abnormalities that particularly affect cerebellum, and that within this population those who develop schizophrenia have generalized reduced brain volume, which might reflect genetically determined aberrant neurodevelopment.

Effects of imprinting

It has been suggested that, within the VCFS population, additional genetic factors may modulate the neurobehavioral phenotype (Ryan et al., 1997; Swillen et al., 1997; Eliez et al., 2001a). One recent report proposed that parental origin of the deletion impacts brain development (Eliez et al., 2001a). Moreover, other studies, primarily involving subjects transmitted through maternal germ line cells, showed that familial transmission indicates lower cognitive outcomes than de novo cases (Ryan et al., 1997; Swillen et al., 1997). Considered together, these studies could suggest that the greater severity of disabilities may be explained by maternal origin of the deletion rather than by familial transmission, which would imply an imprinting effect due to the parental origin of the deletion. Imprinting is a genetic mechanism in which gene expression is modulated by the parental origin of the chromosome on which the gene is located (Greally & State, 2000). Research on imprinting has shown that parental origin of a genomic deletion can affect the physical and cognitive phenotype of individuals with the genetic disorder (Prows & Hopkin, 1999).

A study (Eliez et al., 2001a) investigated the impact of parental origin of the deletion on brain development among 18 subjects, 11 males and 7 females aged 11.9 ± 3.3 years (ranging 6.3–17.9 years), diagnosed with a 22q11.2 3mb de novo microdeletion. Nine subjects (6 males / 3 females; 12.1 ± 2.9 years old) had a mater-nal origin of the deletion and nine subjects (5 Males / 4 Females; 11.8 ± 3.9 years old) had a paternal origin of the deletion. Eighteen normal control subjects were matched for gender and age (mean age = 12.5 ± 3.8, ranging from 5.8–19.1 years).

Similar to previous studies, total brain tissue volume was approximately 11% smaller in the VCFS group relative to the control group. Both gray and white matter contributed to this difference. When the two parental origin subgroups were compared to the control group, the subgroup with maternal-origin deletions

showed significantly decreased volumes of both gray and white matter compartments. In contrast, the subgroup with deletions of paternal origin showed only
decreased cerebral white matter relative to control subjects. Finally, the follow-up
tests comparing VCFS subgroups (maternal vs. paternal) indicated that children
with the deletion on the maternal chromosome 22 had significantly decreased gray
matter volumes but no significant difference in white matter volume.

Regression analyses indicated that age significantly predicted gray matter
volume decrease only for maternally deleted subjects ($R^2 = 0.58$; $p = 0.017$).
Utilizing a follow-up Fisher r to z transformation, the age/gray matter correlations
of control subjects and subjects with VCFS with the deletion on the maternal
chromosome 22 were compared for the maternally deleted VCFS and control
groups; this comparison reaches statistical significance on a one-tailed comparison. Imprinting and inhibition of the expression of at least one gene affecting
neuronal proliferation or cell death, dendritic arborization, or creation and elimination of synapses is a possible explanation for these results. Because white matter
tissue tends to be reduced independent of parental origin of the deletion, it seems
likely that haploinsufficiency (reduced gene dosage) of another distinct gene(s)
also mapping to chromosome 22q11.2 is responsible for this effect. Clear limita-
tions of this preliminary study resided in the limited sample sizes and the cross-
sectional nature of data.

Discussion

Smaller gray matter volume exhibited by children with maternal deletion origin
may place these subjects at increased risk for childhood or adult-onset schizophrenia. Recent publications in schizophrenia have demonstrated the potential
significance of cortical gray reduction and support the hypothesis of a premorbid
neurodevelopmental etiological process. In a longitudinal study, Thompson et al.
(2001) showed that an alteration of cortical gray matter first developed in the
parietal regions, then progressed towards frontal and temporal lobe, finally resulting in a severe overall gray matter reduction over a course of 4 years. In people with
adult-onset schizophrenia, gray matter volume reduction is already evident at the
first clinical presentation of the disorder, and appears to at least partially explain
the morbid (Gold et al., 1999; Gur et al., 1999; Mohamed et al., 1999; Thompson
et al., 2001) and premorbid cognitive features (Cannon et al., 2002; Fuller et al.,
2002) associated with this condition. Further, differences in the amount of gray
matter volume decrease over time, modulated by parental origin of the deletion as
other factors – yet to be identified – could explain the observed variability in the
age of onset of schizophrenia in the VCFS population. Figure 9.2, concordant with
a developmental model proposed by McGlashan (McGlashan & Hoffman, 2000),

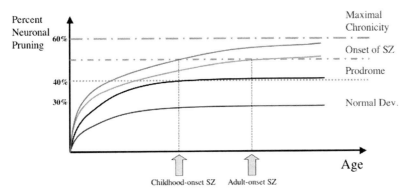

Figure 9.2 Model of reduced synaptic density over time and development of psychosis. The differential pruning rate accounts for the variability of the age of onset and also the course of the psychotic disorder.

illustrates the potential impact of gray matter decrease rate on age-of-onset of clinical symptoms, duration of prodromal phase before the expression of schizophrenia, and age at which the negative symptoms are predominant.

As suggested by McGlashan and other authors, the reduction of gray matter volumes in schizophrenia is principally due to the abnormal dendritic arborization, resulting in excessive pruning, rather than decreased number of neurons. One might speculate that identical neurohistological characteristics are responsible for the gray matter volume decrease observed in individuals with VCFS. To date, no detailed postmortem neuroanatomical and neurohistological studies have been published on human or animal models. These studies also are most needed in order to understand the relation between alteration of white and gray matter compartments: are both compartments separately affected? Is the alteration of the axonal tracts responsible or resulting from abnormal neuronal arborization? What proportion of neuroanatomical changes can be attributed to vascular abnormalities? Is polymicrogyria associated with VCFS secondary to vascular abnormalities or due to another developmental abnormality? Indeed, schizophrenia is increasingly seen by some as a supraregional disorder involving interconnecting white matter tracts (Sigmundsson *et al.*, 2001), and studies using newer neuroimaging techniques such as DTI do report abnormalities of white matter structure (Lim *et al.*, 1999). Most likely answers to these questions will require larger and longitudinal MRI studies as well as neurohistological studies on single-gene knock-out animal models to help us understand the contributions of the different genes, as well as secondary expressed genes, related to the commonly 3MB deleted region.

Ultimately, understanding how specific genes impact brain development and neuronal function will help us to better understand the specific cognitive and psychiatric profile associated with VCFS, and better address the needs of affected individuals and their families. VCFS is a model system for examining the multifaceted nature of behavioral development that will give us insight into pathways leading to schizophrenia. Methodological approaches, developed to study neurogenetic disorders like VCFS, will set a path and make tools available for the investigation of future candidate gene(s) in schizophrenia, mood disorders, or ADHD.

REFERENCES

Andreasen, N. C., Paradiso, S. & O'Leary, D. S. (1998) "Cognitive dysmetria" as an integrative theory of schizophrenia: a dysfunction in cortical-subcortical-cerebellar circuitry? *Schizophr. Bull.*, **24** (2), 203–18.

Barnea-Goraly, N., Menon, V., Krasnow, B. *et al.* (2003) Investigation of white matter structure in velocardiofacial syndrome: a diffusion tensor imaging study. *Am. J. Psychiatry*, **160 (10)**, 1863–9.

Bassett, A. S. & Chow, E. W. (1999) 22q11 deletion syndrome: a genetic subtype of schizophrenia. *Biol. Psychiatry*, **46 (7)**, 882–91.

Bingham, P. M., Lynch, D., McDonald-McGinn, D. *et al.* (1998) Polymicrogyria in chromosome 22 delection syndrome. *Neurology*, **51 (5)**, 1500–2.

Bird, L. M. & Scambler, P. (2000) Cortical dysgenesis in 2 patients with chromosome 22q11 deletion. *Clin. Genet.*, **58 (1)**, 64–8.

Cabelli, R. J., Hohn, A. & Shatz, C. J. (1995) Inhibition of ocular dominance column formation by infusion of NT-4/5 or BDNF. *Science*, **267 (5204)**, 1662–6.

Cannon, M., Caspi, A., Moffitt, T. E. *et al.* (2002) Evidence for early-childhood, pan-developmental impairment specific to schizophreniform disorder: results from a longitudinal birth cohort. *Arch. Gen. Psychiatry*, **59 (5)**, 449–56.

Chow, E. W., Mikulis, D. J., Zipursky, R. B. *et al.* (1999) Qualitative MRI findings in adults with 22q11 deletion syndrome and schizophrenia. *Biol. Psychiatry*, **46 (10)**, 1436–42.

Chow, E. W., Zipursky, R. B., Mikulis, D. J. *et al.* (2002) Structural brain abnormalities in patients with schizophrenia and 22q11 deletion syndrome. *Biol. Psychiatry*, **51 (3)**, 208–15.

Cohen, I. L., Fisch, G. S., Sudhalter, V. *et al.* (1988) Social gaze, social avoidance, and repetitive behavior in fragile X males: a controlled study. *Am. J. Ment. Retard*, **92 (5)**, 436–46.

Cohen, I. L., Vietze, P. M., Sudhalter, V. *et al.* (1991) Effects of age and communication level on eye contact in fragile X males and non-fragile X autistic males. *Am. J. Med. Genet.*, **38 (2–3)**, 498–502.

Devriendt, K., Thienen, M. N., Swillen, A. *et al.* (1996) Cerebellar hypoplasia in a patient with velo-cardio-facial syndrome. *Dev. Med. Child Neurol.*, **38 (10)**, 949–53.

Eliez, S., Schmitt, J. E., White, C. D. *et al.* (2000) Children and adolescents with velocardiofacial syndrome: a volumetric MRI study. *Am. J. Psychiatry*, **157 (3)**, 409–15.

Eliez, S., Antonarakis, S. E., Morris, M. A. *et al.* (2001a) Parental origin of the deletion 22q11.2 and brain development in velocardiofacial syndrome: a preliminary study. *Arch. Gen. Psychiatry*, **58 (1)**, 64–8.

Eliez, S., Blasey, C. M., Menon, V. *et al.* (2001b) Functional brain imaging study of mathematical reasoning abilities in velocardiofacial syndrome (del22q11.2). *Genet. Med.*, **3** (1), 49–55.

Eliez, S., Blasey, C. M., Schmitt, E. J. *et al.* (2001c) Velocardiofacial syndrome: are structural changes in the temporal and mesial temporal regions related to schizophrenia? *Am. J. Psychiatry*, **158** (3), 447–53.

Eliez, S., Schmitt, J. E., White, C. D. *et al.* (2001d) A quantitative MRI study of posterior fossa development in velocardiofacial syndrome. *Biol. Psychiatry*, **49** (6), 540–6.

Feinberg, I. & Guazzelli, M. (1999) Schizophrenia – a disorder of the corollary discharge systems that integrate the motor systems of thought with the sensory systems of consciousness. *Br. J. Psychiatry*, **174**, 196–204.

Filley, M. C. (2001) *The Behavioral Neurology of White Matter*. Oxford: Oxford University Press.

Ford, J. M., Mathalon, D. H., Whitfield, S. *et al.* (2002) Reduced communication between frontal and temporal lobes during talking in schizophrenia. *Biol. Psychiatry*, **51** (6), 485–92.

Friston, K. J. & Frith, C. D. (1995) Schizophrenia: a disconnection syndrome? *Clin. Neurosci.*, **3** (2), 89–97.

Fuller, R., Nopoulos, P., Arndt, S. *et al.* (2002) Longitudinal assessment of premorbid cognitive functioning in patients with schizophrenia through examination of standardized scholastic test performance. *Am. J. Psychiatry*, **159** (7), 1183–9.

Gerdes, M., Solot, C., Wang, P. P. *et al.* (1999) Cognitive and behavior profile of preschool children with chromosome 22q11.2 deletion. *Am. J. Med. Genet.*, **85** (2), 127–33.

Ghariani, S., Dahan, K., Saint-Martin, C. *et al.* (2002) Polymicrogyria in chromosome 22q11 deletion syndrome. *Eur. J. Paediatr. Neurol.*, **6** (1), 73–7.

Giedd, J. N., Blumenthal, J., Jeffries, N. O. *et al.* (1999) Brain development during childhood and adolescence: a longitudinal MRI study. *Nat. Neurosci.*, **2** (10), 861–3.

Gold, S., Arndt, S., Nopoulos, P. *et al.* (1999) Longitudinal study of cognitive function in first-episode and recent-onset schizophrenia. *Am. J. Psychiatry*, **156** (9), 1342–8.

Goldberg, R., Motzkin, B., Marion, R. *et al.* (1993) Velo-cardio-facial syndrome: a review of 120 patients. *Am. J. Med. Genet.*, **45** (3), 313–19.

Golding-Kushner, K. J., Weller, G. & Shprintzen, R. J. (1985) Velo-cardio-facial syndrome: language and psychological profiles. *J. Craniofac. Genet. Dev. Biol.*, **5** (3), 259–66.

Greally, J. M. & State, M. W. (2000) Genetics of childhood disorders: XIII. Genomic imprinting: the indelible mark of the gamete. *J. Am. Acad. Child, Adolesc. Psychiatry*, **39** (4), 532–5.

Grishkat, H. L. & Eisenman, L. M. (1995) Development of the spinocerebellar projection in the prenatal mouse. *J. Comp. Neurol.*, **363** (1), 93–108.

Guerreiro, M. M., Camargo, E. E., Kato, M. *et al.* (1998) Fragile X syndrome. Clinical, electroencephalographic and neuroimaging characteristics. *Arq. Neuropsiquiatr.*, **56** (1), 18–23.

Guerrini, R., Barkovich, A. J., Sztriha, L. *et al.* (2000) Bilateral frontal polymicrogyria: a newly recognized brain malformation syndrome. *Neurology*, **54** (4), 909–13.

Gur, R. E., Turetsky, B. I., Bilker, W. B. *et al.* (1999) Reduced gray matter volume in schizophrenia. *Arch. Gen. Psychiatry*, **56** (10), 905–11.

Hallonet, M. E., Teillet, M. A. & Le Douarin, N. M. (1990) A new approach to the development of the cerebellum provided by the quail-chick marker system. *Development*, **108** (1), 19–31.

Henry, J. C., van Amelsvoort, T., Morris, R. G. *et al.* (2002) An investigation of the neuropsychological profile in adults with velo-cardio-facial syndrome (VCFS). *Neuropsychologia*, **40 (5)**, 471–8.

Holroyd, S., Reiss, A. L. & Bryan, R. N. (1991) Autistic features in Joubert syndrome: a genetic disorder with agenesis of the cerebellar vermis. *Biol. Psychiatry*, **29 (3)**, 287–94.

Ichimiya, T., Okubo, Y., Suhara, T. *et al.* (2001) Reduced volume of the cerebellar vermis in neuroleptic-naive schizophrenia. *Biol. Psychiatry*, **49 (1)**, 20–7.

Jacobsen, L. K., Giedd, J. N., Vaituzis, A. C. *et al.* (1996) Temporal lobe morphology in childhood-onset schizophrenia. *Am. J. Psychiatry*, **153 (3)**, 355–61.

Jacobsen, L. K., Giedd, J. N., Castellanos, F. X. *et al.* (1998) Progressive reduction of temporal lobe structures in childhood-onset schizophrenia. *Am. J. Psychiatry*, **155 (5)**, 678–85.

Kates, W. R., Burnette, C. P., Jabs, E. W. *et al.* (2001) Regional cortical white matter reductions in velocardiofacial syndrome: a volumetric MRI analysis. *Biol. Psychiatry*, **49 (8)**, 677–84.

Kawame, H., Kurosawa, K., Akatsuka, A. *et al.* (2000) Polymicrogyria is an uncommon manifestation in 22q11.2 deletion syndrome. *Am. J. Med. Genet.*, **94 (1)**, 77–8.

Kok, L. L. & Solman, R. T. (1995) Velocardiofacial syndrome: learning difficulties and intervention. *J. Med. Genet.*, **32 (8)**, 612–18.

Kubicki, M., Westin, C. F., Maier, S. E. *et al.* (2002) Uncinate fasciculus findings in schizophrenia: a magnetic resonance diffusion tensor imaging study. *Am. J. Psychiatry*, **159 (5)**, 813–20.

Lenhoff, H. M., Wang, P. P., Greenberg, F. *et al.* (1997) Williams syndrome and the brain. *Sci. Am.*, **277 (6)**, 68–73.

LeVay, S., Stryker, M. P. & Shatz, C. J. (1978) Ocular dominance columns and their development in layer IV of the cat's visual cortex: a quantitative study. *J. Comp. Neurol.*, **179 (1)**, 223–44.

Lim, K. O., Hedehus, M., Moseley, M. *et al.* (1999) Compromised white matter tract integrity in schizophrenia inferred from diffusion tensor imaging. *Arch. Gen. Psychiatry*, **56 (4)**, 367–74.

Lynch, D. R., McDonald-McGinn, D. M., Zackai, E. H. *et al.* (1995) Cerebellar atrophy in a patient with velocardiofacial syndrome. *J. Med. Genet.*, **32 (7)**, 561–3.

Martinez, S. & Alvarado-Mallart, R. (1989) Rostral cerebellum originates from the caudal portion of the so-called 'mesencephalic' vesicle: a study using chick/quail chimeras. *Eur. J. Neurosci.*, **1**, 549–60.

McGlashan, T. H. & Hoffman, R. E. (2000) Schizophrenia as a disorder of developmentally reduced synaptic connectivity. *Arch. Gen. Psychiatry*, **57 (7)**, 637–48.

Merscher, S., Funke, B., Epstein, J. A. *et al.* (2001) TBX1 is responsible for cardiovascular defects in velo-cardio-facial/DiGeorge syndrome. *Cell*, **104 (4)**, 619–29.

Millet, S., Bloch-Gallego, E., Simeone, A. *et al.* (1996) The caudal limit of Otx2 gene expression as a marker of the midbrain/hindbrain boundary: a study using in situ hybridisation and chick/quail homotopic grafts. *Development*, **122 (12)**, 3785–97.

Mitnick, R. J., Bello, J. A. & Shprintzen, R. J. (1994) Brain anomalies in velo-cardio-facial syndrome. *Am. J. Med. Genet.*, **54 (2)**, 100–6.

Mohamed, S., Paulsen, J. S., O'Leary, D. *et al.* (1999) Generalized cognitive deficits in schizophrenia: a study of first-episode patients. *Arch. Gen. Psychiatry*, **56 (8)**, 749–54.

Moore, K. L. & Persaud, T. V. N. (1993) *The Developing Human: Clinically Oriented Embryology*. Philadelphia, PA: WB Saunders Company.

Mostofsky, S. H., Mazzocco, M. M., Aakalu, G. *et al.* (1998) Decreased cerebellar posterior vermis size in fragile X syndrome: correlation with neurocognitive performance. *Neurology*, **50 (1)**, 121–30.

Nicolson, R. & Rapoport, J. L. (2000). Childhood-onset schizophrenia: what can it teach us? In Rapoport, J. L., ed., *Childhood Onset of "Adult" Psychopathology*. Washington, DC: American Psychiatric Press, pp. 167–92.

Nopoulos, P. C., Ceilley, J. W., Gailis, E. A. *et al.* (1999) An MRI study of cerebellar vermis morphology in patients with schizophrenia: evidence in support of the cognitive dysmetria concept. *Biol. Psychiatry*, **46 (5)**, 703–11.

Prows, C. A. & Hopkin, R. J. (1999) Prader Willi and Angelman syndromes: exemplars of genomic imprinting. *J. Perinat. Neonatal. Nurs.*, **13 (2)**, 76–89.

Rajarethinam, R., Miedler, J., DeQuardo, J. *et al.* (2001) Prevalence of cavum septum pellucidum in schizophrenia studied with MRI. *Schizophr. Res.*, **48 (2–3)**, 201–5.

Reiss, A. L., Faruque, F., Naidu, S. *et al.* (1993) Neuroanatomy of Rett syndrome: a volumetric imaging study. *Ann. Neurol.*, **34 (2)**, 227–34.

Reiss, A. L., Abrams, M. T., Singer, H. S. *et al.* (1996) Brain development, gender and IQ in children. A volumetric imaging study. *Brain*, **119 (Pt 5)**, 1763–74.

Reiss, A. L., Eliez, S., Schmitt, J. E. *et al.* (2000) IV. Neuroanatomy of Williams syndrome: a high-resolution MRI study. *J. Cogn. Neurosci.*, **12 Suppl. 1**, 65–73.

Rivkin, P., Kraut, M., Barta, P. *et al.* (2000) White matter hyperintensity volume in late-onset and early-onset schizophrenia. *Int. J. Geriatr. Psychiatry*, **15 (12)**, 1085–9.

Rowitch, D. H., Danielian, P. S., McMahon, A. P. *et al.* (1999) Cystic malformation of the posterior cerebellar vermis in transgenic mice that ectopically express Engrailed-1, a homeodomain transcription factor. *Teratology*, **60 (1)**, 22–8.

Rugg, M. D., Mark, R. E., Walla, P. *et al.* (1998) Dissociation of the neural correlates of implicit and explicit memory. *Nature*, **392 (6676)**, 595–8.

Ryan, A. K., Goodship, J. A., Wilson, D. I. *et al.* (1997) Spectrum of clinical features associated with interstitial chromosome 22q11 deletions: a European collaborative study. *J. Med. Genet.*, **34 (10)**, 798–804.

Schaefer, G. B. & Bodensteiner, J. B. (1999) Developmental anomalies of the brain in mental retardation. *Int. Rev. Psychiatry*, **11**, 47–55.

Schmahmann, J. D. & Pandya, D. N. (1991) Projections to the basis pontis from the superior temporal sulcus and superior temporal region in the rhesus monkey. *J. Comp. Neurol.*, **308 (2)**, 224–48.

Schmitt, J. E., Eliez, S., Warsofsky, I. S. *et al.* (2001) Enlarged cerebellar vermis in Williams syndrome. *J. Psychiatr. Res.*, **35 (4)**, 225–9.

Shadmehr, R. & Holcomb, H. H. (1997) Neural correlates of motor memory consolidation. *Science*, **277 (5327)**, 821–5.

Shallice, T., Fletcher, P., Frith, C. D. *et al.* (1994) Brain regions associated with acquisition and retrieval of verbal episodic memory. *Nature*, **368 (6472)**, 633–5.

Shenton, M. E., Dickey, C. C., Frumin, M. *et al.* (2001) A review of MRI findings in schizophrenia. *Schizophr. Res.*, **49 (1–2)**, 1–52.

Shprintzen, R. J., Morrow, B. & Kucherlapati, R. (1997) Vascular anomalies may explain many of the features in velo-cardio-facial syndrome. *Am. J. Hum. Gene*, **61**, A5.

Sigmundsson, T., Suckling, J., Maier, M. *et al.* (2001) Structural abnormalities in frontal, temporal, and limbic regions and interconnecting white matter tracts in schizophrenic patients with prominent negative symptoms. *Am. J. Psychiatry*, **158 (2)**, 234–43.

Sowell, E. R., Thompson, P. M., Holmes, C. J. *et al.* (1999) In vivo evidence for post-adolescent brain maturation in frontal and striatal regions. *Nat. Neurosci.*, **2 (10)**, 859–61.

Swillen, A., Devriendt, K., Legius, E. *et al.* (1997) Intelligence and psychosocial adjustment in velocardiofacial syndrome: a study of 37 children and adolescents with VCFS. *J. Med. Genet.*, **34 (6)**, 453–8.

(1999) The behavioural phenotype in velo-cardio-facial syndrome (VCFS): from infancy to adolescence. *Genet. Couns.*, **10 (1)**, 79–88.

Taylor, W. D., Payne, M. E., Krishnan, K. R. *et al.* (2001) Evidence of white matter tract disruption in MRI hyperintensities. *Biol. Psychiatry*, **50 (3)**, 179–83.

Thompson, P. M., Vidal, C., Giedd, J. N. *et al.* (2001) Mapping adolescent brain change reveals dynamic wave of accelerated gray matter loss in very early-onset schizophrenia. *Proc. Natl. Acad. Sci. USA*, **98 (20)**, 11650–5.

Ungerleider, L. G. (1995) Functional brain imaging studies of cortical mechanisms for memory. *Science*, **270 (5237)**, 769–75

van Amelsvoort, T., Daly, E., Robertson, D. *et al.* (2001) Structural brain abnormalities associated with deletion at chromosome 22q11: quantitative neuroimaging study of adults with velo-cardio-facial syndrome. *Br. J. Psychiatry*, **178**, 412–19.

van Amelsvoort, T., Daly, E., Henry, J., *et al.* (2004) Brain anatomy in adults with velo-cardio-facial syndrome with and without schizophrenia: preliminary results of a structural magnetic resonance imaging study. *Arch. Gen. Psych.*, (in press)

Vataja, R. & Elomaa, E. (1998) Midline brain anomalies and schizophrenia in people with CATCH 22 syndrome. *Br. J. Psychiatry*, **172**, 518–20.

Worthington, S., Turner, A., Elber, J. *et al.* (2000) 22q11 deletion and polymicrogyria: cause or coincidence? *Clin. Dysmorphol.*, **9 (3)**, 193–7.

Yachnis, A. T. & Rorke, L. B. (1999) Cerebellar and brainstem development: an overview in relation to Joubert syndrome. *J. Child. Neurol.*, **14**, 570–3.

10

Speech and language disorders in velo-cardio-facial syndrome

Karen J. Golding-Kushner

Velo-cardio-facial syndrome Educational Foundation, NJ, USA

Speech, language, and learning problems are among the most common characteristics of velo-cardio-facial syndrome (VCFS) (Shprintzen *et al.*, 1978; Golding-Kushner *et al.*, 1985; Golding-Kushner, 1991; Kok & Solman, 1995; Wang *et al.*, 1998; Scherer *et al.*, 1999; Shprintzen, 2000; D'Antonio *et al.*, 2001), and speech, language, and cognitive patterns in children with VCFS may, in some ways, be unique (Scherer *et al.*, 1999; Eliez *et al.*, 2000a; Shprintzen, 2000; Bearden *et al.*, 2001; D'Antonio *et al.*, 2001). In fact, it is often the speech, language, and learning problems that lead – or should lead – clinicians to suspect a diagnosis of VCFS (Murphy *et al.*, 1998; Carneol *et al.*, 1999; Greenberg & Fifer, 2000). Speech includes the actual production of oral communication: articulation, voice, resonance, and fluency. The term language refers to the symbolic aspects of communication: comprehension and the formulation and expression of ideas and concepts. Our current understanding of speech and language patterns and best treatment practices for individuals with VCFS will be described in this chapter.

Language

As many as 98% of children with VCFS have developmental delay (Shprintzen, 1999) and speech and language delays are usually apparent from the onset of language (Shprintzen *et al.*, 1978; Scherer *et al.*, 1999; Solot *et al.*, 2000). In the first descriptive cross-sectional study on language and psychological skills of preschool, young school-aged, and older children with VCFS, Golding-Kushner *et al.* (1985) reported delays in comprehension and use of vocabulary and syntax in early childhood and increasing difficulty with abstract reasoning as language demands increased with age. Expressive language and speech skills tended to be disproportionately low in comparison with receptive skills, and both were lower than expected based on tests of cognitive development. Pragmatic skills, including use of language and social communication were among the most impaired

Velo-Cardial-Facial Syndrome: A Model for Understanding Microdeletion Disorders, ed. Kieran C. Murphy and Peter J. Scambler. Published by Cambridge University Press. © Cambridge University Press, 2005.

communication skills in all age groups. The youngest children, including those with good speech intelligibility, tended to rely on nonverbal communication at home. The older children (11–18 years) used language that was terse and concrete, and missed nuances of meaning typically gleaned from interpretation of one's communication partner's tone of voice, facial expression, and choice of words. Children also demonstrated disproportionately low scores on tests of mathematics and reading comprehension relative to tests of language, but rote or concrete skills, such as spelling and reading decoding were relatively preserved. Perceptual motor and graphomotor skills were delayed with minor coordination deficits at all ages.

The observations made by Golding-Kushner et al. (1985) have been supported by more recent cross-sectional and longitudinal studies (Kok & Solman, 1995; Moss et al., 1999; Scherer et al., 1999; Swillen et al., 1999; D'Antonio et al., 2001; Solot et al., 2001). Early development is often characterized by mild delay in most areas, but with expressive language lagging behind other milestones. Many children with VCFS are essentially nonverbal through 30 months of age (Scherer et al., 1999; D'Antonio et al., 2001), but show dramatic improvement between 3 and 4 years of age (Shprintzen, 2000; Solot et al., 2001). By school age, expressive language and speech improve, perhaps as a result of intervention, but specific language impairment (SLI) persists (Nayak & Sell, 1998; Solot et al., 2001; Scherer, 2002). Further, higher order receptive language skills involving abstract thinking remain poorly developed, affecting both communication and academic skills.

Golding-Kushner (2001) noted that, in VCFS, young children's expressive language may appear uneven and cyclic as they are developing conversational skills. This may be part of their step-wise approach to learning and, in some cases, may represent an early manifestation of psychiatric disorder (Shprintzen, 1993). For example, during a behavioral cycle in which they are shy and withdrawn, they may produce terse sentences. The same child may then go through a cycle during which their behavior is more animated and they speak constantly. These cycles are unpredictable and may last for hours or weeks.

Less information is available on communication skills of adults with VCFS. A recent study of 19 adults with VCFS indicated that, compared with age-, gender-, and IQ-matched controls, adults with VCFS had significant impairments in visuo-perceptual ability, problem solving and planning, and abstract and social thinking (Henry et al., 2002). Visuo-spatial cognition and memory, processing new information, reasoning, and mathematics pose the greatest challenges throughout development and problems in these areas seem to persist into adulthood in VCFS (Swillen et al., 1999; Bearden et al., 2001). This is discussed in more detail in Chapter 8.

Several studies have sought to determine the cause of language delays and disorders in children and adults with VCFS. Sensorineural hearing loss was reported in about 9–15% of patients with VCFS and conductive hearing loss in about 45% (Digilio *et al.*, 1999; Shprintzen, 1999). However, the nature of the language disturbance in VCFS is different from patterns of those with hearing loss as a primary etiology, and very few children with VCFS seem to have speech or language problems directly attributable to hearing problems (Golding-Kushner, 1991). On the contrary, there is evidence that the pattern of communication disorders in VCFS is syndrome-specific. To study this, the speech and language of children with VCFS has been compared with that of children with idiopathic developmental delay, children with Down syndrome, and children with nonsyndromic cleft palate. Glaser *et al.* (2002) compared 27 subjects with VCFS between 6 and 19 years old with age-, gender-, and IQ-matched controls with idiopathic developmental delay (DD). Receptive language scores were significantly below expressive language scores for VCFS group, but not for the DD group. This was especially true for children over age nine years, with whom tasks of reasoning were included. These findings suggest that speech and language in VCFS is syndrome-related, and not simply a reflection of cognitive or developmental problems. Furthermore, subjects with VCFS of maternal origin (gene inherited from the mother) scored significantly lower on receptive tasks than subjects with VCFS of paternal origin (Eliez *et al.*, 2001a; Glaser *et al.*, 2002).

Scherer *et al.* (1999) showed that the vocabulary and speech sound inventories of children with VCFS were profoundly impaired in comparison to children with cleft lip and palate or isolated cleft palate. In a subsequent study, they found that the communication patterns of children with VCFS also differed qualitatively and quantitatively from children with Down syndrome (Scherer *et al.*, 2001). They considered children with Down syndrome an important comparison group because of similarities in early developmental issues such as hypotonia, otitis media, feeding difficulties, and developmental delay. The children with Down syndrome presented with speech and language skills that were consonant with their cognitive skills. In contrast, articulation, vocabulary, and early syntax in young children with VCFS were depressed relative to their cognitive level. Results of these studies add support to the idea that the communicative profile of children with VCFS is distinctive to the syndrome.

Brain imaging research, especially functional brain imaging, has provided insight into the neural mechanisms underlying the linguistic and mathematical deficits seen in VCFS. Structural differences in the VCFS brain including a small left parietal lobe may explain difficulty with arithmetic and mathematic processing (Eliez *et al.*, 2000b, 2001b; Kates *et al.*, 2001). The parietal lobe also has an essential role in memory, particularly working memory, which is also poor in VCFS (Eliez *et al.*, 2000b). This is described in more detail in Chapter 9.

There is no question that VCFS poses a serious risk for speech and language deficits. Because of their severe deficits in expressive language and speech sound production, infants and toddlers with VCFS should receive aggressive early intervention services (Golding-Kushner et al., 1985; Shprintzen & Goldberg, 1995; Carneol et al., 1999; Havkin et al., 2000; Shprintzen, 2000; Golding-Kushner, 2001; Solot et al., 2001). Golding-Kushner (1995, 2001) and Golding-Kushner & Shprintzen (1998) strongly advocated an oral language approach with a focus on establishing a functional, spoken vocabulary and on speech sound production. Others (Scherer & D'Antonio, 1998; Solot et al., 2001) suggest teaching sign language as a "bridge" to facilitate communication with caregivers. Evidence to date is primarily anecdotal, but suggests that intensive articulation and language therapy (without diverting therapy time to signs) is effective in teaching oral speech and also conveys to the child the value of learning to talk. Instead of teaching parents sign, clinicians teach them how to model, stimulate, and reinforce vocalization and verbalization – speech and language. All toddlers (and adults, for that matter) gesture and point to help communicate their wants and needs, and children with VCFS are no exception. It would seem that if the only goal is communication, a total communication approach combining teaching of speech and formal signs is a reasonable strategy. However, if the goal is normal speech, the focus should be on speech and oral expressive language. There is no evidence to suggest that children with VCFS who are first taught sign language have better language skills than children who are not, or that they speak earlier. Intervention with older children may also need to include training in social communication.

Children with VCFS learn differently than other children with cleft palate and the clinician and parents must adjust their expectations accordingly. Even if it appears that the child is not responding, they should continue stimulating speech and language. Improvement is often slow, but does occur. The learning curve of children with VCFS may be more stepwise than smooth, and it is important not to become discouraged by the plateaus (Golding-Kushner, 2001). One of the learning characteristics of children with VCFS is that their ability to learn and retain information on a single presentation is limited. Therefore, sessions should be frequent and short in order to provide maximum repetition. The speech and language pathologist must train parents to provide a daily home program that supplements therapy. Home programs are especially advantageous for babies with VCFS who may have difficulty coping with changes in environment (Golding-Kushner, 2001).

Speech

Children with VCFS are at very high risk for speech disorders, higher than children with nonsyndromic cleft palate and many other syndromes. It has been reported that as many as 75% of children with VCFS have cleft palate, 74% are hypernasal, 62% have severe articulation disorder, and 22% are hoarse (Shprintzen, 1999).

In contrast, Hall & Golding-Kushner (1989) and others have reported that only 14% of nonsyndromic cleft patients were hypernasal after primary palate repair. This is discussed in more detail in Chapter 4. Studies suggest that the predominant speech patterns in children with VCFS are not simply due to a delay in speech sound acquisition but, rather, are uncharacteristic of both normal and delayed speech development (Van Lierde et al., 2001) and are also different from the pattern of sound acquisition in other children with cleft palate and VPI (Golding-Kushner, 1991; D'Antonio et al., 2001). In fact, like the language profile, the speech patterns in VCFS may be syndrome-specific. Many of the voice and resonance characteristics prevalent in VCFS may be attributed to morphologic and physiologic features of the syndrome (Table 10.1). However, that relationship is not straightforward (D'Antonio et al., 2001).

Voice

Phonation is the production of sound at the larynx resulting in voice. The three primary aspects of voice – pitch, quality, and volume – are determined by physical characteristics of the vocal folds, the way in which the vocal folds respond to muscle tension and displacement, and respiration. As a general rule, vocal pitch corresponds to the frequency of vocal fold vibration, quality corresponds to the completeness of contact of the inner margins of the vocal folds during their closed cycle and regularity of the vibratory cycles, and volume corresponds to respiratory effort and laryngeal tension.

Elevated vocal pitch has been reported in 28% of subjects with VCFS (Golding-Kushner, 1991). In at least some cases, this can be attributed to laryngeal web (Figure 10.1a). Laryngeal web is a relatively rare finding in the general population with an estimated incidence of 1 in 10 000 births (Chong et al., 1997). They account for only 5% of all congenital laryngeal anomalies (http://www.vcfsef.org), but have been reported in as many as 13% of children with VCFS (Drevensek et al., 2002). The presence of a laryngeal web shortens the vibrating length of the vocal folds and may result in increased vocal pitch. Webbing may also cause asynchronous movement of the vocal folds, causing hoarseness. Hoarseness affects about 22% of children with VCFS (Shprintzen, 1999). Laryngeal anomalies, such as unilateral vocal fold paralysis (Figure 10.1b) and laryngeal asymmetry have been reported in VCFS (Shprintzen, 2000). These may result in incomplete vocal fold adduction during the vibratory cycle, resulting in hoarseness. However, these laryngeal anomalies are infrequent findings and less prevalent than hoarseness. Vascular anomalies, such as medial displacement of the internal carotid artery, may also affect laryngeal function. Shprintzen (2003) and Mortelliti et al. (2004) described patients in whom prominent pulsations of the internal carotid caused

Table 10.1. Phenotype of VCFS and potential effect on speech

Morphologic features	Possible physiological result	Possible effect on voice
Laryngeal web	Shortened vibrating length of vocal folds	High pitch Hoarseness
Unilateral vocal fold paralysis Laryngeal asymmetry Vascular anomalies	Incomplete glottal closure	Hoarseness
Tonsilar hypertrophy with tonsilar base adjacent to epiglottis or larynx	Irritation of larynx causing chronic coughing or gagging	Hoarseness
		Possible effect on resonance
Adenoid hypoplasia	Velopharyngeal	Hypernasality (nasal resonance)
Platybasia and increased pharyngeal depth	insufficiency	
Overt or occult submucous cleft palate		
Thin pharyngeal tissue with abnormal histology and histochemistry	Pharyngeal hypotonia	Hypernasality
Tonsilar hypertrophy	Decreased posterior oral cavity space	"Hot potato" oral resonance
		Possible effect on articulation
	Velopharyngeal insufficiency	Obligatory errors: nasal emission, nasal rustle, reduced intraoral pressure Compensatory errors such as glottal stops

the pharyngeal wall to contact the epiglottis, triggering coughing which, in turn, caused vocal fold irritation and chronic hoarseness. They also reported that infero-posterior displacement of hypertrophic tonsils had a similar detrimental effect on the larynx and vocal quality.

Disorders of vocal pitch in VCFS are not easily treated therapeutically, especially when caused by a morphological deviation. In fact, attempting to lower the pitch in such cases could actually precipitate a disorder of vocal quality in the same way as other types of vocal abuse may cause changes in vocal fold morphology and cause hoarseness. Large laryngeal webs are typically resected to

anterior laryngeal web

unilateral vocal cord
paresis and atrophy

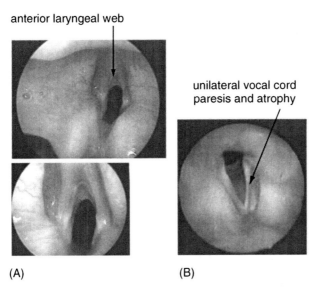

(A)   (B)

Figure 10.1 Endoscopic view of anterior laryngeal web (A) and (B) unilateral vocal fold paresis and atrophy in VCFS. Photographs courtesy of Robert J. Shprintzen, Ph.D.

alleviate airway obstruction, resulting in normalization of vocal pitch. Smaller webs may go unnoticed if they do not cause airway obstruction and their effect on vocal pitch would be less significant. However, they may cause unanticipated difficulty during intubation for surgery (Chong *et al.*, 1997). Therefore, examination of children with VCFS should include careful laryngeal examination to identify the presence of a laryngeal web, even in the absence of speech or respiratory symptoms.

Speech pathologists use a variety of procedures to treat disorders of vocal quality, depending on the cause of hoarseness. If hoarseness is due to a paralyzed or paretic vocal fold, pushing and other exercises that increase vocal effort and elicit increased movement of the unaffected vocal fold are used. If hoarseness is caused by vocal fold hyperfunction, exercises to decrease vocal effort are implemented. As with any voice disorder, selection of the appropriate therapeutic technique is fully dependent upon accurate diagnosis and direct examination of the vocal folds during phonation. Once that has been accomplished, the procedures applied to the treatment of hoarseness in VCFS are the same as those for patients without VCFS.

Resonance

Once air has passed through the glottis and acquired the vocal characteristics of pitch, volume, and quality, the air resonates through the upper airway, or vocal tract. The speech signal is modified as a result of its passage through the vocal tract and acquires the characteristic referred to as resonance. Normal resonance is perceived when the speech signal contains a balance of oral and nasal resonance. The amount of nasal resonance imposed on the speech signal is determined by velopharyngeal activity. Inadequate velopharyngeal closure, or velopharyngeal insufficiency (VPI) causes speech to sound hypernasal and nearly 75% of individuals with VCFS are hypernasal, even after palatal repair (Golding-Kushner, 1991; Shprintzen, 1999). This is significantly higher than the 16–20% prevalence of hypernasality reported following repair of non-syndromic cleft palate (Hall & Golding-Kushner, 1989). In addition, hypernasality is severe in about 80% of cases (Golding-Kushner, 1991). Why are children with VCFS so much more likely to be hypernasal than other children with cleft palate? There is evidence that several morphological factors may be responsible.

Velopharyngeal closure in children is velo-adenoidal, rather than velo-pharyngeal. Children with VCFS often have a small or absent adenoid which might be expected to increase the risk of VPI (Arvystas & Shprintzen, 1984; Havkin et al., 2000). Golding-Kushner (1991) studied the correlation between adenoid size and severity of VPI in a series of children with VCFS. All of the subjects with a small or absent adenoid (occupying less than 15% of the vocal tract area at the level of VP closure) had severe or gross VPI. On the other hand, every subject with relatively good velopharyngeal movement and only mild VPI had a large adenoid (filling 40% or more of the vocal tract at the level of VP closure). However, every subject with a large adenoid did not have good VP closure, indicating that other factors interacted with adenoid size to determine VP function.

Individuals with VCFS have platybasia, or an obtuse cranial base angle. Glander (1990) reported a mean cranial base angle in VCFS of 133° degrees and Golding-Kushner (1991) reported a mean of 138° (median 140°). Both were significantly more obtuse than the mean cranial base angle for normal subjects, which is 130° (Riolo et al., 1974). Because the cranial base is the skeletal framework from which the pharynx is suspended, platybasia results in an increased palate-to-posterior pharyngeal wall distance. An increased distance could be expected to increase the likelihood of VPI. Golding-Kushner (1991) compared the cranial base angle and pharyngeal depth (palate to posterior pharyngeal wall) in VCFS and van der Woude syndrome (VDWS), another genetic cleft-palate syndrome characterized by platybasia and increased velopharyngeal depth. The median cranial base angle in VDWS was 135.5 degrees, less obtuse than in VCFS, but the pharyngeal depth at the level of the palatal plane was 23 mm, larger than the depth of 20 mm in VCFS and 16 mm in normal development. In spite of this, the prevalence and severity of VPI in VDWS were significantly lower than in VCFS. Golding-Kushner (1991) also observed, via endoscopy and frontal-view videofluoroscopy, that the lateral pharyngeal walls (LPWs) were more widely spaced in VCFS, so widely spaced that VCFS was the only syndrome she studied in which both LPWs could not be seen at the same time in any endoscopic view. Thus, although an obtuse cranial base angle and increased pharyngeal depth alone would appear to be insufficient explanations for the frequency and severity of VPI in VCFS, overall pharyngeal volume could be a factor.

Pharyngeal "hypotonia" without a diagnosed neurological disorder has also been suggested as a cause of increased VPI in VCFS. Lateral pharyngeal wall motion in VCFS tends to appear hypotonic and deficient, and was completely absent in half of Golding-Kushner's subjects (1991, 1995). Also, some individuals with VCFS establish velopharyngeal closure on sustained fricatives /s, f/ or during production of single words but do not sustain closure during connected speech, with closure seeming to "pulse" open and close (Golding-Kushner, 2001). Golding-Kushner (2001) measured soft tissue thickness of the velum and posterior pharyngeal wall at several vertical levels by tracing lateral cephalographs. As seen in Figure 10.2, soft tissue of the velum and pharyngeal walls was significantly thinner in people with VCFS compared with normal subjects. Tissue thinning was present in each of the VCFS subjects, of whom 20% had repaired overt cleft palate, 46% had submucous cleft palate, and 34% had occult submucous cleft palate (OSMCP). She hypothesized that reduced velar and pharyngeal thickness and muscle bulk contributed to hypotonic velopharyngeal motion and were significant morphological factors predisposing individuals with VCFS to severe velopharyngeal insufficiency and hypernasality. Golding-Kushner questioned if the occult submucous cleft palate diagnosed in VCFS might actually be a contiguous paucity of muscle tissue suggesting a velar abnormality of different embryonic origin than cleft palate.

A few years later, Zim *et al.* (2003) conducted a histological investigation of the superior constrictor muscle in the area of the velopharyngeal region of subjects with VCFS and normal subjects matched for age and gender. They identified a significant deficiency of muscle tissue confirming Golding-Kushner's radiographic findings, and also noted deviations in the histology and histochemistry of the muscle in patients with VCFS. They concluded that the differences probably contributed to pharyngeal hypotonia and hypernasal speech in VCFS. Hypernasality in general, and certainly in VCFS, cannot be treated directly with speech therapy. Unfortunately, speech clinicians have a long history of trying to increase velopharyngeal closure and eliminate or reduce hypernasality with activities such as blowing (bubbles, horns, whistles), whistling, gagging, and performing oral-motor exercises designed to "strengthen" the palate or to increase its range of motion. Studies using these techniques were reviewed by Ruscello (1982) and later by Peterson-Falzon *et al.* (2001). They confirmed that the exercises are of no clinical value in improving speech or velopharyngeal function. Unfortunately,

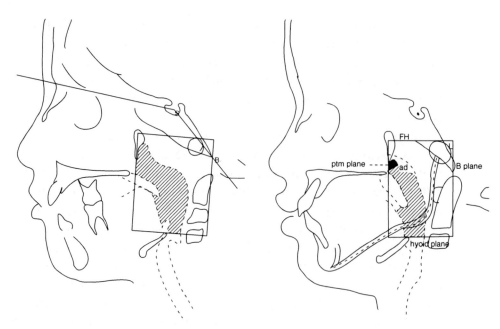

Figure 10.2 Tracing of cephalographs of a child with VCFS (left) compared with tracing of a gender- and age-matched normal child (right). Note obtuse cranial base angle, thin tissue of velum and posterior pharyngeal wall, and large airway volume (shaded) in VCFS (reprinted from Golding-Kushner, 1991).

in spite of evidence against their effectiveness, these practices continue today, resulting in great waste of therapeutic resources, time, energy, and finances, and resulting in great frustration for patients, parents, and clinicians. Children who are subjected to blowing exercises learn to blow, and nobody would argue against teaching a child to do so in order to blow out the candles on his or her birthday cake, which is a functional skill and a source of great anxiety for some parents and grandparents. However, this skill does not result in better velopharyngeal motion during speech or in decreased hypernasality. On the contrary, these exercises may result in increased respiratory and laryngeal effort, a source of vocal abuse that may lead to hoarseness, a disorder of vocal quality described in the previous section.

Treatment of VPI should occur only after velopharyngeal function during speech has been examined directly, that is, after nasopharyngoscopy and multi-view videofluoroscopy during connected speech. Therefore, assessment and treatment of VPI cannot occur until the child produces two and three-word utterances and cooperates for direct examination. Some 3-year-old children and most 4-year-old children meet these criteria. Use of a nasometer, a computer-based instrument to quantify resonance and diagnose hypernasality (but not VPI), has become popular because of its apparent objectivity. However, it is widely accepted that perceptual evaluation, reliance on the ear of the clinician, is the gold standard for assessment of hypernasality (Kuehn & Moller, 2000). Also, even if they were reliable and valid, nasometry results do not provide information about the location, size, configuration, and variability of a velopharyngeal gap, information that is necessary for appropriate therapeutic and surgical planning. Therefore, nasopharyngoscopy and multi-view videofluoroscopy are the techniques on which treatment decisions about VPI should be based (Karnell, 1994).

The most common treatment for hypernasality in VCFS is surgery, usually pharyngeal flap (see Chapter 4). Other surgical procedures have been used with varying degrees of success as discussed elsewhere in this text. It must be kept in mind that the sole purpose of these procedures is to eliminate velopharyngeal insufficiency. In other words, the only expected outcome of surgery is the elimination of nasal escape of air during speech. The procedure is not designed to change abnormal patterns of articulation. Surgery can be performed safely and effectively in VCFS, resulting in elimination of VPI (Golding-Kushner, 1993; Golding-Kushner et al., 1994; Tatum et al. 2002). Elimination of VPI results in immediate elimination of hypernasality without any speech therapy.

Speech-bulb appliances offer a nonsurgical option for treatment of VPI. Shaping of the bulb portion of the appliance that will occlude the velopharyngeal area requires the coordinated efforts of a dentist, speech pathologist, and endoscopist. However, as with a pharyngeal flap, if the appliance is fit correctly, it completely eliminates VPI and results in elimination of hypernasality.

In addition to hypernasality, another disorder of nasal resonance is hyponasality or denasality. In this disorder, there is insufficient nasalization of nasal consonants and adjacent vowels. It is how most people sound with nasal congestion. Hyponasality is caused by nasal or nasopharyngeal obstruction and is rare in VCFS, except after pharyngeal flap surgery. Hyponasality is a common finding following pharyngeal flap, especially in individuals with VCFS who have poor lateral pharyngeal wall motion and require very wide flaps (Golding-Kushner, 1993; Golding-Kushner et al., 1994). Post-flap hyponasality tends to improve over a period of time and is almost always gone within 6–12 months. In some instances, hyponasality persists longer. Unlike hypernasal speech, hyponasal speech is fully intelligible, and therapy may not be needed, even if hyponasality persists. In severe cases, a minor revision to the pharyngeal flap may be done to open the lateral ports a little. Speech therapy may be useful to decrease hyponasality by teaching the patient to increase the duration of nasal consonants (Golding-Kushner, 2001). Hypernasality and hyponasality are disorders of nasal resonance. Individuals with VCFS may also have a disorder of oral resonance referred to as "potato-in-the-mouth" or "marshmallow-mouth" resonance. The speaker sounds as if he or she was about to swallow a large marshmallow and started talking while the marshmallow was at the back of the mouth but not swallowed. This is usually the result of tonsillar hypertrophy, even in the presence of an absent or small adenoid. The hypertrophied tissue acts as an absorbent material in the vocal tract and has a damping effect on the speech signal, reducing the clarity of speech. Interestingly, there does not seem to be a correlation between tonsil size and adenoid size in VCFS. Examination of the tonsils may not suggest any pathology other than enlargement, and is often dismissed as unimportant. However, the enlarged tissue mass may extend beyond the posterior faucial pillar and inferiorly as low as the larynx. This may not be visible on oral examination but is easily visualized endoscopically or radiographically (Traquina *et al.*, 1990). Hypertrophied tonsils may also result in sleeping and eating disturbances by contacting the epiglottis or aryepiglottic folds and resulting in stimulation of the larynx on every swallow, the same mechanism that may cause hoarseness, as described above (Shprintzen, 2005; Mortelliti *et al.*, 2005).

Tonsillectomy is indicated when hypertrophic tonsils cause speech, sleep, or eating disturbance. The tonsils do not play a role in speech production. Therefore, their removal poses little risk to speech.

Articulation

Articulation is the physical production (pronunciation) of speech sounds. Children with VCFS may have four different classes of articulation errors: developmental, phonological, obligatory, or compensatory. Correct classification of errors is essential in order to determine treatment goals and the sequence of application of different treatment modalities.

Developmental errors are speech mistakes in which sounds are produced in a way that is typical at an earlier stage of speech development. Examples of developmental errors include "fum" for "thumb" (a substitution), distorted s (a distortion), and "top" for "stop" (omission of a sound). Developmental errors are not in any way caused by cleft palate or VPI. These errors are very common in children without cleft palate or VCFS, and respond well to traditional articulation therapy techniques. Children with VCFS respond best when therapy progresses according to a logical sequence, following a hierarchy from simple to complex sounds and word contexts, and when therapy includes a lot of repetition and practice.

When a child exhibits multiple articulation errors, speech pathologists look beyond the individual mistakes to identify patterns that could account for the errors. In some children, the presence of multiple errors reflects an underlying problem in the organization of the child's sound system. For example, a child who omits the last consonant of most words does not necessarily have difficulty producing the individual sounds that were omitted. Rather, he or she may be following a pattern – or phonological rule – according to which words must end in vowels. Phonology is the study of the organization of sounds in a language and phonological disorders are actually a language disturbance, not a speech disturbance. Like developmental articulation errors, phonological errors are unrelated to cleft palate or VPI and do not appear to be any more prevalent in VCFS than in other clinical populations. Procedures to treat phonological disorders are different than those for treating developmental articulation disorders and include listening to correct production without specific demands or practice producing words correctly. These procedures are highly effective in treating typical phonological disorders but may be problematic for children with VCFS because, as concrete thinkers, they learn poorly using "discovery" approaches and need direct instruction in small groups or individually (Golding-Kushner *et al.*, 1985; Landsman, 2001). The effectiveness of auditory bombardment and other strict phonological approaches is based on a child's ability to discover a pattern, extract a rule, and apply the rule to his or her own speech production. Therefore, strict phonological approaches may not be effective in correcting phonological disorders in children with VCFS. Because they are concrete thinkers, and because they rely on repetition and rehearsal to learn, their therapy must include simple verbal explanations and production practice. Therefore, for children with VCFS, hybrid approaches that combine elements of phonological strategies (teaching related phonemes in groups rather than separately), and articulation strategies (teaching production and not relying only on auditory stimulation), are best for elimination of phonological processes in children with VCFS (Golding-Kushner, 2001).

Unlike developmental and phonological errors, obligatory articulation errors are directly caused by VPI. Because of the direct relationship between obligatory errors and VPI, obligatory errors cannot be corrected using speech therapy but disappear completely when VPI is eliminated. Obligatory errors include nasal emission or nasal escape of air, nasal turbulence, and reduced intraoral air pressure. Nasal emission may be audible, sounding like a rush of air through the nose that is most noticeable during production of high-pressure consonants. Sometimes nasal emission is inaudible during normal speech but may be detected using a mirror, stethoscope, straw, or other instrument held beneath the nostrils. Nasal turbulence or nasal rustle is nasal emission that passes some type of constriction causing noise to be imposed on the nasal air escape. This is most often heard during production of high-pressure consonants, but may also be heard during nasal-to-oral and oral-to-nasal sound transitions within words. Of importance is the fact that both nasal emission and nasal turbulence are the result of a passive air leak, directly caused by VPI, oronasal fistula, or both. Production of most consonants requires a build-up of intraoral air pressure that is blocked or released gradually during the articulation gesture. Because of the constant loss of air through the VP port, speakers with VPI experience a reduction in the amount of oral air pressure that can be impounded during articulation. This loss of intraoral air pressure results in production of consonants that are weak and may become so distorted that they sound like nasal consonants. For example, "bye" may sound like "my" and "dada" like "nana." Again, obligatory errors cannot be corrected using speech therapy and can only be treated by physical elimination of VPI using surgery or prosthetics. Therefore, speech therapy to correct obligatory errors is contraindicated.

The most common class of errors produced by children with VCFS is the category of compensatory errors. This category includes errors often called "cleft palate speech" because they are errors unique to individuals with a history of cleft palate, VPI, or both. With the production of these errors, the child is attempting to produce sounds at a location in the vocal tract instead of in the mouth, and inferior to the velopharyngeal region, so as to complete the articulatory gesture before air pressure is lost. There are several types of maladaptive compensatory errors including pharyngeal fricatives, nasal snorting, and others (Trost, 1981).

Hall & Golding-Kushner (1989) reported that the prevalence of compensatory articulation disorders among 500 children with nonsyndromic cleft palate at a single institution was 16%. In a subsequent study of children with syndromic cleft palate at the same institution, Golding-Kushner (1991) found that the prevalence of compensatory speech disorders in children with VCFS was 88%. In contrast, she reported that compensatory errors were produced by 40% of children with van der Woude syndrome, 37% with Stickler syndrome, and 10% with Treacher–Collins syndrome. More recent studies of subjects obtained from a broader referral base have suggested that the prevalence of compensatory speech in VCFS is closer to 62% (Shprintzen, 1999). Clearly, a diagnosis of VCFS significantly increases the risk of cleft palate speech.

The most commonly produced compensatory error in VCFS is the glottal stop (Golding-Kushner et al., 1985; Shprintzen, 2000; D'Antonio et al., 2001). Glottal stops are produced by abrupt approximation and release of the vocal folds. Persons with VPI produce glottal stops most often as a substitute for other plosive consonants /b, p, d, t, g, k/. However, children with VCFS tend to produce glottal stops as a substitute for all sounds, including fricatives (s, z, th, v, f, sh) and even nasal sounds (n, m, ng), the latter of which are almost never glottalized by others with cleft palate speech (Golding-Kushner, 1991; Shprintzen, 1993, 2000; D'Antonio et al., 2001). When a glottal stop is produced, lip and tongue movement that would normally occur during production of the sound is often neglected because it is superfluous, the sound having been made in the larynx instead of in the mouth. Glottal stop substitutions are often misperceived as consonant omissions. This impression is supported by the obvious lack of movement of the articulators. It is likely for this reason that glottal speech is frequently misdiagnosed as apraxia, which is actually a neurological disorder. Invariably, misdiagnosis leads to inappropriate and ineffective treatment.

Compensatory articulation errors increase the perception of hypernasality. In some individuals with cleft palate, eliminating compensatory articulation errors results in increased velopharyngeal motion (Golding-Kushner, 1981; Henningsson & Isberg, 1986). However, eliminating compensatory errors does not seem to have any effect on velopharyngeal closure in individuals with VCFS (Golding-Kushner, 2001). Elimination of glottal stops and other compensatory errors increases the speech intelligibility of children with VCFS but unlike with other children, does not result in increased velopharyngeal motion or decreased hypernasality. This is further evidence that the speech disorder associated with VCFS is syndrome-specific.

Articulation therapy is effective in eliminating compensatory articulation disorders in children with VCFS. However, treatment must be intensive, frequent, individual, concrete, and highly organized. Treatment involves direct training in the production of oral consonants. The errors should be approached as what they are: errors in place of articulation (glottal stops substituted for oral stops) and manner of articulation (glottal stops substituted for fricative or nasal consonants). Compensatory errors are not caused by oral-motor dysfunction, and oral exercises do not result in elimination of these errors. Golding-Kushner (2001) described modifications of traditional articulation approaches that follow a logical hierarchy and have proven effective with children with VCFS. Therapy should begin as early as possible because compensatory errors are not "outgrown." They are easily eliminated at any age but, as with any "habit," the longer the incorrect pattern is used, the more difficult it is to generalize the corrected articulation patterns to automatic speech. A tendency to glottal speech can be detected as early as 8 months of age when a child starts babbling, even before true words are produced. Early intervention can prevent the development of glottal speech.

Summary

Children with VCFS are at very high risk for communicative impairment. Further, the communication skills of children with VCFS may be syndrome-specific and are typically characterized by severe VPI, hypernasality, and a glottal stop articulation disorder. Onset of language is typically delayed with receptive language developing more rapidly than expressive and with severe deficits in early vocabulary acquisition and speech sound production. Speech and expressive language show rapid improvement between age 3 and 4 years but specific language impairment persists and, even as language continues to improve, working memory, reasoning, abstract thinking, and social language present challenges. Individuals with VCFS respond well to direct teaching in therapy and academics, but intensive and frequent repetition is necessary for mastery and application of new skills and concepts. The combination of aggressive articulation therapy and surgical correction of VPI results in normal speech and resonance. Language therapy and a need for academic support typically continue throughout the school years.

REFERENCES

Arvystas,M. & Shprintzen, R. (1984) Craniofacial morphology in velo-cardio-facial syndrome. *J. Craniofacial Genet. Dev. Biol.*, **4**, 39–45.

Bearden, C., Woodin, M., Wang, P. *et al.* (2001) The neurocognitive phenotype of the 22q11.2 deletion syndrome: selective deficit in visual-spatial memory. *J. Clin. Exp. Neuropsych.*, **23**, 447–64.

Carneol, S., Marks, S. & Weik, L. (1999) The speech-language pathologist: key role in the diagnosis of velocardiofacial syndrome. *Am. J. Speech Lang. Pathol.*, **8**, 23–32.

Chong, Z., Jawan, B., Poon, Y. *et al.* (1997) Unsuspected difficult intubation caused by a laryngeal web. *Br. J Anaesthes.*, **79**, 396–97.

D'Antonio, L., Scherer, N., Miller, L. *et al.* (2001) Analysis of speech characteristics in children with velocardiofacial syndrome (VCFS) and children with phenotypic overlap without VCFS. *Cleft Pal-Craniofacial J.*, **39**, 455–67.

Digilio, M., Pacifico, C., Tieri, L. *et al.* (1999) Audiological findings in patients with microdeletion 22q11 (di George/velocardiofacial syndrome). *Br. J. Audiol.*, **33**, 329–33.

Drevensek, S., Purcell, A., van Doom., *et al.* (2002) Velo-cardio-facial syndrome: communication features and surgical outcomes. Annual meeting of the Velocardiofacial Syndrome Educational Foundation, Brisbane, Australia.

Eliez, S., Palacio-Espasa, F., Spira, A. *et al.* (2000a) Young children with velo-cardio-facial syndrome (CATCH-22): psychological and language phenotypes. *Eur. Child Adolesc. Psychiatry*, **9**, 109–15.

Eliez, S., Schmitt, E., White, C. *et al.* (2000b) Children and adolescents with velocardiofacial syndrome: a volumetric MRI study. *Am. J. Psychiatry*, **157**, 409–15.

Eliez, S., Antonarakis, S., Morris, M. *et al.* (2001a) Parental origin of the deletion 22q11.2 and brain development in velocardiofacial syndrome. *Arch. Gen. Psychiatry*, **58**, 64–8.

Eliez, S., Blasey, C., Menon, V. *et al.* (2001b) Functional brain imaging study of mathematical reasoning abilities in velocardiofacial syndrome (del22q11.2). *Genet. Med.*, **3**, 49–55.

Glander, K. (1990) A comparison of the craniofacial characteristics of two syndromes associated with Pierre Robin sequence. Unpublished orthodontic thesis, Department of Dentistry, Montefiore Medical Center and the Albert Einstein College of Medicine, Bronx, NY.

Glaser, B., Mumme, D., Blasey, C. *et al.* (2002) Language skills in children with velocardiofacial syndrome (deletion 22q11.2). *J. Pediatr.*, **140**, 753–8.

Golding-Kushner, K. (1981) Articulation and velopharyngeal insufficiency: A rational for pre-surgical speech therapy. Fourth International Congress of Cleft Palate and Craniofacial Anomalies, Acapulco, Mexico.

(1991) *Craniofacial Morphology and Velopharyngeal Function in Four Syndromes of Clefting.* Unpublished doctoral dissertation, The Graduate School and University Center, New York.

(1993) Pharyngeal flaps in patients with velo-cardio-facial syndrome. Society for Ear, Nose, and Throat Advances in Children. Pittsburgh, PA.

(1995) Treatment of articulation and resonance disorders associated with cleft palate and VPI. In Shprintzen, R. J. & Bardach, J., eds. *Cleft Palate Speech Management: a Multidisciplinary Approach.* St. Louis: C.V. Mosby, pp. 327–51.

(2001) *Therapy Techniques for Cleft Palate Speech and VPI.* San Diego, CA: Singular Publishing Group.

Golding-Kushner, K. & Shprintzen, R. (1998) To sign or not to sign? VCFSEF Newsletter, November.

Golding-Kushner, K., Weller, G. & Shprintzen, R. (1985) Velo-cardio-facial syndrome: language and psychological profiles. *J. Craniofacial Genet. Dev. Biol.*, **5**, 259–66.

Golding-Kushner, K., Argamaso, R. V. & Mitnick, R. (1994) Pharyngeal flaps in patients with velo-cardio-facial syndrome. American Cleft Palate-Craniofacial Association. Toronto, Canada.

Greenberg, I. & Fifer, R. (2000) Evidence that the association between hypernasality and 22q11 deletion syndrome still goes undetected. *Am. J. Speech Lang. Pathol..*, **9**, 197–201.

Hall, C. & Golding-Kushner, K. J. (1989) Long-term follow-up of 500 patients after palate repair performed prior to 18 months of age. Sixth International Congress on Cleft Palate and Related Craniofacial Anomalies. Jerusalem, Israel.

Havkin, N., Tatum, S. & Shprintzen, R. (2000) Velopharyngeal insufficiency and articulation impairment in velo-cardio-facial syndrome: the influence of adenoids on phonemic development. *Int. J. Ped. Otolaryngol.*, **54**, 103–10.

Henningsson, G. & Isberg, A. (1986) Velopharyngeal movements in patients alternating between oral and glottal articulation: a clinical and cineradiographical study. *Cleft Palate J.*, **23**, 1–9.

Henry, J., Amelsvoort, T., Morris, R. *et al.* (2002) An investigation of the neuropsychological profile in adults with velo-cardio-facial syndrome (VCFS). *Neuropsychologia*, **40**, 471–8.

Karnell, M. (1994) *Videoendoscopy: from Velopharynx to Larynx.* San Diego, CA: Singular Publishing Group.

Kates, W., Burnette, C., Jabs, E. *et al.* (2001) Regional cortical white matter reductions in velocardiofacial syndrome: a volumetric MRI analysis. *Biol. Psychiatry*, **49**, 677–84.

Kok, L. & Solman, R. (1995) Velocardiofacial syndrome: learning difficulties and intervention. *J. Med. Genet.*, **32**, 612–18.

Kuehn, D. & Moller, K. (2000) The state of the art: speech and language issues in the cleft palate population. *Cleft Pal-Craniofacial J.*, **37**, 348.

Landsman, D. (2001) Educating the Child with Velo-Cardio-Facial Syndrome: A Handbook for Parents and Professionals. http://vcfsef.org/vcfs_education.html.

Mortelliti, A., Tatum, S., Havkin, N. *et al.* (2005) Posterior displacement of the tonsils can cause chronic cough and symptoms typically associated with reflux. *Int. J. Ped. Otorhinolaryngol* (in press).

Moss, E., Batshaw, M., Solot, C. *et al.* (1999) Psychoeducational profile of the 22q11.2 microdeletion: a complex pattern. *J. Pediatr.*, **134**, 193–8.

Murphy, K. C., Jones, R., Griffiths, E. *et al.* (1998) Chromosome 22q11 deletions: an under-recognized cause of idiopathic learning disability. *Br. J. Psychiatry*, **172**, 180–3.

Nayak, J. & Sell, D. (1998) Communication disorders in VCFS: A clinical audit. Fourth Annual Meeting of the Velocardiofacial Syndrome Educational Foundation, Boston, MA.

Peterson-Falzon, S., Hardin-Jones, M. & Karnell, M. (2001) *Cleft Palate Speech.* St. Louis, MO: Mosby.

Riolo, M., Moyers, R., McNamara, J. *et al.* (1974) *Atlas of Cranial Growth.* University of Michigan Center for Human Growth and Development. Ann Arbor, MI:

Ruscello, D. (1982) A selected review of palatal training procedures. *Cleft Palate J.*, **18**, 181–93.

Scherer, N. (2002) Language impairments and school success. VCFSEF News, **8**, 4.

Scherer, N. & D'Antonio L. (1998) To sign or not to sign? VCFSEF Newsletter, November.

Scherer, N., D'Antonio, L. & Kalbfleish, J. (1999) Early speech and language development in children with velocardiofacial syndrome. *Am. J. Med. Genet.*, **88**, 714–23.

Scherer, N., D'Antonio, L. & Rodgers, J. (2001) Profiles of communication disorder in children with velocardiofacial syndrome: comparison to children with Down syndrome. *Genet. Med.*, **3**, 72–8.

Shprintzen, R. (1993) Genetics, syndrome delineation, and communicative impairment. In Minifie, F., ed., *Introduction to Communication Sciences and Disorders.* San Diego, CA:, Singular Publishing Group, pp. 439–80.

(1999) Clinical data base project. http://vcfsef.org/pp/vcf_facts/sld001.htm.

(2000) *Syndrome Identification for Speech-Language Pathology.* San Diego, CA: Singular Publishing Group.

(2003) Velo-cardio-facial syndrome. In Cassidy, S., & Allanson, J., eds., *Management of Genetic Syndromes,* 2nd edn. New York: John Wiley & Sons, pp. 615–632

Shprintzen, R. & Goldberg, R. (1995) The genetics of clefting and associated syndromes. In Shprintzen, R. J. & Bardach, J. eds., *Cleft Palate Speech Management: A Multidisciplinary Approach.* St. Louis: C.V. Mosby, pp. 16–43.

Shprintzen, R., Goldberg, R., Lewin, M. *et al.* (1978) A new syndrome involving cleft palate, cardiac anomalies, typical facies and learning disabilities: velo-cardio-facial syndrome. *Cleft Palate J.*, **15**, 56–62.

Solot, C., Knightly, C., Handler, S. *et al.* (2000) Communication disorders in the 22q11.2 microdeletion syndrome. *J. Commun. Dis.*, **33**, 187–204.

Solot, C., Gerdes, M., Kirschner, R. *et al.* (2001) Communication issues in 22q11.2 deletion syndrome: children at risk. *Genet. Med.*, **3**, 67–71.

Swillen, A., Vandeputte, L., Cracco, J. *et al.* (1999) Neuropsychological, learning and psycho-social profile of primary school aged children with velo-cardio-facial syndrome (22q11 deletion): evidence for a nonverbal learning disability? *Child Neuropsychol.*, **5**, 230–41.

Tatum, S., Chang, J., Havkin, N. *et al.* (2002) Pharyngeal flap and the internal carotid in velocardiofacial syndrome. *Arch Facial Plast. Surg.*, **4**, 73–80.

Traquina, D., Golding-Kushner, K. J. & Shprintzen, R. J. (December 1990) Comparison of tonsil size based on oral and nasopharyngoscopic observation. Society of Ear Nose and Throat Advances in Children, Washington, DC.

Trost, J. (1981) Articulatory additions to the classical description of the speech of persons with cleft palate. *Cleft Palate J.*, **18**, 193–203.

Van Lierde, K., Van Borsel, J., Van Cauwenberge, P. *et al.* (2001) Speech patterns in children with velo-cardio-facial syndrome: two case studies. *Fol. Phoniatr. Logopaed.*, **53**, 213–21.

Wang, P., Solot, C., Moss, E. *et al.* (1998) Developmental presentation of 22q11.2 deletion (DiGeorge/velocardiofacial syndrome). *J. Dev. Behav. Ped.*, **19**, 342–5.

Zim, S., Schelper, R., Kellman, R. *et al.* (2003) Thickness, histology, and histochemistry of the superior pharyngeal constrictor muscle in velocardiofacial syndrome. Annual Meeting of the Velocardiofacial Syndrome Educational Foundation, San Diego, CA.

11

Genetic counseling

Donna M. McDonald-McGinn and Elaine H. Zackai

22q and You Center, The Children's Hospital of Philadelphia, PA, USA

The 22q11.2 deletion has been identified in the majority of patients with DiGeorge syndrome (de la Chapelle *et al.*, 1981; Kelley *et al.*, 1982; Scambler *et al.*, 1991; Driscoll *et al.*, 1992a), velo-cardio-facial syndrome (VCFS) (Driscoll *et al.*, 1992b, 1993) and conotruncal anomaly face syndrome (Burn *et al.*, 1993; Matsouka *et al.*, 1994) and in some patients with autosomal dominant Opitz G/BBB syndrome (McDonald-McGinn *et al.*, 1995; Fryburg *et al.*, 1996; LaCassie & Arriaza, 1996) and Cayler cardiofacial syndrome (Giannotti *et al.*, 1994; Bawle *et al.*, 1998). These diagnoses were originally described as individual entities by a number of subspecialists who were concentrating on one particular area of interest. For example, Dr. Angelo DiGeorge, an endocrinologist, first reported the combination of hypoparathyroidism and immune deficiency in children and this syndrome later came to bear his name. However, those syndromes are now collectively referred to by their chromosomal etiology – the 22q11.2 deletion. This phenomenon was previously likened to the old adage of a group of nearsighted veterinarians trying to identify an elephant by each examining a separate part (Figure 11.1). Each person was accurate in describing his own area of interest, but none was able to see the big picture. So too is the case with the 22q11.2 deletion. It was not until Fluorescence in situ hybridization (FISH) studies were available and we could identify a submicroscopic deletion in these patients that the etiology of the previously described separate entities was elucidated. Furthermore, it was not until this point that we could truly appreciate the magnitude of this disorder (McDonald-McGinn *et al.*, 1996). Thus, the 22q11.2 deletion is now thought to be the most common microdeletion syndrome with an estimated incidence of 1 in 4000 live births (Wilson *et al.*, 1992). It is so common, in fact, that there are reports of affected relatives within families who have the deletion by chance alone. For example, we have identified affected first cousins (Figure 11.2) with the 22q11.2 deletion. Parent of origin studies revealed that the deletions arose as independent de novo events in the patients' unrelated mothers. Thus, the deletion occurred randomly in both cousins by chance alone. Furthermore, there have been a number of patients

Velo-Cardial-Facial Syndrome: A Model for Understanding Microdeletion Disorders, ed. Kieran C. Murphy and Peter J. Scambler. Published by Cambridge University Press. © Cambridge University Press, 2005.

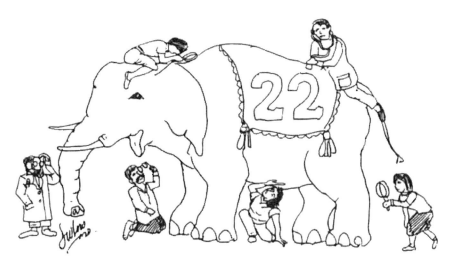

Figure 11.1 We have likened this phenomenon to the old adage of a group of nearsighted veterinarians trying to identify an elephant by each examining a separate part. Each person was accurate in describing his/her own area of interest, but none was able to see the big picture. So too was the case of the 22q11.2 deletion.

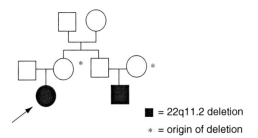

■ = 22q11.2 deletion
* = origin of deletion

Figure 11.2 This pedigree highlights the frequency of the deletion with affected first cousins occurring by chance alone. Parental FISH studies were normal. Parent of origin studies revealed maternally inherited deletions which arose as independent de novo events in the unrelated mothers' germ cells.

identified with both the 22q11.2 deletion and concomitant diagnoses including familial single gene disorders such as Marfan syndrome (Stewart, personal communication), neurofibromatosis (Coleman, personal communication) an *FGFR3* mutation (Reardon *et al.*, 1997), and Ehlers–Danlos syndrome (McDonald-McGinn *et al.*, 2002b), as well as additional sporadic cytogenetic abnormalities including a patient with both the 22q11.2 deletion and trisomy 8 mosaicism (McDonald-McGinn *et al.*, 2002b). Once again, these patients serve to emphasize the frequency of the 22q11.2 microdeletion and to highlight the importance of screening for other diagnoses in a child with the 22q11.2 deletion who happens to have additional features which are not known to be associated with the deletion.

Mortality

In contrast to the early reports of DiGeorge syndrome, the 22q11.2 deletion is far from a uniformly lethal diagnosis. In fact, we recently reported a mortality rate of 5% in 460 patients identified by FISH where the median age of death was 4 months (McDonald-McGinn et al., 2002a). The majority of patients who did expire succumbed to complications of congenital heart disease. These numbers reflect the relatively recent advances in both palliative cardiac care and the treatment of infectious disease. Moreover, they suggest that there will likely be an increase in the prevalence of the 22q11.2 deletion due to the decreasing mortality of the diagnosis, as well as the minimal impact on reproductive fitness. It is important to mention, however, that although systematic investigation has not yet occurred, anecdotally, it appears as though some patients with the clinical diagnosis of DiGeorge syndrome, without the 22q11.2 deletion, do have an increased mortality rate due to thymic aplasia/hypoplasia with significant immune compromise (Sullivan, personal communication).

Variability

In addition to the fact that the 22q11.2 deletion is quite common, it is also extremely variable. This includes the presence of abnormalities traditionally known to be associated with the deletion such as cardiac disease (Goldmuntz, 1998), palatal involvement (McDonald-McGinn et al., 1997b), immune deficiency (Sullivan et al., 1999), hypoparathyroidism, neurologic involvement (Lynch et al., 1995), and speech and learning disabilities (Wang et al., 1998; Gerdes et al., 1999; Moss et al., 1999; Solot et al., 2000, 2001). As well as new findings such as feeding problems (Eicher et al., 2000), growth hormone deficiency (Weinzimer et al., 1998) and autoimmune disorders (Keenan et al., 1997; Sullivan et al., 1997, 1998; Kawame et al., 2001). Furthermore, there is wide inter- and intrafamilial variability even among identical twins (Figure 11.3) (Driscoll et al., 1995a; McDonald-McGinn et al., 1997a, 1999b, 2001a; Ryan et al., 1997).

Parent of origin

In our cohort of 460 patients with the deletion, 49% are male and 51% are female, demonstrating that males and females are equally likely to be affected by the deletion (McDonald-McGinn, 2002a). Furthermore, we have found that the

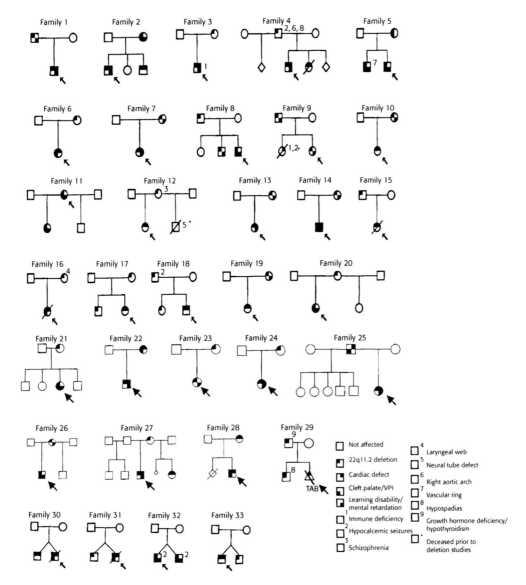

Figure 11.3 Twenty-nine nuclear families identified with the 22q11.2 deletion in a cohort of 460 patients and four sets of presumed monozygotic twins (parental FISH studies were negative but monozygosity studies were not performed). The 42 unselected patients are represented here along with their affected proband parent, child, or sibling. Note both interfamilial and intrafamilial variability.

deletion is equally likely to occur either in the egg or sperm cells in de novo cases (McDonald-McGinn, 2001a).

In a subset of our cohort, the parent of origin in de novo cases does not appear to affect the phenotype. Specifically, we reviewed the medical records of 51 de novo cases where the parent of origin was established. We noted the presence and severity of congenital heart disease, definitive palatal anomalies, presence of hypocalcemia, structural brain abnormalities, and learning disabilities and we found no statistical significance from the expected $1:1$ ratio based on Chi-square analysis. In addition, immunologic profile findings including CD3, CD4, CD8, CD19, and NK cells and the presence of articulation errors and delays in emergence of language in these patients appears to be independent of the parent of origin based on standard deviation calculations (McDonald-McGinn, 2001b).

Inheritance

In looking at the inheritance of the 22q11.2 deletion, it is clear that the majority of cases occur as a de novo event (Figure 11.4). This is reportedly due to the inherent structure of the deletion. Specifically, a number of low copy repeats make this region especially susceptible to rearrangements (Edelman *et al.*, 1999; Shaikh *et al.*, 2000). To establish the true incidence of familial cases, we prospectively screened the parents of 30 consecutive affected children for the 22q11.2 deletion regardless of the family history and identified two previously unrecognized affected parents. This yielded a 7% familial incidence of the deletion, which is consistent with our previous reports of between 6% and 14% depending on our ascertainment (McDonald-McGinn *et al.*, 2001a). These two newly identified parents included a 20-year-old mother with a history of a repaired VSD and a learning disability (Figure 11.5), as well as a completely normal father (Figure 11.6) who was found to have mosaicism both on an initial study (13% of cells with a deletion) and on a repeat study (12% of cells deleted) (McDonald-McGinn *et al.*, 2002a, 2002b). These findings, therefore, support parental FISH studies in *all* families with an affected child in order to identify mildly affected parents and to rule out mosaicism, which has also been reported previously (Consevage *et al.*, 1996). Also, there are reports of germline mosaicism in the literature (Hatchwell *et al.*, 1998; Sandrin-Garcia *et al.*, 2002), so in addition, clinicians must now caution non-deleted parents regarding the risk of germline mosaicism.

Recurrence risk

The 22q11.2 deletion is a contiguous deletion syndrome with a recurrence risk for an affected individual of 50% (Figure 11.7). Although the pattern of inheritance is similar to that seen in an autosomal dominant condition (i.e., the trait appears in every generation with no skipping; the occurrence and transmission are not influenced by sex; any child of an affected parent has a 50% chance of inheriting the trait and unaffected persons do not transmit the trait to their offspring

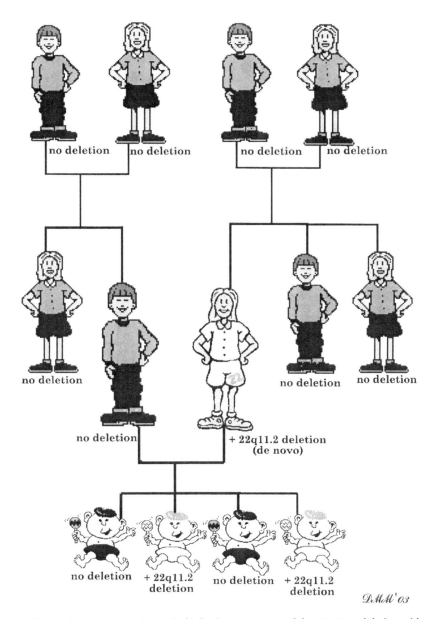

Figure 11.4   Pedigree demonstrating the typical inheritance pattern of the 22q11.2 deletion with most cases occurring as de novo events followed by a 50% recurrence risk for subsequent offspring of affected individuals.

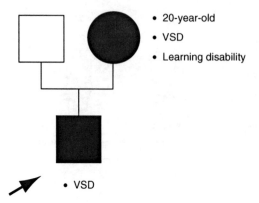

Figure 11.5 Mildly affected parent identified following the birth of an affected child.

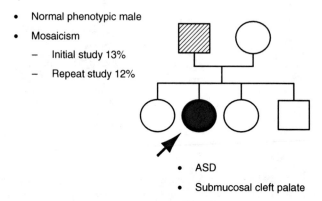

Figure 11.6 Normal phenotypic male, found to have mosaicism for the 22q11.2 deletion following
identification of the deletion in his affected daughter.

(Thompson & Thompson, 1986), the use of the term autosomal dominant is a
misnomer, as there are many genes involved in the 22q11.2 microdeletion syndrome, as opposed to a single gene disorder.

Genetic counseling

Genetic counseling for an adult with the 22q11.2 deletion is often quite difficult due,
in part, to the wide inter- and intrafamilial variability of the deletion. Furthermore,
reporting the risk for medically relevant findings such as congenital heart disease is
complicated by ascertainment bias. For example, in our own cohort of 460 patients
with the 22q11.2 deletion, 75% were found to have congenital heart disease, most
often tetralogy of Fallot (TOF) (McDonald-McGinn et al., 2002a). However, our
ascertainment is within a large tertiary care facility which acts as a referral center for
children with critical cardiac defects. Therefore, the optimal way to obtain data for

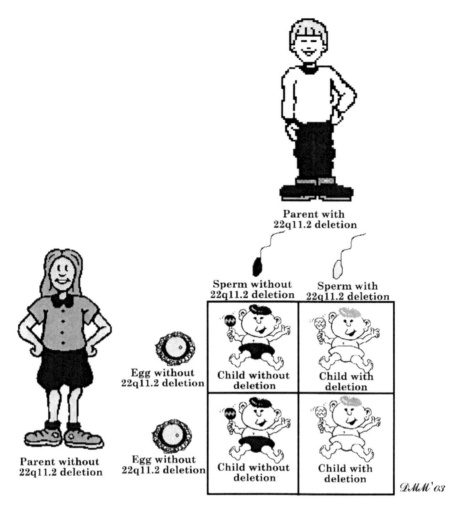

Figure 11.7 Punnett square demonstrating 50% recurrence risk when one parent has the 22q11.2 deletion.

counseling purposes is to prospectively observe the phenotype in individuals identified via an affected relative or through a newborn screening study.

In looking at our own cohort, we previously identified 30 affected persons following the diagnosis in their relative (McDonald-McGinn *et al.*, 2001a). We have subsequently diagnosed 12 additional individuals, increasing the total to 42. Of this group, 28 are parents of affected children and 14 are children born before or after an affected parent was diagnosed. Four of these children were in fact diagnosed prenatally via amniocentesis. Of this group of 42 individuals, 55% have no findings including 68% of affected parents and 29% of children. Of the remaining individuals with abnormalities, the findings include congenital heart disease in 17%, overt

Table 11.1. Findings in unselected patients with the 22q11.2 deletion (n = 42)

	Adults (28)	Children (14)
Congenital heart disease	2	5
Overt cleft palate	2	2
Hypocalcemic seizures	1	0
Hypocalcemic seizures/hypospadias	1	0
Hypospadias	0	1
Laryngeal web	1	0
VPI and vascular ring	0	1
Neural tube defect	0	1
Growth hormone deficiency/hypothyroidism	1	0
Schizophrenia	1	0
Normal	19 (68%)	4 (29%)

cleft palate in 10%, hypocalcemic seizures in 5%, hypospadias in 5%, laryngeal web in 2%, VPI/vascular ring in 2%, a neural tube defect in 2%, growth hormone deficiency/hypothyroidism in 2%, and schizophrenia in 2% (Table 11.1).

In reviewing the educational background of 20 of these adults with the deletion, 70% are high school graduates. However, 30% reported the need for significant learning support while in high school. Many of these adults are currently working. Occupations include: chef, farmer, security guard, maintenance worker, delivery person, office worker, and homemakers (McDonald-McGinn et al., 2001a). Despite the high graduation rate and relatively mild phenotype in this adult population, we believe that, in general, parents with the 22q11.2 deletion have more difficulty understanding the ramifications of the diagnosis and in complying with treatment recommendations than their nondeleted counterparts.

For this reason, using a written questionnaire, we assessed the differences in parental medical knowledge and compliance between familial and de novo cases of the deletion following genetic counseling. When compared with de novo families, in general we find that parents with the 22q11.2 deletion have a lack of understanding regarding their recurrence risk (77% of unaffected parents responded correctly when asked about recurrence risk as compared with 27% of affected parents) and sub-optimal medical compliance for themselves, as well as for their affected child/children. For example, 95% of children with de novo deletions have undergone neuropsychology evaluations and 85% have been evaluated by immunology compared with 50% and 40% of offspring of affected parents respectively. Therefore, we strongly suggest the utilization of a social safety net for these families, perhaps in the form of a social worker or nondeleted relative (Tonnesen et al., 2001). In fact, in many familial cases, the care of the affected proband is often managed by the unaffected grandparent/grandparents. Many of these caregivers have expressed concern over their situation, having struggled to raise one child with complex medical and/or educational needs and now feeling obligated to provide the same resources for an affected grandchild. They also express worry over their own life expectancy as it relates to the care of their grandchild once they are no longer able to provide such support.

Guidelines for prenatal diagnosis

Based on our current knowledge of the 22q11.2 deletion, guidelines for the prenatal detection of the 22q11.2 deletion can be divided into three groups: (1) those couples where one partner has the deletion; (2) couples who have an affected child with a de novo deletion; and (3) the general population.

For the first group, the options are relatively straightforward (Table 11.2). Knowing that the couple has a 50% recurrence risk, the first option involves the least invasive prenatal monitoring. This would include a Level II ultrasound at approximately 16 weeks gestation followed by fetal echocardiography, often serially, beginning at about 18 weeks through 22 weeks gestation. If an abnormality were found, the couple could then decide whether or not to proceed with an invasive prenatal study such as amniocentesis or percutaneous blood sampling depending on when in the pregnancy the abnormality was found. It is important for the couple to understand that a normal level II ultrasound and fetal echocardiogram are not definitive diagnostic tests and that normal results from these studies do not assure that the fetus is unaffected. Alternatively, a couple could choose a more direct and definitive approach, where the mother would undergo amniocentesis utilizing FISH for the 22q11.2 deletion at approximately 16 weeks gestation with an estimated miscarriage rate of approximately 1/200 or chorionic villus sampling (CVS) at 11–12 weeks gestation utilizing FISH for the 22q11.2 deletion with an estimated miscarriage rate of 1/100. Both amniocentesis and CVS would provide diagnostic results early enough in the pregnancy so that a therapeutic termination could be considered. An alternative to prenatal testing involves donor sperm or oocytes. If the 22q11.2 deletion is paternal, the couple may choose artificial insemination by donor. Using an anonymous donor, the woman is inseminated and the 50% recurrence risk is reduced to that of the general population. This procedure is relatively simple and inexpensive. If the deletion is maternal, the same concept may be invoked utilizing donor eggs. However, in this case, in vitro fertilization (IVF) is necessary in that the donor eggs would need to be fertilized in vitro using the partner's sperm. This raises the cost of the procedure substantially but also circumvents the 50% recurrence risk. More recently, strides are being made in the area of preimplantation diagnosis (PID). Utilizing IVF with

Table 11.2. Prenatal diagnostic/preconception options when one parent has the 22q11.2 deletion

Option 1:
Minimal non-invasive prenatal monitoring
   Level II Ultrasound
   Fetal Echocardiogram
If abnormal, consider direct prenatal monitoring

Option 2:
Direct prenatal monitoring
   Chorionic villus sampling (CVS)
      (11–12 weeks gestation)
         or
   Amniocentesis (amnio)
      (16 weeks gestation)
         or
   Percutaneous umbilical blood sampling (PUBS)
      (generally performed in late pregnancy/third trimester)

Option 3:
Donor sperm or eggs (oocytes)
   Father has the 22q11.2 deletion: donor sperm
   Mother has the 22q11.2 deletion: donor oocytes with in vitro fertilization

Option 4:
Preimplantation genetic diagnosis (PGD)

---

the biological parents' eggs and sperm, embryos are screened for the deletion at a very early stage. Those embryos which are found not to have the cytogenetic abnormality are then implanted into the woman's uterus. The procedure is quite costly and currently has limited availability. However, it is a viable alternative for those couples who would not consider a termination of pregnancy or donor gametes.

In counseling couples who have had a child affected with the 22q11.2 deletion we would recommend parental studies, as discussed previously, in an effort to ascertain mildly affected individuals and also to rule out low-level mosaicism. Following normal parental chromosome studies, the recurrence risk for this group is close to zero (Figure 11.8). However, since germline mosaicism is a true, but ill-defined risk (Hatchwell et al., 1998; Sandrin-Garcia et al., 2002), the couple may choose to monitor a subsequent pregnancy utilizing either noninvasive techniques, including Level II ultrasonography and fetal echocardiography as outlined above, or couple these studies with a definitive diagnostic test such as amniocentesis using FISH specifically for the 22q11.2 deletion. The latter is often most

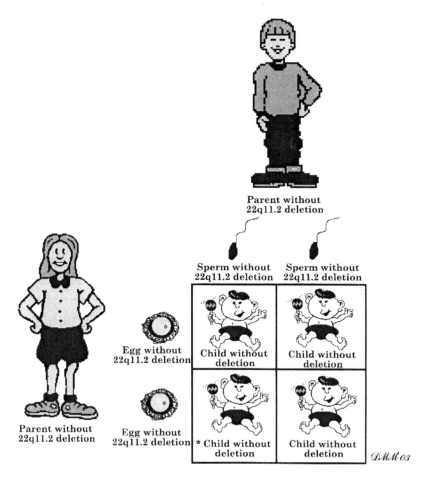

Figure 11.8 Punnett square demonstrating recurrence risk when neither parent has the 22q11.2 deletion.

justifiable when amniocentesis or chorionic villus sampling is already being considered for another reason such as advanced maternal age. However, in many instances, parental anxiety is enough to support these studies. Genetic counseling for the general population is more complicated and should be considered on a case-by-case basis when anatomic abnormalities are seen on fetal ultrasonography, or following significant findings from a careful family history. As stated previously, the estimated incidence of the 22q11.2 deletion is 1/4000 at minimum (Wilson *et al.*, 1992) making it the second most frequent chromosome aberration significantly associated with cardiac malformations after Down syndrome (Schinzel, 2001). With this in mind, FISH studies to rule out the

Table 11.3. Congenital heart disease in patients with a 22q11.2 deletion (n = 440)

Normal	106 (24%)
Tetralogy of Fallot	87 (20%)
Ventricular septal defect	61 (14%)
Interrupted aortic arch	58 (13%)
Truncus arteriosus	28 (6%)
Vascular ring	25 (5.5%)
Atrial septal defect/ventricular septal defect	17 (4%)
Atrial septal defect	15 (3.5%)
Other*	43 (10%)

*Transposition of the great vessels, bicuspid aortic valve, pulmonary valve stenosis, isolated right pulmonary artery atresia, hypoplastic left heart syndrome, aortic root dilatation, A-V canal/heterotaxy.

deletion should be considered in any fetus with congenital heart disease, especially those with conotruncal cardiac anomalies. Goldmuntz *et al.* (1998) reported the incidence of the 22q11.2 deletion in a prospective evaluation of 251 children with conotruncal cardiac anomalies. They found the deletion in 50% of children with interrupted aortic arch, 35% of children with truncus arteriosus, and 16% of children with tetralogy of Fallot (TOF). Conversely, when looking at our cohort of 440 patients with the 22q11.2 deletion who have had cardiac evaluations, 74% have congenital heart disease, most often TOF (Table 11.3) (McDonald-McGinn *et al.*, 2002b). This is important because many prenatal diagnostic centers routinely offer amniocentesis to rule out aneuploidy, such as trisomy 21, when TOF is noted by ultrasound and/or fetal echocardiography. However, it should also be noted that the incidence of TOF in the 22q11.2 deletion is 20% (McDonald-McGinn *et al.*, 2002b) as compared with 4% in children with Down syndrome (Freeman *et al.*, 1998) and, therefore, 22q11.2 deletion studies are equally, if not more, justifiable in a fetus noted to have TOF (see Chapter 3 for more details).

In addition to congenital heart disease, we have observed a number of findings in patients with the 22q11.2 deletion that are often identifiable prenatally which may support intrauterine deletion studies when found on a level II ultrasound. These include overt cleft palate, renal anomalies, polyhydramnios, polydactyly, congenital diaphragmatic hernia, and neural tube defects (McDonald-McGinn *et al.*, 2002a, 2002b).

We have observed overt cleft palate in 10% of our 460 patients while cleft lip and palate is seen in 1% (McDonald-McGinn *et al.*, 2002a, 2002b). These numbers are similar to those figures reported in the large European collaborative study (Ryan *et al.*, 1997) and are significantly greater than the general population incidence of cleft palate (1/2500) and cleft lip and palate (1/800) (Fraser, 1980). It is important to note, however, that in prospectively screening 50 consecutive children with isolated cleft palate, we found no children affected with the deletion and, therefore, a cleft palate alone may not warrant deletion studies in an otherwise normal child or fetus (Driscoll *et al.*, 1995b).

In reviewing renal ultrasounds on 85 patients with the 22q11.2 deletion, we found structural abnormalities in 31%, including renal agenesis in 12%, hydronephrosis in 5%, and multicystic/dysplastic kidneys in 4% (Wu *et al.*, 2002). Similar findings have been reported previously, including bilateral renal agenesis (Devriendt *et al.*, 1996).

We noted polyhydramnios in 16% of 320 pregnancies (McDonald-McGinn *et al.*, 2002a, 2002b). This is 16-fold greater than the general population incidence of polyhydramnios and may be attributable to the presence of fetal palatal anomalies, swallowing difficulties, or esophageal atresia (Digilio *et al.*, 1997; Eicher *et al.*, 2000).

We previously reported limb anomalies following the review of records in our initial 104 patients. We identified pre- and postaxial polydactyly of the hands in 4% of patients and postaxial polydactyly of the feet in 1%. This is at least 10-fold greater than the general population incidence of polydactyly in both Caucasians and African-Americans (Ming *et al.*, 1997). Additional limb defects which have been reported and may be identifiable on fetal ultrasonography include: radial aplasia (Digilio, 1997); symbrachydactyly (Devriendt *et al.*, 1997); absent/hypoplastic thumb (Cormier-Daire *et al.*, 1995); tibial hemimelia, clubfoot (Prasad *et al.*, 1997), and a terminal transverse defect of the upper extremity (personal observations).

We have identified congenital diaphragmatic hernia (CDH) in 1% of 460 patients with the 22q11.2 deletion which is 20-fold greater than the general population incidence of CDH (Russell *et al.*, 2000; McDonald-McGinn *et al.*, 2002a, 2002b). Like polyhydramnios, this is a newly recognized association which is often identifiable prenatally. As with congenital heart disease, the identification of CDH in a fetus frequently prompts consideration of prenatal cytogenetic studies in order to rule out aneuploidy, in particular, tetrasomy 12p (Bergoffen *et al.*, 1993).

Neural tube defects (NTDs) have occasionally been reported in patients with the 22q11.2 deletion (Nickel & Magenis, 1996). We have identified 1 of 460 patients with both the deletion and a myelomeningocele. This suggests that NTDs may occur more frequently in patients with the 22q11.2 deletion than in the general population.

Thus, prenatal sonographic findings including overt cleft palate, renal anomalies, polyhydramnios, polydactyly, congenital diaphragmatic hernia, and neural tube defects, in combination or in the presence of congenital heart disease, should prompt consideration of intrauterine deletion studies in order to provide appropriate prenatal counseling and clinical management. Furthermore, should any of these findings lead to prenatal chromosome analysis to rule out aneuploidy (i.e., polydactyly in a fetus may prompt consideration of amniocentesis to rule out trisomy 13), one might consider the addition of 22q11.2 deletion FISH studies as an adjunct to standard cytogenetics.

It is also imperative to stress the importance of a careful family history in the prenatal setting. For example, we recently diagnosed a 24-week premature infant with the 22q11.2 deletion in the newborn period. Prenatal history revealed an intrauterine diagnosis of TOF but no cytogenetic studies were performed at that time. We subsequently identified a deletion in her mother as well. The mother's past medical history revealed a repaired TOF and a learning disability. Despite these findings and the association of the 22q11.2 deletion and TOF, the mother's history had not prompted further evaluation in the prenatal setting. The proband later succumbed to complications of prematurity. The mother has subsequently delivered another affected child who was diagnosed prenatally with both a large VSD and the 22q11.2 deletion. This family highlights the importance of a careful family history with particular attention to any of the following findings in the parents: congenital heart disease, palatal anomalies including velopharyngeal incompetence, hypoparathyroidism, learning disability or mental retardation, psychiatric illness, and minor facial dysmorphisms. The adult facies most often includes some combination of the following: hooding of the eyelids, hypertelorism, auricular anomalies, a nasal dimple or crease, malar flatness, a small mouth, or asymmetric crying facies (Gripp et al., 1997; McDonald-McGinn et al., 1997a). However, we have found a paucity of these facial features in non-Caucasian individuals and, therefore, the facies may be less helpful in African-Americans and Asian patients (McDonald-McGinn et al., 1996b; McDonald-McGinn, 2003). One should also be mindful of less common structural anomalies which may be present in parents, such as scoliosis, genitourinary anomalies including hypospadias and unilateral renal agenesis (McDonald-McGinn et al., 1995; Wu et al., 2002), craniosynostosis (McDonald-McGinn, 1999a), and laryngeal abnormalities (McDonald-McGinn et al., 1995), as well as associated autoimmune disorders (i.e., ITP, JRA, psoriasis, vitiligo, Graves disease) (Keenan et al., 1997; Sullivan et al., 1997, 1998; Kawame et al., 2002) especially in conjunction with a learning disability. This is particularly important in nonCaucasian parents (McDonald-McGinn et al., 1996). Lastly, families such as the one described above again highlight the likely increase in the prevalence of the 22q11.2 deletion due to the decreasing mortality rate associated with the diagnosis and the minimal impact on reproductive fitness.

REFERENCES

Bawle, E. V., Conard, J., Van Dyke, D. L. *et al.* (1998) Letter to the Editor: seven new cases of Cayler cardiofacial syndrome with chromosome 22q11.2 deletion, including a familial case. *Am. J. Med. Genet.*, **79**, 406–10.

Bergoffen, J., Punnett, H., Campbell, T. J. *et al.* (1993) Diaphragmatic hernia in tetrasomy 12p mosaicism. *J. Pediatr.*, **122** (**4**), 603–6.

Burn, J., Takao, A., Wilson, D. *et al.* (1993) Conotruncal anomaly face syndrome is associated with a deletion within chromosome 22. *J. Med. Genet.*, **30**, 822–4.

Consegave, M. W., Seip, J. R., Belchis, D. A. *et al.* (1996) Association of a mosaic chromosomal 22q11 deletion with hypoplastic left heart syndrome. *Am. J. Cardiol.*, **77**, 1023–5.

Cormier-Daire, V., Iserin, L., Theophile, D. *et al.* (1995) Upper limb malformations in DiGeorge syndrome. *Am. J. Med. Genet.*, **56**, 39–41.

de la Chapelle, A., Herva, R., Koivisto, M. *et al.* (1981) A deletion in chromosome 22 can cause DiGeorge syndrome. *Hum. Genet.*, **57**, 253–6.

Devriendt, K., Swillen, A., Fryns, J. P. *et al.* (1996) Renal and urological tract malformations caused by a 22q11 deletion. *J. Med. Genet.*, **33**, 349.

Devriendt, K., de Smet, L., de Boeck, K. *et al.* (1997) DiGeorge syndrome and unilateral symbrachydactyly. *Genet. Counsec.*, **8**, 345–7.

Digilio, M. C., Giannotti, A., Marino, B. *et al.* (1997) Radial aplasia and chromosome 22q11 deletion. *J. Med. Genet.*, **34**, 942–4.

Driscoll, D. A., Budarf, M. L. & Emanuel, B. S. (1992a) A genetic etiology for DiGeorge syndrome: consistent deletions and microdeletions of 22q11. *Am. J. Hum. Genet.*, **50**, 924–33.

Driscoll, D. A., Spinner, N. B., Budarf, M. L. *et al.* (1992b) Deletions and microdeletions of 22q11.2 in velo-cardio-facial syndrome. *Am. J. Med. Genet.*, **44**, 261–8.

Driscoll, D. A., Salvin, J., Sellinger, B. *et al.* (1993) Prevalence of 22q11 microdeletions in DGS and VCFS: implications for genetic counseling and prenatal diagnosis. *J. Med. Genet.*, **30**, 813–17.

Driscoll, D. A., Chen, P., Li, M. *et al.* (1995a) Familial 22q11 deletions: phenotypic variability and determination of deletion boundaries by FISH. *Am. J. Hum. Genet.*, **57**, 92 (abstr).

Driscoll, D. A., Randall, P., McDonald-McGinn, D. M. *et al.* (1995b) Are 22q11.2 chromosomal deletions a major cause of isolated cleft palate? 52nd Annual Meeting, American Cleft Palate-Craniofacial Association, Tampa, FL.

Edelman, L., Pandita, R. K. & Morrow, B. E. (1999) Low-copy repeats mediate the common 3-Mb deletion in patients with velo-cardio-facial syndrome. *Am. J. Hum. Genet.*, **64**, 1076–86.

Eicher, P. S., McDonald-McGinn, D. M., Fox, C. A. *et al.* (2000) Dysphagia in children with a 22q11.2 deletion: unusual pattern found on modified barium swallow. *J. Pediatr.*, **137** (**2**), 158–64.

Emanuel, B. S., Budarf, M. L., Shaikh, T., *et al.* (1998) Blocks of duplicated sequence define the endpoints of DGS/VCFS 22q11.2 deletions. *Am. J. Hum. Genet.*, **63**, A11(abstr).

Fraser, F. C. (1980) The genetics of cleft lip and palate: Yet another look. In Pratt, R. M. & Christiansen, R. L., eds., *Current Research Trends in Prenatal Craniofacial Development*. Amsterdam: Elsevier Publishers.

Freeman, S. B., Taft, L. F., Dooley, K. J. *et al.* (1998) Population-based study of congenital heart defects in Down syndrome. *Am. J. Med. Genet.*, **80** (**3**), 213–17.

Fryburg, J. S., Lin, K. Y. & Golden, E. F. (1996) Chromosome 22q11.2 deletion in a boy with Opitz oculo-genito-laryngeal syndrome. *Am. J. Med. Genet.*, **62**, 274–5.

Gerdes, M., Solot, C., Wang, P. P. *et al.* (1999) Cognitive and behavioral profile of preschool children with chromosome 22q11.2 microdeletion. *Am. J. Med. Genet.*, **85** (**2**), 127–33.

Giannotti, A., Diglio, M. C., Marino, B. *et al.* (1994) Cayler cardiofacial syndrome and del 22q11: part of the CATCH22 phenotype. *Am. J. Med. Genet.*, **30**, 807–12.

Goldmuntz, E., Clark, B. J., Mitchell, L. E. *et al.* (1998) Frequency of 22q11 deletions in patients with conotruncal defects. *J. Am. Coll. Cardiol.*, **32**, 492–8.

Gripp, K. W., McDonald-McGinn, D. M., Driscoll, D. A. *et al.* (1997) Nasal dimple as part of the 22q11.2 deletion syndrome. *Am. J. Med. Genet.*, **69**, 290–2.

Hatchwell, E., Long, F., Wilde, J. *et al.* (1998) Molecular confirmation of germ line mosaicism for a submicroscopic deletion of chromosome 22q11. *Am. J. Med. Genet.*, **78**, 103–6.

Kawame, H., Adachi, M., Tachibana, K. *et al.* (2001) Graves' disease in patients with 22q11.2 deletion. *J. Pediatr.*, **139** (**6**), 892–5.

Keenan, G. F., Sullivan, K. E., McDonald-McGinn, D. M. *et al.* (1997) Letter to the editor: arthritis associated with 22q11.2: more common than previously suspected. *Am. J. Med. Genet.*, **71**, 488.

Kelley, R. I., Zackai, E. H., Emanuel, B. S. *et al.* (1982) The association of the DiGeorge anomalad with partial monosomy of chromosome 22. *J. Pediatr.*, **101**, 197–200.

LaCassie, Y. & Arriaza, M. I. (1996) Letter to the Editor: Opitz GBBB syndrome and the 22q11.2 deletion syndrome. *Am. J. Med. Genet.*, **62**, 318.

Lynch, D. R., McDonald-McGinn, D., Zackai, E. H. *et al.* (1995) Cerebellar atrophy in a patient with velocardiofacial syndrome. *J. Med. Genet.*, **32**, 561–3.

Matsouka, R., Takao, A., Kimura, M. *et al.* (1994) Confirmation that the conotruncal anomaly face syndrome is associated with a deletion within 22q11.2. *Am. J. Med. Genet.*, **53**, 285–9.

McDonald-McGinn, D. M., Driscoll, D. A., Bason, L. *et al.* (1995) Autosomal dominant "Opitz" GBBB syndrome due to a 22q11.2 deletion. *Am. J. Med. Genet.*, **59**, 103–13.

McDonald-McGinn, D. M., Emanuel, B. S., Zackai, E. H. (1996) Letter to the Editor: Autosomal dominant "Opitz" GBBB syndrome due to a 22q11.2 deletion. *Am. J. Med. Genet.*, **64**, 525–6.

McDonald-McGinn, D. M., Driscoll, D. A., Emanuel, B. S. *et al.* (1996) The 22q11.2 deletion in African-American patients: an underdiagnosed population. *Am. J. Hum. Genet.*, **59**, A20.

McDonald-McGinn, D. M., LaRossa, D., Goldmuntz, E. *et al.* (1997a) The 22q11.2 deletion: screening, diagnostic workup, and outcome of results; report on 181 patients. *Genetic Testing*, **1**, 99–108.

McDonald-McGinn, D. M., Driscoll, D. A., Emanuel, B. S. *et al.* (1997b) Detection of a 22q11.2 deletion in cardiac patients suggests a risk for velopharyngeal incompetence. *Pediatrics*, **99**, 1–5.

McDonald-McGinn, D. M., Kirschner, R., Gripp, K. *et al.* (1999a) Craniosynostosis: another feature of the 22q11.2 deletion syndrome. American Cleft-Palate Craniofacial Association 56th Annual Meeting and Conference Symposium, Scottsdale, AZ.

McDonald-McGinn, D. M., Kirschner, R., Goldmuntz, E. *et al.* (1999b) The Philadelphia Story: The 22q11.2 Deletion: Report on 250 Patients. *Genetic Counseling*, **10** (**1**), 11–24.

McDonald-McGinn, D. M., Tonnesen, M. K., Laufer-Cahana, A. *et al.* (2001a) Phenotype of the 22q11.2 deletion in individuals identified through an affected relative: cast a wide *FISH*ing net! *Genet. Med.*, **3**, 23–9.

McDonald-McGinn, D. M., Driscoll, D. A., Tonnesen, M. *et al.* (2001b) Parent of origin does not determine phenotype in the 22q11.2 deletion. *Am. J. Hum. Genet.*, **69**, 285 (A597).

McDonald-McGinn, D. M., Tonnesen, M. K., Saitta, S. *et al.* (2002a) The Philadelphia Story: Update on our Population of Patients with a 22q11.2 deletion. Deletion 22q11.2 Third International Meeting, Rome, Italy, June 7–8.

McDonald-McGinn, D. M., Driscoll, D. A., Saitta, S. *et al.* (2002b) Guidelines for prenatal detection of the 22q11.2 deletion. *Am. J. Hum. Genet.*, **71** (**4**), 198 (A173).

Ming, J. E., McDonald-McGinn, D. M., Megerian, T. E. *et al.* (1997) Skeletal anomalies in patients with deletions of 22q11. *Am. J. Med. Genet.*, **72**, 210–15.

Moss, E. M., Batshaw, M. L., Solot, C. B. *et al.* (1999) Psychoeducational profile of the 22q11.2 microdeletion: A complex pattern. *J. Pediatr.*, **134**, 193–8.

Nickel, R. E. & Magenis, R. E. (1996) Neural tube defects and deletions of 22q11. *Am. J. Med. Genet.*, **66**, 25–7.

Prasad, C., Quackenbush, E. J., Whiteman, D. *et al.* (1997) Limb anomalies in DiGeorge and CHARGE syndromes. *Am. J. Med. Genet.*, **68**, 179–81.

Reardon, W., Wilkes, D., Rutland, P. *et al.* (1997) Craniosynostosis associated with FGFR3 pro250arg mutation results in a range of clinical presentations including unisutural cranio-synostosis. *J. Med. Genet.*, **34**, 632–6.

Russell, K. L., McDonald-McGinn, D. M., Mahle, W. *et al.* (2000) Congenital diaphragmatic hernia in the 22q11.2 deletion. Presentation, Second International 22q11.2 Deletion Meeting, June 22–25, Philadelphia, PA.

Ryan, A. K., Goodship, J. A., Wilson, D. I. *et al.* (1997) Spectrum of clinical features associated with interstitial chromosome 22q11 deletions: a European collaborative study. *J. Med. Genet.*, **34**, 798–804.

Sandrin-Garcia, P., Macedo, C., Martelli, L. R. *et al.* (2002) Recurrent 22q11.2 deletion in a sibship suggestive of parental germline mosaicism in velocardiofacial syndrome. *Clin. Genet.*, **61**, 380–3.

Scambler, P. J., Carey, A. H., Wyse, R. K. *et al.* (1991) Microdeletions within 22q11 associated with sporadic and familial DiGeorge syndrome. *Genomics*, **10** (**1**), 201–6.

Schinzel, A. (2001) In *Catalogue of Unbalanced Chromosome Aberrations in Man.* New York: Walter de Gruyter, Inc., pp. 846–57.

Shaikh, T. H., Kurahashi, H., Saitta, S. C. *et al.* (2000) Chromosome 22-specific low copy repeats and the 22q11.2 deletion syndrome: genomic organization and deletion endpoint analysis. *Hum. Mol. Genet.*, **9**, 489–501.

Solot, C., Knightly, C., Handler, S. *et al.* (2000) Communication disorders in the 22q11.2 microdeletion syndrome. *J. Comm. Dis.*, **33**, 187–204.

Solot, C. B., Gerdes, M., Kirschner, R. E. *et al.* (2001) Communication issues in 22q11.2 deletion syndrome: children at risk. *Genet. Med.*, **3**, 67–71.

Sullivan, K. E., McDonald-McGinn, D. M., Driscoll, D. A. *et al.* (1997) JRA-like polyarthritis in chromosome 22q11.2 deletion syndrome (DiGeorge anomalad/velocardiofacial syndrome/conotruncal anomaly face syndrome). *Arthritis Rheumatism*, **40**, 430–6.

Sullivan, K. E., Jawad, A. F., Randall, P. *et al.* (1998) The frequency and severity of immuno-deficiency in chromosome 22q11.2 deletion syndromes (DiGeorge syndrome/Velocardiofacial syndrome). *Clin. Immunol. Immunopathol.*, **86**, 141–6.

Sullivan, K. E., McDonald-McGinn, D., Driscoll, D. A. *et al.* (1999) Longitudinal analysis of lymphocyte function and numbers in the first year of life in chromosome 22q11.2 deletion syndrome (DiGeorge syndrome/Velocardiofacial syndrome). *Clin. Diagn. Lab. Immunol.*, **6**, 906–11.

Thompson, J. S. & Thompson, M. W. (1986) *Genetics in Medicine,* 4th Edn. Philadelphia, PA: W. B. Saunders Company.

Tonnesen, M., McDonald-McGinn, D. M., Valverde, K. *et al.* (2001) Affected parents with a 22q11.2 deletion: the need for basic and ongoing educational health, and supportive counseling. *Am. J. Hum. Genet.*, **69** (4), 223 (A241).

Wang, P., Solot, C., Gerdes, M. *et al.* (1998) Developmental presentation of 22q11.2 deletion. *Dev. Behav. Pediatr.*, **19**, 342–5.

Weinzimer, S. A., McDonald-McGinn, D. M., Driscoll, D. A. *et al.* (1998) Growth hormone deficiency in patients with a 22q11.2 deletion: expanding the phenotype. *Pediatrics*, **101**, 929–32.

Wilson, D. I., Cross, I. E., Goodship, J. A. *et al.* (1992) A prospective cytogenetic study of 36 cases of DiGeorge syndrome. *Am. J. Hum. Genet.*, **51**, 957–63.

Wu, H-Y., Rusnack, S. L., Bellah, R. D. *et al.* (2002) Genitourinary malformations in chromosome 22q11.2 deletion. *J. Urology*, **168**, 2564–5.

12

Family issues

Julie Squair

The 22q11 Group, Milton Keynes, UK

Impact of initial diagnosis

Why us?

After 9 months of pregnancy, most parents expect to leave hospital with their little "bundle of joy" and never anticipate their child having any kind of medical condition. Heart problems are often deemed to be something "which happens to other people." The impact on the whole family is so great that it takes years to come to terms with the devastating effects, although some parents do not realize initially that they are affected; they are running on automatic pilot and are trying to make the best of what life has thrown at them. So how does it affect different families, personalities, and cultures to find out that their child has been diagnosed with velo-cardio-facial syndrome (VCFS)?

Those diagnosed early with VCFS, after being born with severe heart defects such as interrupted aortic arch (IAA) or tetralogy of Fallot (TOF) may nowadays have the benefit of early intervention in their medical, social, and educational needs. However, the impact on the family on finding that their newborn is going to need a lot more care and attention than other children puts a huge strain on everyone involved. Everyone's needs at this time are different.

The mother

The baby's mother, recovering after the birth, often feels guilty and thinks that maybe she did something wrong during her pregnancy. Most mothers towards the end of pregnancy just want to give birth and get to know their babies at a time when they are also finding it difficult to carry out their normal, everyday chores. However, when the baby is born, and is sick, the mother may have an overwhelming urge to somehow turn back time. When she realizes this is not possible, the trauma and guilt continue to repeat hour after hour, day after day. Patience and understanding at this time is very important to ensure a good recovery from the birth and allow the normal maternal instincts and bonding to follow through.

Velo-Cardial-Facial Syndrome: A Model for Understanding Microdeletion Disorders, ed. Kieran C. Murphy and Peter J. Scambler. Published by Cambridge University Press. ⓒ Cambridge University Press, 2005.

The father

The father, expecting to be the bearer of good news to family and friends, is as devastated as the mother but also worries about the effects on his partner and other children in the family. It is perfectly normal to feel quite helpless at this stage. The father normally has the added burden of having to go back to work, but finds it impossible while his family needs him so much. Some employers are understanding whilst others are quite strict in the amount of leave they will allow. This puts an added social strain on the family structure.

Some fathers react in a completely different way and completely shut down and find it hard to express their grief. This may have a detrimental affect on the family unit as his wife might not feel supported, thus increasing further the strain on her and on the family unit.

Siblings

Brothers and sisters have usually been prepared for the new baby for many weeks or months. Most parents will talk to their other children about what will happen when Mummy goes into hospital to have their new brother or sister and how life might be when the baby comes home. What nobody is ever prepared for is a baby who doesn't come straight home or who has to undergo major surgery at such a young age. It is easy not to involve siblings when their baby brother or sister is very sick, but this can have a damaging effect on them if they don't feel included, or if they only hear whispers and odd words which can make them feel frightened and alone. Even small children can be given some simple explanations that help them formulate their own questions and feel more secure.

The grandparents

Throughout the pregnancy and the birth, the grandparents may be extremely involved with the whole family. Their role should not be underestimated, especially once the new baby has come into the world. The grandparents are often the first people the new parents turn to for support, emotionally and practically. For the grandparents, this can be a very difficult time for them as they feel their role is to support their "children," yet they too have fears and anxieties and a feeling of helplessness. Most grandparents realize that their children need to look after *their* own children and are ultimately responsible for decision-making. This does not mean that they won't have the urge to be more involved – maybe causing friction. This could add to the burden already being carried by the parents.

Some grandparents react totally differently. They find that they are so upset and frightened by what is happening that they just shut down completely – *if I don't get involved, then it's not really happening!* Many grandparents were brought up at a time when people were not given explanations about medical conditions and readily accepted whatever they were told. They may feel that their children should do the same. Many children surviving major cardiac surgery today would not have lived even 15 years ago! This is very different for other generations to comprehend and accept. In fact, many of the older generation believe that sick babies should not be kept alive – incomprehensible in this day and age to most of us but still a very real concept.

What happens while the baby is still in hospital?

First of all, life becomes a day-to-day existence away from the reality of normal life. The parents have to survive on hospital food and often feel acutely aware of a lack of privacy. They don't get to know their "little bundle of joy" intimately, although most hospitals actively encourage parental support in the care of their baby. In reality for the parents, it usually feels like they are allowed to care for their child as long as they abide by the hospital rules. This is fine for the hospital who have to have rules and regulations with regard to hygiene and security, but it is a very false situation for parents who long to do things their way, whilst still being afraid to handle their baby too much and worry that they might not actually be able to care for their child properly at home.

Issues for children and adults with VCFS

Social implications

The social implications for the VCFS child or adult are enormous. As babies they are often small and developmentally delayed but do not look out of place in a pram/pushchair even at the toddler stage. Some babies have feeding problems and need to be tube fed or fed small amounts regularly. This may cause some distress for families who have to take these issues into account when carrying out the simplest activity or outing.

As the children mature, they usually appear "normal" at first sight to those who do not know them although some displays of immature social behavior are often noted. This can make everyday life difficult for the parents who want to be just like any other family.

The VCFS child in school can perform well in the structured environment but may find any slight change in routine confusing and difficult to deal with. This may lead to crying in class or angry outbursts, depending on how the child usually reacts to this kind of situation. The younger VCFS child may be "mothered" by others in the class when they are upset, but this will happen less and less as they grow up as their peers mature at a different rate to them.

Adolescents in general may find they are living life on a roller coaster. Therefore, the VCFS child will probably find adolescence even more challenging as the large school environment and the amount of work they have to deal with can pose more difficulties than usual and cause the child to feel overwhelmed. Many VCFS adolescents have been reported to "shut down" completely when they have too much to cope with both at home and at school. This does not apply solely to their schoolwork but also to their friendships, which are often the root of many of their difficulties. Most children will make and break friendships with several others in their lifetime but will usually get over their disappointments quite quickly. The VCFS child finds it difficult to communicate easily with more than one person at a time and can easily fall out with a friend over something trivial because of their language deficits and communication difficulties. When this is the only friend they have – or believe they have – it can cause a major upset in their lives, which is not easy to overcome. Children with VCFS have also been heard to say that they have lots of friends when in actual fact they just believe that everyone in their class is a friend. The social implications accompanying this kind of trust are huge. The children will often do anything for a treat and could get themselves into dangerous situations without an understanding of the risks involved.

Many parents learn which button to press to change the mood of their child but once they are teenagers it is not always as easy to do. As teenagers, VCFS children need very careful handling with regard to their self-esteem as problems with anxiety and mood swings may be noted. Any signs of depression need to be handled sensitively in any child, but more so in the VCFS child. They get upset at what people say and do not take kindly to jokes aimed at them. Their literal viewpoint can make them believe that people are laughing at them and this could lead to anxieties and depression which in turn could lead to further teasing when they respond in an odd or unusual fashion. Many families find that the odd social behavior is most likened to children with autistic tendencies and it seems to help when they are treated as such in school.

Personality

It is the experience of The 22q11 Group (UK) that children with VCFS appear to have lots of similarities in their personality (A Parents' Guide – Everything You Need to Know About Velo-Cardio-Facial Syndrome/Di George Syndrome *The 22q11 Group (Charity No 1046847 Registered in the United Kingdom)* – extract from unpublished data.). If they decide they want something they will consistently ask for it time and time again, ignoring the fact that they have been told 'no'. They will appear to be obsessive about things, e.g., they will watch the same video over and over again or repeatedly ask for the same type of food. This obsession will suddenly stop as if it had never occurred, but will be replaced by something else. This can be even more frustrating if you actually give in and say 'yes' because they will not want it anymore and will ask for something else. Children with VCFS always seem to be concerned with what is going to happen next week rather than what is happening now. They are friendly with older children and adults but easily fall out with their peers. They appear not to listen to the current conversation, changing the subject to whatever is on their mind. They very quickly become disrupted by a change in routine. Good periods of being relaxed and happy can change very quickly to periods of agitation and moodiness. They often binge on food and can often appear to be constantly opening the fridge door. They can get over-excited about events like birthdays and Christmas and often worry excessively about little things.

Medical

Many babies diagnosed with VCFS have quite a difficult start to life. Life seems to be a constant round of surgery and feeding difficulties, which seem to take up most of the first year. Although a very small number of babies do not survive the heart surgery (see Chapter 3), and many have compromised immune systems (see chapter 6), the majority start to show signs of great improvement after only a few weeks or months. It is very difficult for families to imagine they will ever get through this period but, more often than not, they get there in the end. There will always be some children of course who continue to have major medical problems, but it is important to stress to families that the outlook is generally very positive medically. This is where it is advantageous to point out the benefits of the support group. Families will find it easier to comprehend when they speak to others who have been in a similar situation to them and survived!

As the child begins to reach the normal milestones – usually a little later than normal – the question comes up with regard to speech and whether surgery on the palate is necessary (see Chapter 4). It is extremely frustrating for families to have a child who cannot communicate his needs verbally and be told by doctors that they cannot see anything wrong with the palate. Further investigations need to be carried out by a cleft palate team, but only once the child has had some speech therapy for articulation. A clear and sympathetic understanding on the part of the physician and a full explanation of the risks and benefits of the various treatment options available is very important to ease the pain and frustration that many parents and other family members experience.

Communication and education

Velo-cardio-facial syndrome is a communication disorder that affects two-way social interaction, verbal and nonverbal communication (see Chapter 10). VCFS children often have difficulty accepting and dealing with change. This can show in changes of mood, behavior, hyperactivity, or withdrawal. They can be very inflexible in their thought – narrow minded with a focus on just one topic. This reflects in their conversation which is often one-sided, talking about what they want to talk about with an unfailing ability to butt in and change a conversation to their own desired topic.

Children with VCFS may have all-absorbing narrow areas of interest and often appear obsessional about certain things; videos, books, games they like and their routines. If their routines are broken they can become upset and out of sorts for days.

They are usually good at learning by rote, but some individuals may have problems retaining information, so learning often has to be repeated and continued throughout school holidays.

Socially, they find making friends difficult and are often immature for their age (see Chapter 7). They often do not instigate "normal" conversation or join in the banter within a group of children. In addition, they frequently do not understand or cannot tell jokes.

VCFS children often misread body language and facial expressions. They are frequently unaware of "personal space" between themselves and others and will often stand too close or too far away.

When a group of children are "hanging out," the VCFS child will try to single out one child to talk to (or at). Their use of language can appear odd, especially to other children their own age, and they often take the literal meaning of what is said or read.

Generally, VCFS children love and react very well to praise, but find criticism difficult to cope with. Bad behavior and mood changes often stem from their inability to communicate their frustrations and anxieties. They need love, tenderness, care, patience, and understanding. They do not need negative criticism and bullying, which are upsetting for any child but even more so for them.

They can FLOURISH, they can LEARN, and they can be HAPPY!

The difficulties with communication that many VCFS children experience can easily affect education. As children with VCFS cannot readily ask appropriate questions and often appear not to be listening or responding, the teacher needs to be aware of the disorder to make the child's education more achievable. Parents often take on the role of intermediary between the school and the medical community. This can be very tiring for the family so it is crucial that the child's needs are fully met through an individual education plan (IEP) which clearly outlines the following:

- their performance at the time of the planning
- the aims and objectives to get them to reach their potential
- how progress will be measured.

These needs ought to include social skills and language help as most problems can be eased if the child understands their role in the classroom and knows what is expected of them in a typical day. This help is not always given through special education services (Statement of Special Educational Needs in the UK) with an individual education plan (IEP) but it generally helps to have it formalized in some way.

Once the VCFS child is in senior school (from about the age of 12 years), they need to think also about organizational skills along with all the extra work they have to do. Computers and palmtops can help in this respect as work can be kept and changed as necessary and transferred from school to home and vice versa with the aid of a disk. Lack of organizational skills and a work overload adds unnecessary stress to the VCFS child who may already be struggling with the growing up process and this in turn can lead to emotional difficulties. Therefore, it is wise to try and make their working day as organized and stress-free as possible and watch out for any signs of withdrawal or changes in mood. Parents often struggle to help their child with homework. Our experience suggests that it is fine to help as long as the child understands what the work is about and does not just expect the parents to do it for them. In some of the more abstract subjects, VCFS children are often only happy if they know it is done and don't realize that they should also know what it was about. In instances such as these it would be helpful if the child was excused from doing the homework as it does nothing more than cause added stress to the already busy family life. The 22q11 Group (UK) has found that some parents find this makes life much easier at home and means the child does not get as tired or worried.

How physicians can help individuals with VCFS and their families

First and foremost, families need early support from all healthcare professionals working with their child. When a child is born with a heart condition needing immediate surgery, the surgeon and his team are normally the first real contact for the parents and have to give details of what is involved in the surgery. They have the very difficult job of explaining the risks involved in cardiac surgery (see Chapter 3) yet are the part of the medical community who seem to be able to communicate best with parents at this stage. The 22q11 Group experience is that parents cope much better knowing the truth, even though it may frighten them or they may not fully understand what they are being told. This acceptance that families "need to know" is often difficult for physicians who sometimes believe that too much medical information worries families. The 22q11 Group knows from experience that it does shock families to have to take so much on board initially but gradually they will feel armed with enough information to move on, learn about and deal with their child's problems. Some parents of course will shut down completely and either refuse to accept it, or be incapable of taking in the information. This does not mean that they won't at some time decide they are ready to learn more. The medical community could help parents more by not taking it upon themselves to decide whether the parents should know or not. Most parents, without any experience, seem to find an inner strength and capability to understand that springs from nowhere when given the opportunity. They cannot learn overnight; it is a gradual process which begins the day their child is born.

Once the child leaves the safe confines of the hospital, the family needs support from a whole group of professionals – beginning with the health visitor and family doctor (GP). Information needs to be shared amongst professionals as a real strain is put on families who have to be the main coordinators when dealing with different doctors who have different areas of expertise.

From a support group point of view, it has been found that medical staff sometimes feel that the family is too upset to take extra information on board from parent groups. Our experience suggests that it is helpful to pass on information and contact details for the family to read when they are ready for it. This could be included in a take-home pack which might be put to one side initially but read through when the family feels more able to cope and talk.

Families sometimes go a long way round the system to try and find somebody to talk to and find it frustrating that they could have had the information at an earlier date, not just when they are desperate. For families who would like to find a contact in their part of the world they can always find information through The VCFS Educational Foundation (www.vcfsef.org), a nonprofit-making foundation set up to educate people with VCFS, their families, and healthcare professionals about velo-cardio-facial syndrome. They hold an annual conference in different locations over a period of three days and find that the mix of parents and professionals allows for a wonderful exchange of ideas and information.

Although not always practical in a syndrome which affects so many parts of the body, it would be really helpful for all concerned to have services centralized. The child would have his/her needs taken care of by a group of professionals who could easily communicate locally; there would be less time taken out of school and parents would not have to travel too far or take time off work as frequently so there would be less stress on everybody.

How else might the physician help?

A sympathetic ear usually makes the world of difference. Many parents who have either had a child with a severe congenital cardiac defect or with no diagnosis yet several problems, are sometimes labelled as "neurotic" or "over-involved." This only seems to prolong the issues and affect the family emotionally as it is extremely draining to know there is something wrong – *and we all know that a parent's instinct is usually right* – but nobody wants to listen or do anything about it. The way this affects parents extends to the rest of the family and ultimately affects the VCFS child/adult.

It has been shown that early intervention does indeed aid the medical, emotional, and learning outcomes of the individual with VCFS. The family doctor (GP) or pediatrician is usually the primary physician dealing with all aspects of the syndrome and has the wisdom to refer patients to the relevant consultant. Working closely with the family the GP can indeed be the friend they need to help them through what are often difficult times.

Last, but not least, educating themselves on different aspects of the syndrome will have many benefits. The satisfaction from being able to get to know a child with VCFS and understand a little about what makes them tick is a huge benefit, whilst the relief on a parent's face when they know a particular physician is on their side is second to none. The physician needs to understand that just because a child with VCFS has had cardiac surgery, and maybe palate or other surgicial interventions, does not mean that he/she is "fixed." The syndrome has many different faces which may show themselves at different times in the patient's life and in many different ways. VCFS is a genetic condition which will never get better but can be managed. People with VCFS can go on to live a normal life and have a family of their own, albeit with support from family, friends and the medical profession.

Support services

Initially, support services means nurses, doctors, and surgeons in the hospital. However, they work very closely with health visitors who will visit the new family at home and be a listening ear as well as the main link between all kinds of services. These services include the family doctor, social workers and therapists (speech and language, occupational, and physiotherapy for example). The health visitor plays a very important role as he/she will not only visit the family at home but will carry out most of the normal development checks, speech and hearing tests. They are helpful to the family as they will sit and listen to how the whole family is affected and will act accordingly.

Once the child approaches nursery and/or school age, parents are usually just beginning to get over their children's surgeries and find choosing a school a daunting prospect at times. Local Education Authorities (LEAs) do not usually understand the difficulties associated with VCFS, as they are not always apparent from an early age. The learning at school, until about the age of 8–9 years, is quite concrete so the VCFS child can get by in class unnoticed. It is at this point that the support of a good teacher and Special Educational Needs Coordinator (SENCO) is necessary to guide the child through the system to ensure they get the right kind of help so they can move on to a senior school environment at the age of 11–12 years.

Some children will cope reasonably well at the lower end of the class whilst others will find life increasingly difficult. Although learning can be a huge problem – yet not always obviously so – more serious problems may be encountered socially and become more and more apparent as the child reaches and passes puberty. This is a difficult time for most children in some shape or form but the VCFS child is very susceptible to teasing and lack of understanding due to their immaturity. This in turn can lead to them falling behind in some of the more abstract subjects at school.

Family life with a teenager can be fraught with difficulties in any family, but with the mood swings of the VCFS adolescent too, the family may be overwhelmed. At this stage it is natural that the family will begin to look for another kind of support. This may be in the form of a social worker who may be able to help with the supply of respite care or counseling. Sometimes the only kind of help that really works is talking to another parent who has been in the same position. In some circumstances, the family doctor may suggest a referral to a local psychologist or psychiatrist for further support (see Chapter 7)

Conclusions

This chapter on family issues has been written through experience gained whilst working voluntarily for The 22q11 Group in the UK. The group was set up in 1994 by two families whose children were born with similar problems within three days of each other, but in different parts of the country. However, by the time their paths crossed, the children were almost 5 years old. The 22q11 Group went live for the first time in November 1994 and it was a very exciting and rewarding time after having spent a few years feeling alone, a few months working on the project of developing a UK support group for families and professionals, and then the moment when we realized that we had no idea what lay ahead … but could hardly wait to find out!

Since that time more than 700 families and professionals have been in contact and the group has gone from strength to strength. The aim of the group is to provide information, advice and support to families and professionals affected by VCFS/Di George Syndrome. The 22q11 Group can be contacted by writing to P.O. Box 1302, Milton Keynes MK13 0LZ, UK, by telephoning 0870 765 2211 from within the UK or through their website at www.vcfs.net. If you would like to contact and exchange information with other families by email there are currently two listservs running – one based in the UK (email: vcfs-uk@jiscmail.ac.uk) and one in the USA (email: vcfs@maelstrom.stjohns.edu). To subscribe to these listservs (*subscribe means to join – you don't have to pay anything*) enter either 'VCFS-UK' under name of list for the UK listserv then follow instructions, or find VCFS under the online list archives when searching the US listserv and follow instructions.

From very early on in the development of the group, meeting Professor Robert J. Shprintzen when he held the First Annual Meeting of the Velo-cardio-facial

Syndrome Educational Foundation in March 1995 was one of the group's greatest influences. Since that time Professor Shprintzen has been a constant source of knowledge and support to many families all over the world. The VCFS Educational Foundation to date has held annual meetings in the USA and Europe. More information can be found about the work of the Foundation and a support group near you through their website (www.vcfsef.org).

Index

Note: page numbers in *italics* refer to figures and tables

Lightning Source UK Ltd.
Milton Keynes UK
UKOW020627190313

207862UK00007B/285/P